Rehab Clinica

MW00843613

Kimberly A. Sackheim
Editor

Rehab Clinical Pocket Guide

Rehabilitation Medicine

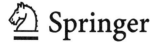 Springer

Editor
Dr. Kimberly A. Sackheim
Rehabilitation Medicine
Pain Medicine and Palliative Care
Beth Israel Medical Center
New York, NY, USA

ISBN 978-1-4614-5418-2   ISBN 978-1-4614-5419-9 (eBook)
DOI 10.1007/978-1-4614-5419-9
Springer New York Heidelberg Dordrecht London

Library of Congress Control Number: 2012954480

© Springer Science+Business Media, LLC 2013
This work is subject to copyright. All rights are reserved by the Publisher, whether the whole or part of the material is concerned, specifically the rights of translation, reprinting, reuse of illustrations, recitation, broadcasting, reproduction on microfilms or in any other physical way, and transmission or information storage and retrieval, electronic adaptation, computer software, or by similar or dissimilar methodology now known or hereafter developed. Exempted from this legal reservation are brief excerpts in connection with reviews or scholarly analysis or material supplied specifically for the purpose of being entered and executed on a computer system, for exclusive use by the purchaser of the work. Duplication of this publication or parts thereof is permitted only under the provisions of the Copyright Law of the Publisher's location, in its current version, and permission for use must always be obtained from Springer. Permissions for use may be obtained through RightsLink at the Copyright Clearance Center. Violations are liable to prosecution under the respective Copyright Law.
The use of general descriptive names, registered names, trademarks, service marks, etc. in this publication does not imply, even in the absence of a specific statement, that such names are exempt from the relevant protective laws and regulations and therefore free for general use.
While the advice and information in this book are believed to be true and accurate at the date of publication, neither the authors nor the editors nor the publisher can accept any legal responsibility for any errors or omissions that may be made. The publisher makes no warranty, express or implied, with respect to the material contained herein.

Printed on acid-free paper

Springer is part of Springer Science+Business Media (www.springer.com)

*To my parents for their love and
support throughout the years.
Also, to my husband, I don't know
what I would do without you.*

Foreword

As a book author myself, I was extremely impressed with the thoroughness and relevance of this clinical pocket guide. Too often, residents struggle to find the appropriate references when managing patients. While this book in no means replaces the need to reference the appropriate rehabilitation texts, it can supplement such learning, providing physiatry residents with an intensified focus on their clinical responsibilities.

Dr. Sackheim has created this pocket guide with the foremost challenges facing residents in the field of physical medicine and rehabilitation in mind. Nonetheless, it will appeal to a much broader audience, as it does not focus solely on residents' needs. Each chapter was written by a specialist in the appropriate field and is diagnosis based, describing in detail pertinent anatomy, symptoms, diagnostics, and treatments needed. It contains detailed rehabilitation prescriptions, order sets for in-patient admissions, and treatment protocols for rehabilitation medical emergencies. For convenience, this book also has specific dosing of medications. However, as is necessary for providing appropriate care, it is highly recommended that you confirm dosing for each patient and take into account his or her personal medical history.

I trust that this pocket guide will soon become an integral component for all physiatry residents during their training and will continue to prove useful throughout their career.

Department of Rehabilitation Medicine,   Dr. Joseph E. Herrera
Mount Sinai Medical Center,
New York, NY, USA

Preface

During my physiatry residency, I often found myself scrambling through the chapters of numerous cumbersome textbooks for the information that I needed to properly manage my patients. These textbooks, while written by experts in their respective fields, often provided me with an overload of details for the task at hand. As a result, I was often unsure of what to focus on and which source was right for each individual rotation. With rotations changing monthly, it became clear that there did not exist a single, transportable, and concise guide that contained all of the relevant clinical information I needed on the rehabilitation unit. At that time I had just finished internship, and despite my excellent training, I was still not at the comfort level necessary to easily take emergency calls in the middle of the night for my rehab patients. All of this, combined with my last-minute decision to enter the field of rehabilitation, only added to an already stressful and overbearing experience. While the ultimate goal was to excel in this field and to be a great doctor to my patients, this aspiration was overshadowed by my struggle for a simple organized clinical approach.

In response to these challenges, I started gathering information into a little book that accompanied me wherever I went. Initially, I diligently entered important facts from lectures, rounds, and books that I needed to succeed in my rotations. These notes grew as I began adding medication dosing, consultant recommendations, specific rehabilitation goals and treatments, and billing details for each diagnosis. Recognizing how useful this information would have been to me at the start of residency, I decided to share these details to help others in similar circumstances succeed more easily in the field rehabilitation medicine.

This book provides all clinical material at your fingertips to properly treat patients and excel in the field of physical medicine and rehabilitation. Appealing to a wide variety of medical occupations from therapists and nutritionists to medical students and physicians, this pocket guide should prove to be an indispensable part of your daily practice. Hopefully, it can help alleviate some level of stress during residency; but at a minimum, I am confident that it will help you to focus, impress your patients and attendings, and further surpass your colleagues.

We are committed to excellence so please e-mail any comments to rehabclinicalpocketguide@gmail.com.

Department of Rehabilitation Medicine,   Dr. Kimberly A. Sackheim
Department of Pain Medicine
    and Palliative Care,
Beth Israel Medical Center,
New York, NY, USA

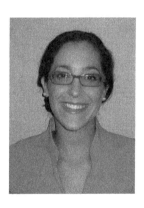

Acknowledgments

I give gratitude to those of you who throughout my training pushed me to strive for excellence. Dr. Jerry Weissman, we truly appreciate your dedication to teaching and to the field of Physical Medicine and Rehabilitation. Also, thank you to all of the amazing authors for their hard work to help the dream of this book become a reality.

Abbreviation List

>	Greater than
<	Less than
5×	5 times
5HT3	Subtype of serotonin receptor
A	Assist
Ab	Antibody
ABC's	Airway, breathing, circulation
ABG	Arterial blood gas
AAROM	Active assistive range of motion
AC	Acromioclavicular
ACE-I	Angitoensin converting enzyme inhibitor
ACL	Anterior cruciate ligament
ACSM	American college of sports medicine
ACTH	Adrenocortictropic hormone
ACPA	Anti-citrullinated peptide antibody
ACR	American college of rheumatology
AD	Autonomic dysreflexia
ADL	Activities of daily living
A. Fib	Atrial fibrillation
Abx	Antibiotics
AC	Anticoagulation
ADH	Antidiuretic hormone
ADM	Abductor digiti minimi
ADMP	Abductor digiti minimi pedis
AED	Antiepileptic drug
AFO	Ankle foot orthosis
AH	Abductor hallucis

AIDP	Acute inflammatory demyelinating polyneuropathy
AIN	Anterior interosseous nerve (in electrodiagnostics), or
AIN	Acute interstitial nephritis
AIS	ASIA impairment scale
aka	Also known as
AKA	Above knee amputation
AKI	Acute kidney injury
AL	Amyloid light chain
ALL	Anterior longitudinal ligament
ALS	Amyotrophic lateral sclerosis
ALT	Alanine aminotransferase
AMI	Arthrogenic muscle inhibition
AMS	Altered mental status
ANA	Antinuclear antibody
Anti-Ds	DNA Anti-double-stranded DNA
Anti-Sm	Anti-smith
AOC	Alteration of consciousness
AP	Anterior–posterior
APB	Abductor pollicis brevis
AROM	Active range of motion
AS	Ankylosing spondylitis
ASA	Aspirin
ASAP	As soon as possible
ASIA	American Spinal Injury Association
ASIS	Anterior superior iliac spine
AST	Aspartate Aminotransferase
ATFL	Anterior talofibular ligament
ATN	Acute tubular necrosis
ATP	Assistive technology professional
AVM	Arteriovenous malformation
AVN	Avascular necrosis
AZT	Zidovudine
β	Beta
BBB	Blood brain barrier
BI	Brain injury
BID	Twice per day
BiPAP	Bilevel positive airway pressure

BKA	Below knee amputation
BM	Bowel movement
BMI	Body mass index
BMP	Basic metabolic panel (aka chem-7)
BP	Blood pressure
BPH	Benign prostatic hypertrophy
BPM	Beats per minute
Bps	Beats per seconds
BR	Brachioradialis
BSS	Brown–Sequard syndrome
BUN	Blood urea nitrogen
C	Celsius
C-collar	Cervical collar
CABG	Coronary artery bypass graft
CAD	Coronary artery disease
CAP	Community acquired pneumonia
CBC	Complete blood count
CBT	Cognitive behavioral therapy
cc	Chief complaint or Cubic centimeter
CCU	Coronary care unit
CD	Compact disc
C diff	Clostridium difficile infection
CESI	Cervical epidural steroid injection
CFN	Common fibular nerve
CG	Contact guard
CHF	Congestive heart failure
CIDP	Chronic inflammatory demyelinating polyneuropathy
CIMT	Constraint induced movement therapy
CK	Creatinine kinase
CKC	Closed kinetic chain
CKD	Chronic kidney disease
CNS	Central nervous system
CMAP	Compound motor action potential
CMBB	Cervical medial branch block
CMP	Comprehensive metabolic panel
CMT	Charcot marie tooth
CMV	Continuous mandatory ventilation
CN	Cranial nerve

CO	Cardiac output
CO2	Carbon dioxide
COPD	Chronic obstructive pulmonary disease
COX	Cyclooxygenase enzyme
CP	Cerebral palsy
CPAP	Continuous positive airway pressure
CPP	Chronic pelvic pain
CTS	Carpal tunnel syndrome
CPC	Carpometacarpal joint
CPK	Creatine phospokinase
CPM	Continuous passive motion
CPP	Cerebral perfusion pressure
CPPD	Calcium pyrophosphate dihydrate
Cps	Cylces per seconds
CR	Cardiac rehabilitation
Cr	Creatinine
CRDs	Complex repetitive discharges
CRP	C Reactive protein
CRPP	Closed reduction percutaneous pinning
CRPS	Complex regional pain syndrome
CRS	Coma recovery scale
CSF	Cerebrospinal fluid
CSF	Cerebrospinal fluid
C-spine	Cervical spine
CSW	Cerebral salt wasting
CT	Computed tomography
CTLSO	Cervico-thoraco-lumbo-sacral orthosis
CTS	Carpal tunnel syndrome
CV	Conduction Velocity, or
CV	Cardiovascular
CVA	Cerebrovascular accident
CVD	Cardiovascular disease
Cx	Culture
CXR	Chest X-ray
D5NS	5 % Dextrose in normal saline solution
D5W	5 % Dextrose in water
d/o	Disorder
DAI	Diffuse axonal injury
DBP	Diastolic blood pressure

DBS	Deep brain stimulator
D/C	Discharge
DC	Direct current
DCS	Double contour sign
Dep	Dependent
DFN	Deep fibular nerve
DI	Diabetes insipidus
DIC	Diffuse intravascular coagulation
DIP	Distal Interphalangeal joint
DJD	Degenerative joint disease
DM	Dermatomyositis-rheum
DM	Diabetes mellitus-cardio
DMARDs	Disease modifying anti-rheumatic drugs
DME	Durable medical equipment
DOE	Dyspnea on exertion
DR	Dorsal root
DREZ	Doral root entry zone lesion
DRG	Dorsal root ganglion
DSD	Detrusor–sphincter dyssynergia
DUC	Dorsal ulnar cutaneous
DVT	Deep vein thrombosis
DWI	Diffusion-weighted imaging
DVT	Deep vein thrombosis
DVT/PE	Deep venous thrombosis/Pulmonary embolism
EAS	External anal sphincter
EBS	Electrical bone growth stimulator
ECG	Electrocardiogram
Echo	Echocardiogram
ECR	Extensor carpi radialis
ECRB	Extensor carpi radialis brevis
EDB	Extensor digitorum brevis
EDL	Extension digitorum longus
EE	Elbow extension
EEG	Electroencephalography
EF	Ejection fraction
eGFR	Estimated glomerular filtration rate
EHL	Extensor hallucis longus
EIP	Extensor indicis proprius

EKG	Electrocardiogram
ELISA	Enzyme-linked immunosorbent assay
EMG	Electromyography
EMG/NCS	Electromyography/Nerve conduction studies
ENT	Ear nose and throat
ER	External rotation
ESI	Epidural steroid injection
ESLD	End stage liver disease
ESR	Erythrocyte sedimentation rate
EST	Exercise stress test
etc	Etcetera
EtOH	Alcohol
eval	Evaluation
EVD	Endoventricular drain
ex.	Example
F	Fahrenheit
FADIR	Flexion, adduction, internal rotation
FAI	Femoralacetabular impingement
FCR	Flexor carpi radialis
FCU	Flexor carpi ulnaris
FDB	Flexor digitorum brevis
FDI	First dorsal interosseus
FDP	Flexor digitorum profundus
FDS	Flexor digitorum superficialis
FE	Finger extension
FENa	Fractional excretion of sodium
FES	Functional electrical stimulation
FEV1	Forced expiratory volume in 1 s
FFP	Fresh frozen plasma
FHB	Flexor hallucis brevis
Fibs	Fibrillation potentials
FIM	Functional Independence Measure
FOOSH	Fall on outstretched hand
FM	Fibromylagia
FPB	Flexor pollicis brevis
FPL	Flexor pollicis longus
FROM	Full range of motion
F/S D	Forequarter/Shoulder disarticulation
FSH	Follicle-stimulating hormone

FSHMD	Facioscapulohumeral muscular dystrophy
FVC	Functional vital capacity
GABA	Gamma-aminobutyric acid
Gallium-Arsenide	(GaAs) lasers
GBS	Guillain–Barre syndrome
GCS	Glasgow coma scale
GFR	Glomerular filtration rate
GH	Glenuhumeral
GI	Gastrointestinal
GMFCS	Gross motor functional classification system
GN	Glomerulonephritis
G-tube	Gastrostomy tube
GU	Genitourinary
h	Hours
H20	Water
HA	Headache
Hb	Hemoglobin
HCA	Hyperechoic cloudy areas
HCTZ	Hydrochlorothiazide
HD	Hemodialysis
HeNe	Helium-neon
HEP	Home exercise program
HHA	Home health aide
HIV	Human immune deficiency virus
HO	Heterotopic ossification
HPI	History of present illness
HR	Heart rate
Hrs	Hours
HTN	Hypertension
HVPC	High volt pulse current
Hz	Hertz
IAS	Internal anal sphincter
IBD	Inflammatory bowel disease
IBM	Inclusion body myositis
IBW	Ideal body weight
IC	Intermittent catheterization
IC	Interstitial cystitis

ICD	Implantable cardiac defibrillator
ICH	Intracranial hemorrhage
ICP	Intracranial pressure
ICU	Intensive care unit
IDEA	Individuals with disabilities act
IDD	Internal disc derangement
IFC	Interferential current
Ig	Immunoglobulin
IGF	Insulin-like growth factor
IL	Interlaminar
IM	Intramuscular
IM	Intramedullary (in ortho chapter)
Ind	Independent
INR	International normalized ratio
IPPV	Intermittent positive pressure ventilation
IQ	Intelligence quotient
IR	Internal rotation
ISIS	International spine intervention society
ISL	Interspinous ligament
ISNY	Icelandic–Swedish–New York
ISO	International Standard Organization
ITB	Iliotibial band, or
ITB	Intrathecal baclofen pump (in SCI/TBI)
IV	Intravenous
IVC	Inferior vena cava
IVF	Intra-venous fluid
IVH	Intraventricular hemorrhage
IVIG	Intravenous immune globulin
JIA	Juvenile idiopathic arthritis
JRA	Juvenile rheumatoid arthritis
Jt	Joint
JVP	Jugular venous pressure
K	Potassium
KAFO	Knee-ankle-foot orthosis
KUB	Kidneys–Ureters–Bladder X-ray
L2	2nd lumbar vertebrae
L3	3rd lumbar vertebrae
L5	5th lumbar vertebrae

LAC	Lateral antecubital cutaneous
LAD	Lymphadenopathy
LAM	Levator ani muscles
lb	Pounds
LBP	Low back pain
LDH	Lactate dehydrogenase
LE	Lower extremity
LEMS	Lambert–Eaton myasthenic syndrome
LESI	Lumbar epidural steroid injection
LF	Ligamentum flavum
LFT	Liver function test
LFTs	Liver function tests
LGMD	Limb girdle muscular dystrophies
LH	Luteinizing hormone
LHBF	Long head of biceps femoris
LLLT	Low-level laser therapy
LMBB	Lumbar medial branch block
LMN	Lower motor neuron
LMWH	Low molecular weight heparin
LN	Ligamentum nuchae
LOC	Loss of consciousness
LP	Lumbar puncture
L-S	Lumbosacral
LT	Light touch
LV	Left ventricular
LVAD	Left ventricular assist device
LVEF	Left ventricular ejection fraction
mA	Milliamperes
MAC	Medial antecubital cutaneous
Mag	Magnesium
MAS	Modified ashworth scale
MAOI	Monoamine oxidase inhibitor
MAP	Mean arterial pressure
MAS	Modified ashworth scale
MB	Medial branch
MBB	Medial branch block
max	Maximum
mcg	Microgram
MCP	Metacarpophalangeal joint
MCS	Minimally conscious state

MCV	Mean corpuscular volume
MD	Muscular dystrophy
MDA	Muscular dystrophy association
MEP	Motor evoked potentials
METs	Metabolic equivalents
mg	Milligram
MG	Myasthenia gravis
MGA	Martin gruber anastomosis
MHz	Megahertz
MI	Myocardial infarction
MMSE	Mini mental status exam
MMT	Manual muscle testing
MNCS	Motor nerve condution studies
MND	Motor neuron disease
MoCA	Montreal cognitive assessment
Mod	Moderate
MPH	Miles per hour
μs	Microseconds
μA	Microamperes
MRADL	Mobility related activity of daily living
MRI	Magnetic resonance imaging
MS	Multiple sclerosis
MSK	Musculoskeletal
MTP	Metatarsophalangeal joint
MTX	Methotrexate
MUA	Manipulation under anesthesia
MUAP's	Motor unit action potentials
mV	Millivolt
uV	Microvolt
MVA	Motor vehicle accident
MVIC	Maximum voluntary isometric contraction
n	Nano, (nm = nanometer, ns = nano seconds)
n/v	Nausea/vomiting
Na	Sodium
NCS	Nerve conduction studies
NG	Naso-gastric
NGT	Naso-gastric tube
NIF	Negative inspiratory force

NIPPVN	Non invasive intermittent positive pressure ventilation
NMES	Neuromuscular electrical stimulation
NMJ	Neuromuscular junction
NMO	Neuromyelitis optica
NMS	Neuroleptic malignant syndrome
NPO	Nil per os (Nothing by mouth)
NPSG	Nocturnal polysomnography
NS	Normal saline (0.9 % NaCl)
NSAID	Non steroidal anti-inflammatory drug
NSAIDS	Non-steroidal anti-inflammatory drugs
NWB	Non-weight bearing
NYHA	New York Heart Association
O&P	Ova and parasites
OA	Osteoarthritis
OI	Obturator internus
OKC	Open kinetic chain
O-Log	Orientation log
OMT	Osteopathic manipulation therapy
OOB	Out of bed
OPB	Opponens pollicis brevis
ORIF	Open reduction internal fixation
OT	Occupational therapy
P	Pulse
PAID	Paroxysmal autonomic instability and dystonia
PBS	Painful bladder syndrome
PBWSTT	Partial body weight supported treadmill training
PC	Pulse current
PCL	Posterior cruciate ligament
PD	Peritoneal dialysis
PDMS-2	Peabody developmental motor scale 2
PE	Pulmonary embolism
PEA	Pulse less electrical activity
PEEP	Positive end-expiratory pressure
PEG	Percutaneous-endoscopic gastrostomy
PEJ	Percuataneous-endoscopic jejunostomy

PEMF	Pulsed electromagnetic fields
PER	Pronation-external rotation
PFD	Pelvic floor dysfunction
PFT	Pulmonary function tests
PFM	Pelvic floor muscles
P-gp	P-glycoprotein
PGP	Pelvic girdle pain
PHR	Peak heart rate
PIN	Posterior interosseus nerve
PIP	Proximal interphalangeal joint
PLL	Posterior longitudinal ligament
PLS	Primary lateral sclerosis
PM	Polymyositis
PMA	Progressive muscular atrophy
PMH	Past medical history
PMR	Polymyalgia rheumatica
PN	Peripheral ner ve
PNA	Pneumonia
PO	Per os (By mouth, oral diet)
POD	Postoperative day
POP	Pelvic organ prolapsed
PP	Pin prick
PPI	Proton pump inhibitor
pps	Pulse per seconds
PQ	Pronator quadrates
PRAFO	Pressure relief ankle foot orthosis
PRD	Pressure relieving device
PRE	Progressive resistive exercises
PRN	As needed
PROM	Passive range of motion
PRP	Platelet rich plasma
PSH	Past surgical history
psi	Pounds per square inch
PSIS	Posterior superior iliac spines
PSWs	Positive sharp waves
PSWD	Pulsed shortwave diathermy
psych	Psychiatric
pt	Patient
PT	Physical therapy
PT	Prothrombin time

PTA	Post-traumatic amnesia
PTB	Patellar tendon-bearing socket
PTS	Post-traumatic seizure
PTSD	Post-traumatic stress disorder
PTT	Partial thromboplastin time
PTX	Pneumothorax
PWB	Partial weight bearing
PVFB	Progressive ventilator-free breathing
PVR	Post-void residual
Q	Every
Q2h	Every 2 h
Q8hrs	Every 8 h
Qac	Before meals
Qhs	Before bed
QD	Daily
QHS	Bedtime
R/o	Rule out
RA	Rheumatoid arthritis
RBCs	Red blood cells
RD	Registered dietitian
RF	Rheumatoid factor or radiofrequency (in interventional pain)
RHR	Resting heart rate
RNS	Repetitive nerve stimulation
ROM	Range of motion
ROS	Review of systems
RPE	Rating of perceived exertion
RR	Respiratory rate
RRMS	Relapsing-remitting multiple sclerosis
RTC	Rotator cuff
S1	1st sacral vertebrae
SACH	Solid ankle cushion heel
SaO_2	Oxygen saturation
SAP	Superior articulating process (in pain), or
SAP	Serum alkaline phosphatase
SBP	Systolic blood pressure
SCD	Sickle cell disease (in rheumatology), or

SCD	Sequential compression devices
SCI	Spinal cord injury
SCM	Sternocleidomastoid
SCS	Spinal cord stimulation
SD	Standard deviation
SEAS	Scientific exercises approach to scoliosis
SER	Supination-external rotation
SFN	Superficial fibular nerve
SHBF	Short head of biceps femoris
SI	Sacroiliac
SIADH	Syndrome of inappropriate anti-diuretic hormone secretion
SIJ	Sacroiliac joint
SIMV	(Synchronized) Intermittent mandatory ventilation
SOB	Shortness of breath
SJS	Steven–Johnson syndrome
SLE	Systemic lupus erythematosus
SLP	Speech language pathologist
SLR	Straight leg raise
SMA	Spinal muscular atrophy
SMART	Sensory modality assessment rehabilitation technique
SNAP	Sensory nerve action potential
SNRI	Serotonin norepinephrine reuptake inhibitor
SNCS	Sensory nerve conduction studies
SPET	Single-photon emission tomography
SSEP	Somatosensory evoked potentials
SSL	Supraspinous ligament
SV	Stroke volume
SLR	Straight leg raise
SS	Sacrospinous
SSRI	Selective serotonin reuptake inhibitor
ST	Sacrotuberous
STIR	Short tau inversion recovery
SubQ or SC	Subcutaneous
SUNA	Short-lasting unilateral neuralgiform headache attacks with cranial autonomic features
SUNCT	Short-lasting unilateral neuralgiform headache attacks with conjunctival injection and tearing
SWD	Short wave diathermy

TA	Tibialis anterior
TAC	Trigeminal autonomic cephalalgias
TBD	To be determined
TBI	Traumatic brain injury
TCA	Tricyclic antidepressant
TDWB	Touch down weight bearing
TEE	Transesophageal echocardiogram
Temp	Temperature
TENS	Transcutaneous electrical nerve stimulation
TES	Total elastic suspension
TFESI	Transformainal epidural steroid injection
TFs	Tube feeds
TFL	Tensor fascia lata
THA	Total hip arthroplasty
THR	Total hip replacement
TH/E D	Transhumeral/Elbow disarticulation
TID	Three times per day
TKA	Total knee replacement
TKR	Total knee replacement
TLSO	Thoraco–lumbo–sacral orthosis
TMA	Transmetatarsal amputations
TNF	Tumor necrosis factor
TON	Third occipital nerve
TP	Transverse process
TPN	Total parenteral nutrition
Trach	Tracheostomy
TR/W D	Transradial/Wrist disarticulation
TSB	Total surface-bearing socket
TSH	Thyroid-stimulating hormone
TT	Tarsal tunnel
TTP/HUS	Thrombotic thrombocytopenic purpura/ hemolytic uremic syndrome
TTWB	Toe touch weight bearing
TV	Tidal volume
UA or U/A	Urinalysis
UCL	Ulnar collateral ligament
UCBL	University of California Berkeley Laboratory
UCx	Urine culture
UE	Upper extremity
UH	Unfractionated heparin

UMN	Upper motor neuron
UOP	Urine output
US or u/s	Ultrasound
U.S.	United States
USP unit	United States Pharmacopeia unit
UTI	Urinary tract infections
VC	Vital capacity
Vent	Ventilator
VGCC	Voltage-gated calcium channel
vit.	Vitamin
VMO	Vastus medialis obliquus
VO_2	Oxygen consumption
VO_2max	Aerobic capacity
VPA	Valproic acid
VPS	Ventriculoperitoneal shunt
VS	Vegetative state
Vs.	Versus
VTE	Venous thromboembolism
w/	With
w/c	Wheelchair
W/cm^2	Watts/cm squared
WBAT	Weight bearing as tolerated
WBC	White blood count
WE	Wrist extension
WNL	Within normal limits
XR	X-ray
Yrs	Years
ZPP	Zone of partial preservation

Contents

Contributors

Shan Babeendran, D.O. Department of Rehabilitation Medicine, New York University Langone Medical Center, New York, NY, USA

Naimish Baxi, M.D. Department of Rehabilitation Medicine, Mount Sinai Medical Center, New York, NY, USA

Jaclyn Bonder, M.D. Department of Rehabilitation Medicine, New York University Langone Medical Center, New York, NY, USA

Anureet Brar, D.O. Department of Rehabilitation Medicine, Mount Sinai Medical Center, New York, NY, USA

David N. Bressler, M.D. Department of Rehabilitation Medicine, Elmhurst Hospital, Elmhurst, NY, USA

Gregory Burkard Jr., D.O. Department of Rehabilitation Medicine, New York University Langone Medical Center, New York, NY, USA

Richard G. Chang, M.D., M.P.H. Department of Rehabilitation Medicine, Mount Sinai Medical Center, New York, NY, USA

Nayeema Chowdhury, D.O. Department of Rehabilitation Medicine, New York University Langone Medical Center, New York, NY, USA

Jeffrey Cohen, M.D. Department of Rehabilitation Medicine, New York University Langone Medical Center, New York, NY, USA

Donna G. D'Alessio, M.D. Department of Physical Medicine and Rehabilitation, Mount Sinai Medical Center, New York, NY, USA

Houman Danesh, M.D. Department of Anesthesiology, The Mount Sinai Hospital, New York, NY, USA

Isaac Darko, M.D. Department of Rehabilitation Medicine, Mount Sinai Medical Center, New York, NY, USA

Andres Deik, M.D. Department of Neurology, Beth Israel Medical Center, New York, NY, USA

Jeffrey Heckman, D.O. Department of Rehabilitation Medicine, New York University Langone Medical Center, New York, NY, USA

Joyce Ho, M.D. Department of Anesthesiology, University of California, Irvine, CA, USA

Aziza Kamani, M.D. Department of Rehabilitation Medicine, Mount Sinai Medical Center, New York, NY, USA

Sarah Khan, D.O. Department of Physical Medicine and Rehabilitation, Mount Sinai Medical Center, New York, NY, USA

Natalie Kretzer, R.D., C.D.N. Department of Clinical Nutrition, Mount Sinai Medical Center, New York, NY, USA

Paul Lee, P.T. Department of Physical Medicine and Rehabilitation, Beth Israel Medical Center, New York, NY, USA

Jenny Lieberman, M.S.O.T. Department of Rehabilitation Medicine, Mount Sinai Hospital, New York, NY, USA

Emerald Lin, M.D. Department of Anesthesiology, The Mount Sinai School of Medicine, New York, NY, USA

Daniel MacGowan, M.D., M.R.C.P.I. Department of Neurology, Beth Israel Medical Center, New York, NY, USA

Colette Maduro, D.O. Department of Physical Medicine and Rehabilitation, Elmhurst Hospital, Elmhurst, NY, USA

Alex Moroz, M.D. Department of Rehabilitation Medicine, New York University Langone Medical Center, New York, NY, USA

Sandia A. Padavan, M.D. Department of Rehabilitation Medicine, Mount Sinai Medical Center, New York, NY, USA

Sagar S. Parikh, M.D. Department of Rehabilitation Medicine, Mount Sinai Medical Center, New York, NY, USA

Michelle Robalino-Sanghavi, M.D. Department of Rehabilitation Medicine, Mount Sinai Medical Center, New York, NY, USA

John-Ross Rizzo, M.D. Department of Rehabilitation Medicine, New York University Langone Medical Center, New York, NY, USA

Rosanna C. Sabini, D.O. Department of Physical Medicine and Rehabilitation, North Shore – Long Island Jewish as Southside, Bay Shore, NY, USA

Christopher Sahler, M.D. Department of Physical Medicine and Rehabilitation, Mount Sinai Medical Center, New York, NY, USA

Jennifer Sayanlar, D.O. Pain Management and Palliative Care, Pain and Wellness Center, Englewood Hospital, Englewood, NJ, USA

Samia Sayegh, D.O. Department of Rehabilitation Medicine, New York University Langone Medical Center, New York, NY, USA

Yolanda Scott, M.D. Department of Physical Medicine and Rehabilitation, Mount Sinai Medical Center, New York, NY, USA

Avniel Shetreat-Klein, M.D., Ph.D. Department of Physical Medicine and Rehabilitation, Mount Sinai Medical Center, New York, NY, USA

Jason W. Siefferman, M.D. Department of Anesthesiology, The Mount Sinai School of Medicine, New York, NY, USA

Lauren Stern, M.D. Department of Medicine and Nephrology, Boston University School of Medicine, Boston, MA, USA

Crystal D. Thomas, D.P.T. Outpatient Orthopedic Private Physical Therapy Practice, Sports Physical Therapy of New York, New York, NY, USA

Joe Vongvorachoti, M.D. Sports Medicine and Spine, Hospital for Special Surgery, New York, NY, USA

Part I
Inpatient Clinical Care

Chapter 1
Brain Injury

Jason W. Siefferman and Rosanna C. Sabini

Four forms of Brain Injury

I. Intracranial Hemorrhage

Bleeding in or around the brain (Intracranial hemorrhage, ICH) that may occur as a primary or secondary process, *classified by location*:

1. **Epidural**—Between the dura and the skull

   Etiologies:
   - Primarily traumatic (MVA, fall, assault)
   - 85% Arterial (i.e., middle meningeal), 75–95% associated with skull fracture, occur in 1–4% of traumatic head injuries
   - Mean age 20–30, rare in ages >50 [1, 2]

   Clinical: "Lucid Interval"—regaining brief consciousness but hematoma continues to expand; also known as the "talk, walk and die syndrome"

J.W. Siefferman, M.D. (✉)
Department of Anesthesiology, The Mount Sinai School of Medicine,
1 Gustave L. Levy Place, Box 1010, New York, NY 10029, USA
e-mail: jsiefferman@gmail.com

R.C. Sabini, D.O.
Department of Physical Medicine and Rehabilitation,
North Shore – Long Island Jewish at Southside Hospital, Bay Shore, NY, USA

K.A. Sackheim (ed.), *Rehab Clinical Pocket Guide:*   3
Rehabilitation Medicine, DOI 10.1007/978-1-4614-5419-9_1,
© Springer Science+Business Media, LLC 2013

Imaging:
- **CT**: Lens-shaped or biconvex appearance. Blood collection is limited by dural attachments at suture margins [3]

2. **Subdural**—between the dura and arachnoid membranes

   Etiologies [3–5]:
   - Tear in bridging veins at surface of the brain and dural sinuses
   - 20–30% are arterial due to cortical artery injury
   - Intracranial hypotension, leading to traction on supporting structures

   Risk Factors: Cerebral atrophy (elderly), EtOH abuse, antithrombotic agents (warfarin > ASA > heparin) [4, 6]

   Timeframe:
   - Acute (1–2 days after onset)
   - Subacute (3–14 days)
   - Chronic (15+ days)

   Clinical: Typically presents with altered consciousness, but can develop slowly and present many days to weeks after onset [4]

   Imaging:
   - **CT**: Crescent shaped, not limited by dural attachments to skull [3]

3. **Subarachnoid**—between the arachnoid layer and pia mater, leaking into CSF [7]

   Etiologies:
   - Ruptured saccular aneurysm
   - Trauma
   - Arteriovenous malformations (AVM)
   - Drug use [7]

   Risk Factors: Cigarette smoking, HTN, EtOH, genetics/family history, sympathomimetics, estrogen deficiency, antithrombotics, statins

   Clinical:
   - Meningeal signs—headache, photophobia, seizure, nausea/vomiting, neck/back pain
   - Mortality rate = 51% [8]

Complications: Rebleeding (73% within first 72 hrs) [9], vasospasm/ischemia, hydrocephalus, increased intracranial pressure, seizures, hyponatremia, cardiac arrhythmias, hypothalamic/pituitary dysfunction [7]

Imaging:
- **CT**: Blood in subarachnoid space seen in 92% of cases within 24 hrs of onset. Intracerebral extension in 20–40% [10]

4. **Intracerebral or Intraparenchymal**—within the neural tissue

Etiologies:
- Hypertensive vasculopathy
- Amyloid angiopathy
- Vascular malformations
- Septic embolism
- Tumor
- Bleeding disorder
- Vasculitis
- Stimulant drug use
- Conversion of ischemic stroke [11]

Risk Factors: HTN, elderly, EtOH abuse, male sex, African-American ethnicity, low cholesterol or triglycerides [12, 13]

Clinical: Gradual onset of neurological symptoms over minutes to hours, which may include: headache, vomiting, altered consciousness, seizures, cardiac arrhythmias [11]

Imaging:
- MRI up to 100% sensitive, superior to CT for chronic hemorrhage [11]

II. Stroke

Two types:

1. **Hemorrhagic**
   - 20% of cases [14]
   - See Intracerebral and Subarachnoid hemorrhage

2. **Ischemic**
   - 80% of cases [14]
   - 3 general causes:
   - **Thrombotic**—focal lesion due to clot formation

- **Embolic**—one or multiple lesions, heart is the primary source for clots (A. Fib)
- **Systemic hypoperfusion**—affects watershed zones

    1. **Anterior** → proximal muscle weakness (shoulders, hips, thighs)
    2. **Posterior** → cortical blindness or visual loss
    3. May also see altered mental status or impaired short-term memory

Imaging:
- **CT** sensitivity within 6 hrs of onset: $61 \pm 21\%$; early CT signs associated with poor functional outcome [15]
- **MRI** with diffusion-weighted imaging (DWI) is superior to CT for diagnosis of acute ischemic stroke within the first 12 h [16]

III. Space-Occupying Lesions

May include:
- Primary brain tumors
- Metastases
- Infectious processes (i.e., abscess, neurocysticercosis)

    Clinical: Patients may present with headache, focal neurological findings, impaired cognition, altered mental status and/or seizures, and workup may reveal hemorrhage and/or edema in addition to lesion. Patients are typically medically complex with chemotherapy, antibiotics, radiation therapy, corticosteroids to control vasogenic edema, and possible postsurgical complications.

    Imaging:
    - MRI with contrast is superior to CT [17]

IV. Traumatic Brain Injury

Classified by:

1. Mechanism of injury (blunt vs. penetrating head trauma vs. blast exposure)

2. Severity, based on [18]:
   (a) Glasgow Coma Scale (GCS)
   (b) Duration of loss of consciousness (LOC)
   (c) Duration of posttraumatic amnesia (PTA) Table 1.1

Table 1.1 Severity of TBI [18]

Mild	Moderate	Severe
Alteration of consciousness or LOC < 30 min	LOC > 30 min	LOC > 24 h
GCS 13–15	GCS 9–12	GCS 3–8
PTA < 24 h	PTA > 24 h	PTA > 7 days

Pathophysiology and clinical presentation:

1. **Diffuse axonal injury** (**DAI**): Shearing of axons at gray–white matter junction due to rapid change in velocity on impact, rotational forces and differences in tissue density between the white and gray matter.

   Clinical: Coma, alteration of consciousness, amnesia, apraxia, hypoarousal, inattention, sleep disturbance, vertigo, anosmia

   Imaging:
   • MRI with diffusion tensor imaging (DTI) may show impaired axonal transport [19]
   • CT may show multiple punctate areas of hemorrhage throughout the brain tissues, primarily in the white matter areas.

2. **Cerebral contusions**: Cout-contracout injury involving rapid acceleration/deceleration, primarily affecting the orbitofrontal and anterior temporal lobes.

   Clinical: Focal neuro deficits, frontal signs (disinhibition), temporal signs (seizures, vertigo, impaired emotional processing), visuoperceptual deficits

   Imaging:
   • CT for large contusions and hemorrhages visualized
   • MRI: petechial hemorrhages better seen

3. **Penetrating injury**: Gunshot or other foreign object

   Clinical: Deficits involving the area of injured tissue unless another mechanism of injury also involved. Monitor for seizures (very high risk) and hemorrhage.

Imaging:
- Use CT, avoid MRI if retained foreign bodies are metal

4. **Hypoxia/Anoxia**: Generally secondary to another traumatic process, prolonged elevation of intracranial pressure, myocardial infarction or large thrombus/embolus.

Clinical: Poor level of consciousness, disorientation, short-term memory loss and motor planning deficits. Neurological impairments are difficult to predict considering wide spread effect of hypoxia. More severe cases associated with coma, quadraparesis and spasticity.

Imaging:
- To rule out secondary pathology; no prognostic benefit [20]

Epidemiology:
- 1.7 million new cases/year in US
- 78% treated in ER only, 15% hospitalized, 3% fatal [21, 22]
- 1.1% of US population lives with long-term disability due to traumatic brain injury (TBI) [23].

Mechanism: Fall (primarily in elderly) > MVA > Struck by/against > Violence

Risk Factors:
- Age 0–4, 15–24, and 65+ years
- Male sex for all categories
- Low socioeconomic status [21]

Brain Injury Assessment

I. Patient/family interview and medical record review

HPI:

For traumatic:
- Logistics/mechanics of injury (clear story of what happened)
- Preventative measures used (seat belt, helmet)
- Confounding factors (Substance use such as EtOH, prior TBI, psychiatric history, and delay in extrication)
- Coexisting injuries, such as SCI, fractures, and respiratory insufficiency (possible anoxia)

For non-traumatic:
- Mechanism of injury

- Complicating factors (anticoagulation, uncontrolled HTN, prior stroke)
- Was there any secondary trauma? (i.e., fall, fractures, hematoma)
- What were the subjective complaints immediately post-injury?
- LOC duration?
- Alteration of consciousness (AOC) duration?
- PTA (Inability to form new memories after injury) duration?
- Memory of events leading up to the injury (retrograde), memory of events since injury (anterograde)
- Describe the treatment course to date, including initial ER presentation, initial GCS and interventions including intubation/sedation and/or surgeries.
- Current Issues:
  1. Focal Motor or Sensory deficits
  2. Pain—may be multiple types of pain, including headaches (for each: location, quality, intensity, radiation, aggravating/alleviating factors)
  3. Spasticity—location, severity, prior and current treatment, effect on sleep, function
  4. Dizziness—quality and aggravating factors (orthostasis vs. vertigo vs. central)
  5. Hearing—tinnitus or decreased hearing
  6. Vision—full visual fields in both eyes, blurriness, diplopia, photophobia, nystagmus, accomodation or convergence disorders
  7. Alteration in smell or taste
  8. Balance Deficits
  9. Diet—i.e., dysphagia, PEG or G-tube, current modified diet such as thickened liquids
  10. Respiratory—on vent or history of vent, trach size, last changed, downgraded, any capping trials, speaking valve trials
  11. Attention, Memory, and Concentration—vacant stare, inability to focus, delayed response, easily interrupted or distracted, able to finish tasks
  12. Communication deficits—word-finding difficulty, slurred speech, hoarse voice, reading difficulty
  13. Psych—symptoms of adjustment d/o or PTSD: flashbacks to event, nightmares, anxiety, depression, disrupted sleep
  14. Behavioral—agitation, aggression, confusion, out-of-proportion reactions, apathy, depression
  15. Sleep—delayed onset, decreased or increased in duration, frequent interruption, dreams or nightmares (may also be PTSD)

PMH: include all risk factors, including prior stroke or TBI, Primary Care Provider and Specialist contact information

PSH: include dates of procedures, surgeons, and hospitals, including craniectomy, shunt placement (VPS), PEG, and trach

Medications and drug allergies.

Social History:
- With whom do they live with?
- Home access (type of dwelling, steps to enter, elevator, wheelchair accessibility)
- Social support—who can assist at home, or provide financial support
- Educational level
- Prior employment
- Substance use
- Hobbies

Prior function:
- Mobility—i.e., ambulated w/walker, cane, wheelchair how far? (three blocks, or only in home)
- ADLs—Could they care for themselves or did they require assistance?
    - With what? (feeding, bathing, dressing, grooming, toileting)
    - Who helped them? (family or home health services)

Current (**Admission**) **function** (best functional exam is from most recent PT and OT notes)

Review of Systems: Review all other organ systems, specifically asking about nausea/vomiting and bowel/bladder dysfunction

II. **Physical Examination**
In addition to the standard medical physical examination, the Brain Injury exam should contain the following elements:

Mental Status: GCS (if appropriate, see Table 1.2)
Mental Function: Mini Mental Status Exam (MMSE), O-Log, or Montreal Cognitive Assessment (MoCA)
Speech: dysarthria, dysphonia; signs of aphasia (expressive or receptive), naming, repetition
HEENT: eye movements, visual fields, jaw range of motion; presence of rhinorrhea (r/o CSF leak)

Muscle Tone: spasticity, graded with the modified Ashworth scale (MAS, see Table 1.3)

Strength: using manual muscle testing, active and passive range of motion, atrophy or asymmetry (see Table 1.4)

Sensation: light touch, pin, vibration, proprioception, ability to extinguish simultaneous stimulation

Neurological: Cranial nerves (especially CN1 for impaired smell)

Reflexes: biceps, patellar, heel; Babinski and Hoffmann; primitive reflexes, if appropriate

Coordination: Finger-to-nose, heel-to-shin, rapid alternating movement, Rhomberg, pronator drift; differentiate coordination deficits from poor balance

Skin: Presence of breakdown (scapulae, sacrum, heels, occiput, hips and elbows) or infection, evaluate surgical sites, catheders, lines, trach site, feeding tube

Table 1.2 Glasgow coma scale (GCS) [24]

Score	Motor	Verbal	Eye
6	Obeys commands	–	–
5	Localized pain response	Oriented	–
4	Generalized pain response	Confused	Spontaneous eye opening
3	Flexor posturing to pain	Inappropriate	Opens eyes to speech
2	Extensor posturing to pain	Incomprehensible	Opens eyes to pain
1	No pain response	Nonverbal	No eye opening

Table 1.3 Modified Ashworth scale (MAS) [25]

0	No increase in tone
1	Slight increase in muscle tone, manifested by a catch and release or minimal resistance at the end of the ROM when the affected part(s) is moved in flexion or extension
1+	Slight increase in muscle tone, manifested by a catch, followed by minimal resistance throughout the remainder (less than half) of the ROM
2	More marked increase in muscle tone through most of the ROM, but affected part(s) easily moved
3	Considerable increase in muscle tone, passive movement difficult
4	Affected part(s) rigid in flexion or extension

Table 1.4 Grading of manual muscle testing (MMT)

0	Total paralysis—no active contraction
1	Palpable or visible contraction
2	Active movement, full range of motion, gravity eliminated
3	Active movement, full range of motion, against gravity
4	Active movement, full range of motion, against gravity and provides some resistance
5	Active movement, full range of motion, against gravity and provides normal resistance

Functional: Bed mobility, sitting/standing balance, and ambulation if able

Admission Orders

Admit to: Inpatient rehabilitation

Referring Physician: Obtain name, hospital and contact information

Diagnosis: Type of Brain Injury (traumatic, nontraumatic, stroke)

Condition: Stable/Fair

Prognosis: Good/Fair/Poor

Nursing:
- Vitals: Q Shift. If unstable, requires more frequent checks
- Turn patient Q2 h if patient unable to turn self
- Glucose fingersticks if on TPN, steroids, or known diabetic
- Tracheostomy care orders (i.e., clean site with hydrogen peroxide then wash with NS)
- Trach suctioning as needed, Chest PT during day Q6 h
- PEG or other feeding tube site care orders (i.e., flush with 30 mL of water before and after meds, clean site daily). If NPO, ensure adequate hydration, 250 mL Q4 to Q6 h.

Observation:
- Impulsive patients at risk for fall may require 1:1 supervision. Use enclosure beds if available

- Patients with frequent needs may require Q15 minute checks, if available.

Restraints:
- Patients interfering with their care (i.e., pulling trach, IV, PEG, Foley) may require mittens in addition to observation.
- Pharmacological restraints are discouraged due to cognitive and motor side effects.

Diet:
- Continue prior diet unless there is a decline in function
- Bolus feeds are recommended 5× daily. Continuous feeds are problematic during therapy and should be minimized. Nutritionist should assist in providing adequate caloric intake.
- Some patients have special needs, such as gluten free diets or religious restrictions.
- If dysphagia is suspected and there is no prior speech evaluation, consider NPO until evaluated.

Allergies: Environmental (latex), medications or food

Medications:
- Acetaminophen 650 mg PO Q4–6 h prn Temp > 100.4 or mild pain (check LFTs)
- Trazodone 25–50 mg PO QHS for sleep, if indicated by history/exam, not suitable for those with cardiac problems, as can cause QT prolongation.
- Colace 2–3× daily, Senna QHS as indicated
- DVT prophylaxis if not contraindicated (check with neurology, neurosurgery). This can include venous compression boots while in bed and TEDs during day.
- Seizure prophylaxis (phenytoin for first 7 days after TBI) [26]

Bladder:
- Indwelling Foley catheter should be removed to encourage bladder function and minimize infections.
- Complete voiding should be confirmed by checking post-void residual volumes with bladder scan or intermittent catheterization.
- If volumes <200 mL for 24 h, patient may use Texas catheter (if male), diaper, or void on commode.

- If greater >400 mL, patient may need Q4–6 intermittent catheterization or bladder medication.
- Begin bladder training—start Q2 h, before bedtime and after meals and modify to patient needs.

DVT Prophylaxis:
- DVT Prophylaxis varies with each patient with a brain injury. (See also section on DVT)
- A screening lower extremity Doppler is indicated to assess for deep venous thrombosis on admission.
- Sequential compression devices (SCDs) may be used if there is no leg trauma or suspected DVT.
- Many trauma patients may have had an inferior vena cava (IVC) filter placed, offering some protection from pulmonary embolism, but DVT prophylaxis is still necessary.
- Aspirin, warfarin, heparin or low-molecular weight heparin should be discussed with the treating neurologist or neurosurgeon prior to initiation.

Skin: Turn Q2 h, wound care management. Consider Zinc, Vit C and MVI supplements if poor wound healing

Labs: CBC, BMP, LFTs weekly but may need more frequently; may also consider Vitamin B12 if h/o EtOH, TSH, and drug-levels (dilantin, valproate). Pre-albumin to assess nutritional status. Screening UA and UCx, especially if had history of having a Foley in place

Imaging Studies:
- Obtain prior diagnostic imaging, including head CT, MRI and lower extremity Dopplers (CD is best as radiology can use to compare future images)
- Baseline Head CT and imaging of other injuries/fractures
- Lower extremity dopplers for DVT (unless previously done and negative)

Therapy:
- **Precautions**: Craniectomy (must wear helmet out of bed at all times), fall, orthosis wearing schedule (to prevent skin breakdown), weight-bearing status. Heart rate and BP precautions
- **Long-Term Goals**: Specify timeframe with target discharge date and determine possible level of independence that can be achieved
- **Short-Term Goals**: timeframe usually half of projected length-of-stay

Physical Therapy: Lower extremity strengthening, ROM, Bed Mobility, Transfers, Mobility (Ambulation vs. Wheelchair). Specify distance, assistive devices required

Occupational Therapy: Upper extremity strengthening, ROM, tone-reducing techniques, ADLs, functional transfers, fine motor and functional tasks, adaptive device eval, home eval, visual and perceptual testing and training

Speech: Assess for dysphagia and silent aspiration, cognitive remediation and needs for communication tools

Nutrition: Increased caloric requirements acutely after brain injury; plan enteral feeding regimen

Psychology/Neuropsychology:
- Eval and supportive therapy for patient and family; consideration of premorbid psych d/o
- Assessment of PTA, cognitive testing, compensatory techniques (day planners, etc.)

Recreational and Vocational Therapy: for community reintegration, identifying outpatient services for returning to work, support groups

Social Work/Case Manager: Evaluate current living environment and support available for discharge planning, including third-party coverage of home health aide, visiting nurse, and home PT/OT/Speech/neuropsychology as indicated.

Sequelae and Complications of Brain Injury

Disorders of Consciousness

Clinical:

1. **Coma**—results from injury to brainstem, midbrain, or both hemispheres [27]
   - Lack of wakefulness and sleep–wake cycles on EEG, eyes remain closed
   - No spontaneous purposeful movement or ability to localize noxious stimulus
   - No evidence of language comprehension or expression

2. **Vegetative State (VS)**—results from diffuse cortical injury, often involving the thalamus bilaterally, often secondary to hypoxia [20, 27]

- Evidence of sleep–wake cycles on EEG
- Eyes may open spontaneously or in response to noxious stimulus
- Startle reflex may be present, but no localization of stimulus
- Variability in cranial nerve and spinal reflexes

3. **Minimally Conscious State** (**MCS**)—for patients who do not meet criteria for VS [20, 27]
   - Evidence of self- or environmental awareness
   - Purposeful, consistently reproducible behaviors, such as yes/no responses or simple commands
   - May respond differently to different people and responses are consistent and not automatic
   - Signs of emergence from MCS: consistency in following commands, communication, and performing functional tasks.

Standardized Assessments of Consciousness:
- JFK coma recovery scale (CRS)
- Western neuro-sensory stimulation profile
- Coma/near coma scale
- Sensory modality assessment rehabilitation technique (SMART)
- Wessex head injury matrix

Important point to consider:
Clinical decline, even small, may indicate presence of medical complications (i.e., UTI) and should be worked up.

Treatment:

1. **Therapy**—benefits patients at all stages of recovery
   - Early rehabilitation helps optimize outcomes when the patient is transitioned to acute rehabilitation.
   - Prevention of secondary complications: Contractures, Skin breakdown, Heterotopic Ossification, Cardiopulmonary (edema, atelectasis, pneumonia)
     - Maintain ROM with positional stretches
     - Need to frequently monitor and adjust positioning, including use of splinting to decrease spasticity and minimize contractures
     - Wheelchair positioning

- Increase sitting/standing tolerance with standing Frame, tilt table, manual assistance, knee ankle foot orthosis, body weight-supported gait devices
- Sensory stimulation may affect the reticular activating system and increase arousal and attention (controversial, not evidence based).
- Tactile, auditory, visual, vestibular, gustatory, and olfactory stimulation
- Educate and provide written instructions for family and nursing regarding ROM, positioning, and splinting schedules.

2. **Medication**—neurostimulants may improve cognitive and behavioral responses
   - **Dopamine Agonists:**
     - **Amantadine**—100 mg po daily, then bid if tolerated. May take 1 week to see response, then may increase to 200 mg bid (max)
     - **Bromocriptine**—1.25 mg po bid, may increase by 1.25 mg every 3–5 days depending on response. Max dose 10 mg/day
     - **Methylphenidate**—5 mg po bid at 7 a.m. and noon, may increase by 5 mg daily depending on response. If no response at 20 mg bid, may be ineffective. Max dose 60 mg/day, or limited by tachycardia, HTN
       Side effects: Can lower seizure threshold, potentiate arrhythmia—use with caution

   - **Acetylcholine Reuptake Inhibitor:**
     - **Donepezil**—5 mg po daily, may increase to 10 mg (max) after 1–2 weeks
       Side effects: Nausea/vomiting/GI intolerance

   - **Other Stimulants**:
     - **Modafinil**—100 mg po qam, may increase by 100 mg every few days to max of 400 mg/day
       Side effects: Can lower seizure threshold, potentiate arrhythmia—use with caution

Elevated Intracranial Pressure (ICP)

Pathophysiology:
Increased matter in a fixed space increases pressure and reduces cerebral perfusion pressure (CPP). ICP increases with:
- Cerebral edema
- Space-occupying lesions or blood
- CSF flow obstruction
- HTN, vigorous PT, chest PT, supine position
- Fever, hyperglycemia, hyponatremia, seizures
- Suctioning, turning head (L > R), loud noises

Clinical:
- HA, nausea, vomiting
- Confusion, drowsiness, decline in GCS
- Seizures
- Focal neurological deficits (vision, weakness)
- Loss of corneal oculocephalic reflexes
- Breathing changes (tachypnea, pathological patterns)
- Papilledema—more common in chronic stages, usually bilateral

Values (**measured with intracranial monitor**):
- Normal ICP: 2–5 mmHg; <15 mmHg is harmless
- Elevated ICP: >20 mmHg for 5+ min
  - ICP > 40 mmHg - neurological dysfunction and impairment
  - ICP > 60 mmHg - tissue deformation, shifts, herniation, ischemia, tissue damage and death
- CPP = MAP–ICP (~5–15 mmHg)
- Maintain CPP >60 mmHg and MAP 70–90 mmHg

Complications:
Transtentorial temporal (Uncal) herniation of the medial temporal lobe
- *CN III palsy*-Ipsilateral pupillary dilation, ptosis, and ophthalmoplegia
- *Ipsilateral hemiparesis*-pressure on contralateral corticospinal tract
- *Contralateral hemiparesis*-mass effect on the ipsilateral precentral motor cortex

Diagnostic Workup:
CT Scan
- Do ASAP, while patient is hemodynamically stable.

- Clarifies severity, determines need for surgical exploration
- May yield etiology

MRI
- Better defines lesions, but due to increased time, does not affect early decision making
- CSF flow studies with sagittal FIESTA imaging may localize obstruction

Lumbar puncture (LP)
- Only after CT has ruled out mass lesion/outflow obstruction, as it can cause herniation

Treatment:
1. Consult neurosurgery, transfer patient for monitoring
2. Minimize ICP
   (a) Elevate head of bed 30°
   (b) Treat HTN
   (c) Address any causative factors above
   (d) Osmotics/Diuretics (Mannitol, hypertonic saline/Furosemide)
      (i) Improves swelling by diuresis and fluid shift
3. Decrease cerebral metabolic activity/oxygen demand
   (a) Intubate—may hyperventilate for short period in acute setting only, as hyperventilation decreases PCO_2, leading to vasoconstriction and decreased cerebral perfusion.
   (b) Induce barbiturate (thiopental) coma
      (i) Rapidly lowers ICP, suppresses electrical brain activity and slows metabolism to reduce cellular injury
   (c) Hypothermia
4. Ventricular drainage (EVD)/neurosurgical decompression (craniectomy)
5. Steroids have no beneficial effect unless there is vasogenic edema related to an abscess or tumor.

Hydrocephalus

Etiology:
- Non-communicating hydrocephalus:
  – Obstruction in the ventricular system

- Communicating hydrocephalus:
  - Decreased CSF resorption in arachnoid villi, more common after TBI
- Posttraumatic hydrocephalus:
  - May occur as early as 2 weeks or as late as 2 years [28]

Epidemiology:
- Incidence: 3.9–8%
  - 1.6% in acute setting, higher in severe TBI [29]
  - 45% overall, higher in severe TBI [30]
  - 5% of severe TBI patients will require shunt placement

Clinical:
- Altered mental status, mood changes, cognitive decline
- Seizures, vomiting
- Headache, incontinence, ataxia, increased spasticity
- Papilledema if increased ICP

Imaging:
- CT—uniform ventricular dilation, periventricular lucency
- MRI—may demonstrate CSF outflow obstruction—request specifically

Treatment:
- Neurosurgery consultation
- Lumbar puncture (if not contraindicated)
- Shunt placement
- See section on elevated ICP

Post-traumatic Seizures

An initial or recurrent seizure episode not attributable to another obvious cause after a TBI

Etiology:
- Brain injury or other structural abnormalities
- Electrolyte abnormalities (Na+, Ca++, Mg++)
- Genetics, pre-morbid

- Drug withdrawal—alcohol, anti-epileptic, benzodiazepine or baclofen
- Cerebrovascular disease, blood in brain or brain tumors
- Factors that lower seizure threshold
  - Hypoglycemia, infection
  - Insomnia
  - Medications
    ◦ Stimulants (methylphenidate, amphetamines, tricyclic anti-depressants, dopamine agonists)
    ◦ Antibiotics (fluoroquinolones)

Pathophysiology:
- Ferric chloride model: Iron salts and hemoglobin is an irritant to neural tissue
- Kindling: Stimulation in damaged neurons causes hypersensitivity and decreased seizure threshold
- Synaptic plasticity: compensatory collateral axonal sprouting can lead to neural hyperexcitability

Timeframe:
- Immediate/impact: first 24 h; more common in children
- Early: >24 h and less than 7 days
- Late: >7 days

Epidemiology [31]:
- 5% incidence in closed head injuries
- 30–50% incidence in open head injuries. Less frequent in mild TBI/concussion, but possible (slightly greater than the general population)

Risk Factors [32]:
- Penetrating head injury
- Intracranial hematoma
- Early seizures
- Depressed skull fracture
- Prolonged coma or PTA (>24 h)
- Dural tear
- Presence of foreign bodies (metal or bone fragments)
- Focal signs such as aphasia and hemiplegia
- Age (younger)
- History of alcohol abuse
- CT findings

Clinical—Types of Seizures:
- *Partial* (more common after TBI)
  - Simple
    1. No LOC
    2. Affects one specific part of the brain–anatomical location determines clinical presentation
  - Complex
    1. Alteration or LOC
    2. Symptoms can include muscle twitching, repetitive motions, and the appearance of "daydreaming"
- *Generalized*
  - Affects entire brain and causes LOC
  - Symptoms can include blank stares, falling, shaking, and repetitive stiffening and relaxing of muscles.
  - Partial seizures may become generalized seizures
- *Generalized Convulsive Status Epilepticus*
  - >5 min of continuous seizure activity OR recurrent seizures without return to baseline consciousness for >30 min.
  - Overall mortality is 20% (related more to the underlying pathology)
  - Requires emergent medical management, intubation, and monitored setting

Complications:
- Hyperthermia
- Acidosis
- Respiratory failure
- Rhabdomyolysis
- Aspiration

Workup:
- **EEG** (standard, sleep deprived, or 24 h)
  - May identify seizure activity and locate focus
  - Prognosticates severity once documented
- **Prolactin level** (serum)
  - Elevations noted immediately post-ictal, but normal levels do not exclude diagnosis
- **SPET Studies**

Treatment:

Prophylaxis:
Prevent early-onset seizures
- **Phenytoin for 7 days after injury** [26]
  - Start 100 mg po tid and follow serum levels, goal 10–20 µg/ml.
  - More than 7 days does not prevent late-onset seizures and can delay motor and cognitive recovery [26]
  - **Side effects**: delayed allergic reaction, nystagmus, vertigo, CNS depression, LFT elevation, hypernatremia

Active Seizures:
- Call a code and start timing
- Most last from 30 s to 2 min
- Primary responsibility—patient safety
  - Place in safe position, adjust the environment to prevent injury
  - Maintain airway, do not put anything in the mouth
  - Do not restrain the patient down
- **Lorazepam**: 2 mg IV or IM stat, may repeat if seizure does not abate in 3–5 minutes
  - $GABA_A$ agonist, may depress all levels of CNS, including limbic and reticular formation
- **Phenytoin**: load 1,000 mg IV, then dose 100 mg tid and adjust for serum phenytoin levels (10–20 µg/ml)

Post-traumatic Seizures (PTS):
Anticonvulsant medications are usually started once late seizures occur
- In TBI, carbamazepine (for partial seizures) and valproic acid (for generalized seizures) are often preferred.
- Important to treat because seizures reduce employment, increase health care costs, lower quality of life [33] and negatively affect outcomes [34, 35].
- PTS is associated with decreased cognitive performance [36].
- Treatment continued for 1–2 years and then trialed off for need to continue treatment

Medication overview:
- **Phenytoin**:
  - 300–900 mg/day, titrate to serum level of 10–20 µg/ml
  - Good for rapid loading (1,000 mg IV)

- Long-term use has been associated with adverse cognitive effects [26]
- **Side effects**:
  - Cerebellar and vestibular disorders (nystagmus, ataxia, vertigo)
  - Visual disturbances (mydriasis, diplopia, ophthalmoplegia)
  - Behavioral changes (hyperactivity, confusion, hallucination)
  - Gastrointestinal symptoms, gingival hyperplasia, osteomalacia, megaloblastic anemia
  - Transient LFT elevation, decreased ADH (hypernatremia).
  - Steven-Johnson syndrome, lupus, neutropenia, agranulocytosis, thrombocytopenia, lymphadenopathy

- **Carbamazepine**:
  - 600–1,200 mg/day, start 200 mg po bid, increase by 200 mg/day weekly as needed
  - Preferred for treatment of partial seizures
  - **Added benefits**: mood stabilizer and neuropathic pain treatment
  - **Side effects**: sedation, ataxia, diplopia, aplastic anemia, nausea, vomiting, LFT increase, SIADH

- **Valproate**:
  - Start 250–500 mg tid, titrate to serum level of 50–100 µg/ml
  - Max dose = 60 mg/kg/day
  - Preferred treatment of generalized seizures
  - **Added benefits**: mood stabilizer, migraine treatment
  - **Side effects**:
    - GI—anorexia, nausea, vomiting, increased appetite
    - Sedation, ataxia, rash, alopecia, LFT elevation, acute pancreatitis, hyperammonemia

- **Neurontin**:
  - Start 100–300 mg tid, titrate by up to 300 mg/day every 5–7 days
  - Max dose = 3,600 mg/day (theoretical)

- Used for partial seizures
- **Added benefits**: mood stabilizing/anti-anxiety properties, improves sleep architecture, neuropathic pain, and weak anti-spasticity agent.
- **Side effects**: fatigue, dizziness, ataxia

- **Lamotrigine**:
  - Start 25 mg po daily for first 2 weeks, unless on another agent, then adjust dosing as indicated. Titration begins week 3.
  - Max dose = 400 mg/day
  - **Added benefits**: strong mood stabilizing properties, neuropathic pain treatment
  - **Side effects**: dizziness, ataxia, blurred or double vision, n/v, rash, Stevens-Johnson's syndrome, DIC

- **Topiramate**:
  - Start 25 mg qhs or tid, titrate as tolerated up to 100–200 mg bid
  - Max dose = 800 mg
  - **Added benefits**: headache, migraine, and neuropathic pain treatment
  - **Side effects**: confusion, sedation, appetite suppression

Spasticity

Tone: muscle resistance to passive stretch across a joint
Spasticity: velocity-dependent increase in the stretch reflex (UMN)
Rigidity: non-velocity-dependent increase in tone (basal ganglia)

Treatment Objectives:
- Indications/goals for treatment
  - Improve function, mobility, balance, ADLs, positioning, hygiene
  - Decrease pain
  - Prevent contractures
- Address problems which increase spasticity first
  - Infection, pain, constipation, urinary retention
- Spasticity treatment varies by severity, location (generalized vs. focal), age, compliance and comorbidities. General principles:

- Focal treatments for focal spasticity (i.e., botulinum, TENS, orthoses)
- Multiple muscles in more than one limb, consider oral medication in addition to other focal treatments

Therapy:
- Correct positioning, splinting, casting, tone-reducing orthosis
- Stretching, ROM exercises
- Modalities (TENS, FES)

Oral Medication:
- **Baclofen**—$GABA_B$ agonist, pre- and post-synaptic
  - Start 10 mg po bid-tid and titrate by 10 mg as needed, max 80 mg/day (theoretical)
  - **Side Effects**: sedation, seizure with sudden discontinuation

- **Tizanidine**—α_{-2} agonist, inhibits spinal interneurons
  - Start 2 mg tid-qid and titrate by 2 mg as needed, max 36 mg/day
  - **Side effects**: sedation, dry mouth, orthostatic hypotension, elevated LFTs

- **Dantrolene sodium**—blocks Ca^{2+} release from sarcoplasmic reticulum
  - Start 25 mg daily and titrate to 3–4 times a day as needed every 4–7 days, max 400 mg/day
  - Preferred for lack of cognitive and sedative adverse effects
  - **Side Effects**: possible liver toxicity—need to monitor LFTs frequently

- **Benzodiazepines**—$GABA_A$ agonist
  - Use limited due to sedative and cognitive side effects

Interventional:
- **Chemical neurolysis with phenol or alcohol**
  - Lasts 6–9 months, inexpensive
  - **Side Effects**: dysesthesias
- **Botulinum toxin type A and type B**
  - For spasticity in selected muscles
  - Onset 2–3 days, peak 2–3 weeks, duration of effect 3 months.

- **Side Effects**: dysphagia, dyspnea, weakness, fatigue, upper respiratory infections
- **Intrathecal Baclofen Pump (ITB)**
  - Consider for patients with ADL-limiting spasticity uncontrolled on oral medications (less sedating), including those with hemi-spasticity.
  - Less effective for upper extremities
  - **Side Effects**: as above, and pump may fail

Agitation

A subtype of delirium unique to TBI survivors with PTA

Pathophysiology:
- Neurotransmitters—↑Norepinephrine, ↑Dopamine, ↓Serotonin

Risk Factors:
- Structural lesions: Hypothalamus, limbic system (amygdala), frontal neocortex
- Premorbid depression or social dysfunction
- EtOH, drug use, younger age
- Foreign environment
- Medical complications
  - Infection/metabolic disorder
  - Seizures/post-ictal
  - Psychosis/anxiety/depression/sundowning
  - Drug or EtOH withdrawal
  - Insomnia

Clinical:
- Explosive physical and verbal outbursts, emotional lability
- Increased psychomotor activity, impulsivity, disorganized thinking
- Destructive/combative behavior

Conservative and Initial Treatment:
1. Control the situation and calm the patient to identify the cause of hehavior
2. Identify the undesirable behavior for targeted treatment

3. Address any underlying contributing condition (i.e., pain, infection)
4. Educate staff and family
    (a) Can be controlled with changes in the environment and behavior of staff and family
    (b) Often, the mistake is to take the TBI patient's behavior personally
5. Tolerate restlessness when possible
    (a) Allow patient to pace around unit with 1:1 supervision
    (b) Allow confused patient to be verbally inappropriate, but correct them in a calm manner
6. Maintain a safe, structured, low-stimulus environment
    (a) Quiet, low-light, private room (No TV, radio, etc.)
    (b) Remove noxious stimuli (tubes, catheters, restraints)
    (c) Limit number of visitors, conversations
    (d) Provide therapies in patient's room, and use the same therapists for consistency
7. Minimize confusion
    (a) Orient the patient with every interaction
    (b) Always state who you are and why you are there
    (c) One person speaking at a time
8. Protect patient from harming self or others
    (a) Use 1:1 or 2:1 observation if available, fall precautions
    (b) Use floor (Craig bed) or low-boy beds with landing pads
    (c) Avoid taking patient off unit, should be on locked ward
9. Avoid use of restraints unless:
    (a) Danger to self (i.e., pull Foley, PEG, IV)
    (b) Danger to others
    (c) Some restraints (i.e., mittens) may be preferred to medications as there are no cognitive side effects

Pharmacologic treatment: *Start low, go slow*
1. Restore sleep–wake cycles:
    • Trazodone 25 mg po qhs and titrate as needed to 200 mg qhs
    • Sleep log and sleep hygiene

2. Minimize violent outbursts:
    • Lipophilic beta-blockers
        – Propranolol 10 mg tid, titrate by 10 mg as needed [37]
        – Monitor blood pressure and pulse

3. Stabilize mood:
   - Antidepressants [38]
     - Citalopram 10 mg po daily, titrate by 10 mg every week to max of 40 mg
   - Anti-epileptic Drugs (AEDs)
     - Valproate 500 mg po tid, titrate up or down for effect, monitor serum levels for toxicity: max 100 μg/ml
4. Improve attention/cognitive function to minimize confusion:
   - Stimulants
     - Amantadine 100 mg po daily, increase to bid, then 200 mg bid if needed [39, 40]
     - Methylphenidate 5 mg po at 7 a.m. and 12 p.m., increase by 5 mg as needed to max of 30 mg bid
       Side effects: Can lower seizure threshold, potentiate arrhythmia—use with caution
   - Acetylcholine Reuptake Inhibitor:
     - Donepezil—5 mg po daily, may increase to 10 mg (max) after 1–2 weeks
       Side effects: Nausea/vomiting/GI intolerance

5. Suppress disorganized thinking/hallucinations, or sedate patient:
   - Atypical antipsychotics—less preferred due to cognitive side effects
     - Quetiapine 25 mg prn, may titrate to 100 mg if needed
   - Benzodiazepines—not recommended due to cognitive side effects, but may need initially until behavior is more controlled
     - Lorazepam or clonazepam 0.25–1 mg bid-tid prn

Sleep Disturbances

Insomnia
- Difficulty falling asleep (i.e., requiring more than 30 min to fall asleep)
- Difficulty maintaining sleep (i.e., more than 30 min of nocturnal awakening)
- Occurs at least 3 nights/week
- Results in impairment of daytime functioning

Epidemiology:
- Sleep disturbances are 3× more prevalent after TBI than in the normal population
- 30–81% experience sleep difficulties in inpatient and outpatient setting [41]
- Sleep disturbance rates vary based on severity of brain injury [42–44]
  - Higher in milder TBI and lower in more severe TBI (may be unaware of their sleep problems secondary to memory and cognitive difficulties)
- Grossly underestimated because it is minimized by
  - Patients—patients may not remember the quantity or quality of sleep
  - Family/friends—not awake the entire night monitoring
  - Rehabilitation professionals—report sleep for brief period each hour (they may wake them up doing so).
- Difficult to assess in the presence of cognitive and behavioral problems

Risk Factors:
- Premorbid sleep disorder
- Hypothalamic injury (coordinates sleep–wake cycles)
- Pineal injury (melatonin release affected)
- Psychiatric distress: depression, anxiety, confusion, family stress, pain, PTSD
- Medication side effects

Clinical:
- Fatigue, impaired arousal
- Cognitive deficits, confusion, memory difficulties, amnesia
- Aggression, agitation, depression, anxiety, psychosis

Complications
- Abnormal sleep patterns can exacerbate and significantly impact recovery
  - Decrease alertness, attention, participation
  - Increase agitation and behavioral disturbances
  - Increase difficulty with new learning
- TBI patients with a sleep disorder perform worse on a battery of neuropsychological tests, sustained attention, and short-term memory [45]

- Early identification and evaluation of sleep disorders with appropriate environmental and pharmacological intervention can limit cognitive and behavioral sequelae.

Workup:
Subjective measures
- Questionnaires (Insomnia Severity Index, Epworth Sleepiness Scale, Pittsburgh Sleep Quality Index)
- Sleep logs/diaries
- Sleep History (family can help with information)
  - How long? How much?
  - Daytime tiredness?
  - Comments from sleep partner?
  - Initiation of sleep vs. maintenance?
  - History Prior to TBI, Asthma, COPD, GERD, Incontinence, BPH, Anxiety, depression, Pain?
  - Cigarette, caffeine, EtOH use?
  - Current medications? (Over the counter, diet pills, caffeine-containing meds, allergy meds such as pseudoephedrine, prescription)

Objective measures
- Nocturnal polysomnography (NPSG, i.e., sleep study)—Gold standard
  - Records EEG, eye movement, RR, HR/rhythm, muscle movement (EMG), O_2 levels
- Actigraphy—a device worn around the arm, leg, or waist
  - Evaluates sleep–wake patterns, circadian rhythm and effectiveness of treatments
  - Measures activity or movement, therefore must consider patients with motor impairments (SCI, CVA) or behavioral difficulties

Treatment—Behavioral:
Sleep hygiene
- Consistent sleep schedule
- Avoid daytime naps
- No caffeine 4–6 h before bed
- Avoid nicotine (stimulant) and alcohol
- Avoid drinking fluids prior to sleep (nocturnal micturition)
- Modify environment by minimizing light and noise, adjust temperature
- If unable to sleep after 30 min, leave bedroom → stay up → get sleepy → return to bed

Cognitive behavioral therapy:

Psychotherapy to positively change: Behavior, perception, and feelings on sleep

- Require patient compliance and dedication
- Frequent therapy visits
- May be more effective than medication

Chronotherapy
- Shifts patient's sleep schedule
- Restrict the time spent in bed to the actual number of hours spent sleeping
- Slowly increase over consecutive nights

Relaxation therapies
- Breathing exercises, guided imagery

Light therapy
- Lamps emit special wavelengths that mimic sunlight
- Used in the morning to aid arousal
- May lead to eye strain and headaches

Treatment—Medications:

Anti-depressants
- **Trazodone**: 25 mg po qhs, may double dose nightly up to 200 mg
  - **Side effects**: hypotension, ↑QT, MAOI interactions, attention or cognitive impairment
- **Nortriptyline**: start 10–25 mg qhs, may increase by 25 mg every 3–5 days, max 150 mg
  - **Side effects**: arrhythmia, agitation, ataxia, confusion, seizure, constipation
- **Mirtazapine**: start 7.5 mg qhs, may increase by 7.5 mg weekly to max of 45 mg
  - **Side effects**: appetite stimulation, constipation, dizziness

Melatonin agonist
- **Ramelteon**: 4–8 mg po qhs
  - Decreases sleep latency and improved total sleep time
  - **Side effects**: dizziness, fatigue, worsened insomnia

Non-benzodiazepines ("Z" Drugs)

Still CNS depressants, but fewer adverse effects than benzos
- **Zolpidem** (Ambien and Ambien CR): start 5 mg qhs, may increase to 10 mg

- **Zaleplon** (Sonata): start 5 mg qhs, may increase by 5 mg to max of 20 mg
- **Zopiclone** (Lunesta): start 1 mg qhs, may increase by 1 mg to max of 3 mg
    - Short half-life to reduce in next-day residual effects
    - **Side effects**: headache, hallucinations, amnesia, fall risk

Avoid
- Benzodiazepines
    - Interferes with resolution of edema, reduces diaschisis
    - Prevents unmasking and relearning and long-term potentiation
    - Rebound insomnia, dependence, withdrawal
- Diphenhydramine
    - Confusion, daytime lethargy, dry mouth, urinary retention, constipation

Language

Communication difficulties from brain injury may be due to impairments in fluency, comprehension, repetition, or naming. Reading, writing, nonverbal gesturing, and problem-solving may also be affected.

Aphasias classification (Table 1.5)

Other definitions:

Agrammatism—loss of grammatical structure

Apraxia—inability to perform a task by verbal command

Automatic speech—frequent use of common phrases to compensate for word-finding difficulty or poor comprehension (common in dementia)

Circumlocution—describing a word that cannot be recalled

Echolalia—repeating words said by another person

Neologism—new word created by the patient, which only has meaning to the patient

Paraphasia—incorrect substitution of words (may be by similar sound or object type)

Stereotype—meaningless repetition of a single word or nonsense syllable in presence of expressive aphasia

Table 1.5 Aphasia classification

Aphasia	Fluent	Comprehension	Repetition	Naming	Brain location
Normal	+	+	+	+	N/A
Anomia	+	+	+	−	Temporo-parietal, angular gyrus
Conduction	+	+	−	N/A	Parietal operculum (arcuate fasciculus) or insula
Transcortical sensory	+	−	+	N/A	Watershed posterior-inferior temporal lobe
Wernicke's (receptive)	+	−	−	N/A	Post. aspect of dominant (L[a]) first temporal gyrus
Transcortical motor	−	+	+	N/A	Frontal lobe
Broca's (expressive)	−	+	−	N/A	Dominant (L[a]) posterior-inferior frontal lobe
Mixed transcortical	−	−	+	N/A	Border zone of frontal, temporal and parietal lobes
Global	−	−	−	N/A	Perisylvian region (MCA distribution)

[a]95% are L-hemisphere dominant

Recovery:
- Most improvement after stroke at 2–3 months, up to 6 months
- Little improvement after 1 year, although it has been reported with therapy

Pain after Brain Injury

Brain injury contributes to the development of pain. Many pain medications have significant cognitive side effects and must be monitored closely. The general principle is "start low, go slow." Also try to take advantage of the multiple effects of many drugs: i.e., valproate is effective for neuropathic pain, headaches, mood, and seizures. TCAs may help sleep, mood, neuropathic, or chronic musculoskeletal pain.

Primary pain examples:
  Headache (post-traumatic, migraine, tension)
  Thalamic pain syndrome
  Fibromyalgia
Secondary pain examples:
  Shoulder subluxation, impingement, rotator cuff tendinosis
  CRPS type I (including shoulder-hand syndrome)
  Heterotopic ossification
  Nerve impingements

Thalamic Pain Syndrome [46, 47]
Pathophysiology:
- The thalamus processes ascending sensory signals from the spinal cord and provides relevant connections to other brain centers and with injuries to any areas, pain processing is impaired.
- Although neuroplasticity is part of recovery, it can be imprecise and maladaptive. In these cases, the parts of the brain that perceive pain are activated by signals which are not true pain signals.
- Signals from other sensory modalities such as light touch or temperature may be interpreted as pain, leading to allodynia or temperature sensitivity.

Clinical:
Onset: few months, up to 2 years after injury
Symptoms:
- Sensory loss, dysesthesias, allodynia, and hyperalgesia

- Pain may be burning, stabbing, squeezing or freezing in quality
- Area of the body affected varies with lesion

Treatment:
TCAs—amitriptyline or nortriptyline
- Start 10–25 mg qhs, may increase by 25 mg every 3–5 days, max 150 mg

AEDs
- Gabapentin 100 mg po tid, titrate up to total of 3,600 mg/day
- Topiramate 25 mg qhs, titrate as tolerated up to 100–200 mg bid
  Side effects: Confusion, sedation, appetite suppression
  Mexiletine (with cardiac monitoring)
  Spinal cord stimulation

Headache
Common after TBI—74% of mild TBI reported headaches, 45% were diagnosed with migraine, 20% chronic daily headaches [48]

Workup:
- Detailed history (location, onset, quality, evolution, duration, associated symptoms, aggravating/alleviating factors)
- Brain imaging: MRI preferred unless acute process suspected, then CT

Types of headaches:
- **Post-traumatic**
  Clinical: nonspecific, but generally has qualities of migraine (photophobia, vertigo) as well as tension-type (bi-frontal, temporal, or occipital distribution)
  Treatment: acetaminophen or NSAIDs; progress to topiramate or other AED if not helpful, may also consider botulinum toxin to painful areas
- **Migraine**
  Clinical: unilateral, throbbing, usually with aura, photophobia, nausea; may be related to oculomotor dysfunction
  Treatment: Consider neurology consultation. Acetaminophen or NSAIDs at time of aura onset, triptans. If chronic, prevention with propranolol 10 mg tid or an AED such as valproate or topiramate
- **Tension-type**
  Clinical: generally bilateral occipital or temporal, dull constant without aura, photophobia, etc. Associated with muscle tension in

scapular stabilizers, paracervical muscles, and/or temporalis. May coexist with TMJ disorder, or traumatic facet arthropathy.

Treatment: acetaminophen or NSAIDs, PT/daily stretching, may consider trigger point injections, botulinum toxin. Muscle relaxers may be helpful, but cognitive side effects outweigh benefit after brain injury.

- **Other causes to consider**
  - **Subarachnoid hemorrhage**—blood is noxious to meninges → meningeal signs
  - **Intracranial hypotension** with possible CSF leak—onset with supine → sit maneuver
  - **Temporomandibular joint injury**—evaluate for symmetry, ROM, tenderness
  - **Occipital neuralgia** (greater occipital nerve injury)—occiput to temple distribution
  - Check Tinel's midway between mastoid process and occipital protuberance
  - **Trigeminal neuralgia**—usually V_1 or V_2; shooting, aching, burning pain
  - **Trigeminal Autonomic Cephalalgias** (**TAC**), including cluster, SUNCT, SUNA, paroxysmal hemicranias. Associated with autonomic irregularity (tearing, scleral injection, sweating; usually unilateral)

Complex Regional Pain Syndrome, Type I

Pain, autonomic changes (abnormal blood flow, edema, temperature changes), and structural changes (cortical bone lesions, alopecia, waxy appearance of skin) maintained by a dysregulated sympathetic nervous system [49].

Clinical: Neuropathic pain (burning, throbbing with allodynia/hyperalgesia), edema, vasomotor, or sudomotor changes. With chronicity, affected region may expand or involve contralateral side. Skin, nails, hair, bone atrophies. Decreased ROM.

Treatment: *Acute*—oral prednisone 1 mg/kg/day tapered over 2 weeks, topical ketamine, NSAIDs

Subacute/Chronic—TCAs, SNRIs, AEDs, stellate ganglion block, epidural anesthetic infusion, ketamine infusion.

Chronic—Spinal cord stimulation

Cranial Nerve Dysfunction

CN I (Olfactory) → Anosmia, decreased appetite

Pathophysiology: tearing of the nerve filaments at the cribriform plate

– Can result from any injury, but more common with blunt trauma, occipital > frontal injuries

Recovery: 1/3 full, 1/3 partial, 1/3 none

CN II (Optic Nerve) → Blurred vision, homonymous hemianopsia, blindness

– Check consensual light reflex

CN IV > CN III > CN VI → Diplopia, strabismus, impaired depth perception, imbalance

Treatment: Requires eye patch

CN VII (Facial) → Partial or full facial drooping, taste alteration

– Nerve conduction study may help guide rehab

CN VIII (Vestibulocochlear) → Hearing loss, balance difficulty, vertigo

Treatment: Vestibular rehab or anticholinergic agent

– Vestibular therapies not as effective if using anticholinergic
– Meclizine 12.5 mg po tid, titrate up to 25 mg after 1 day if no benefit
– Monitor for CNS depression, constipation, dry mouth
– If positive benefit achieved on meclizine, may convert to scopolamine 72 h patch for easier administration and more steady delivery.

Central Dysautonomia

Paroxysmal Autonomic Instability and Dystonia (PAID)

Etiology: Surge of circulating catecholamines

Risk Factors: Anoxic > Traumatic BI, if <2 weeks post-injury, associated with poor prognosis

Clinical:

– Hyperthermia, diaphoresis
– Hypertension, tachycardia
– Tachypnea
– Rigidity
– Lasts several hours, and can reoccur

Central Fever
- Thermoregulation intact with increase set point of body temperature

Central Hyperthermia
- Thermoregulation defect without change of set point

Etiology: Direct trauma to the autoregulatory centers: hypothalamus and/or cortex

Pathophysiology:
- Direct injury to the rostral hypothalamic region resetting thermostats
- Direct frontal damage interrupt inhibitory pathways to the hypothalamus
- Axonal stretch causing inhibition of release of dopamine

Management:
- Cooling blankets, NGT lavage
- NSAIDs (indomethacin), acetaminophen
- Lipophilic beta-blockers to help with hypertension/tachycardia
  - Propranolol—10 mg tid, may titrate by 10 mg as needed
- Dantrolene sodium to help with muscle contractility
  - Start 25 mg daily and titrate to 3–4 times a day as needed every 4–7 days, max 400 mg/day
- Dopamine agonists:
  - Amantadine—100 mg po daily, then bid if tolerated. May take 1 week to see response, then may increase to 200 mg bid (max)
  - Bromocriptine—1.25 mg po bid, may increase by 1.25 mg every 3–5 days depending on response. Max dose 10 mg/day
- A_2-agonists: Clonidine start 0.1 mg q8 h

Cardiac Complications

EKG changes may be due to brain injury without primary cardiac pathology:
- Sinus bradycardia
- Supraventricular tachycardia
- ST segment changes, T wave inversion

- Tall P waves
- Prolonged QRS, QT, or heart block

Cardiac Changes after TBI:
- Cardiomyopathy
- Hypertension
- Tachycardia
  Epidemiology: 11–25% incidence
  Etiology:
  – Rise in catecholamines/sympathetic hyperactivity
  – Autonomic dysregulation/higher heart rate variability
  Treatment:
  – Usually resolves spontaneously
  – Propranolol 10 mg po tid, titrate dose by 10 mg daily as needed, dose limited by response and side effects

Venous Thromboembolic Disease

Deep vein thrombosis (DVT) and pulmonary embolism (PE)
- Most significant cause of mortality in TBI
- Often clinically silent, with sudden death from PE being the first clinical sign in 70–80%

DVT—Epidemiology:
- Trauma: 50–99%
- Brain tumor: 28–43%
- TBI: ~54% in acute

Risk Factors:
Risk starts within the first day of TBI
- Immobility, paralysis
- Fracture or soft tissue injuries
- Disruption in coagulation and fibrinolysis
- Age >40
  Virchow's triad: Venous stasis, vessel-wall (endothelial) damage and hypercoagulable state

Clinical:
- Physical exam minimally helpful
- Calf circumference asymmetry, edema, tenderness, Homan's sign

Complications:
- Pulmonary embolism (PE)
- Clinical signs and symptoms may be absent, or include dyspnea/oxygen desaturation, fatigability, tachycardia, EKG changes, flash pulmonary edema, chest pain, hypoxic seizure or sudden death.
- Post-thrombotic syndrome
- Additional DVTs

Workup:
- Lower extremity ultrasound
  - Standard of care
  - Can get LE Ultrasound on all admissions to r/o DVT
  - Less sensitive, but not invasive
  - If ordering a CTA Chest for PE, consider LE venography as well

DVT Prophylaxis:
Must weight risks/benefits of any anticoagulation
- Choice of prophylaxis should be patient-specific and based on existing comorbidities, recent surgeries/trauma, and discussion with the treating neurosurgeon or neurologist
- May not be able to use anticoagulation in those s/p cranial surgery or with hematomas
- Start as early as possible, ideally on admission

Mechanical Prophylaxis:
Must first rule out DVT
- Compression stockings
- Sequential compression device

Treatment:
- Bedrest for first 24 h
- Discontinue pneumatic compression device
- Immediate-acting anticoagulant + warfarin, if not contraindicated:
  - Heparin drip (discuss goal with medicine and neurosurgery) or LMWH, i.e., enoxaparin 1 mg/kg q12 h
  - Warfarin 5 mg po daily, goal INR of 2–3
- Treat for 3 or 6 months, discuss with medicine service
- IVC filter when anticoagulation is contraindicated
  - Must start anticoagulation as soon as possible, even after filter placement [50]

Chemical Prophylaxis:
- Unfractionated heparin (UH)—5,000 Units SQ Q8 h or Q12 h
  - Activates antithrombin III, inactivates XA/IIA and PLT
  - Effective, reversible, inexpensive
- Low molecular weight heparin (LMWH)—i.e., enoxaparin 40 mg SQ daily
  - Greater bioavailability at lower doses
  - More predictable
  - Longer half life
  - Less complications, including thrombocytopenia
  - Expensive
- Oral anticoagulants
  - Warfarin [53]
  - Aspirin—limited benefit

Surgical Prophylaxis:
- IVC filters [50–52]
  - Often placed early on for patients at high risk for DVT/PT who are unable to be anticoagulated if they develop a DVT or PE.
  - Invasive, placed by vascular surgery or interventional radiology
  - Removable (up to 6 months after)
  - Does not prevent PEs from UE DVTs, or from clots that form on the filter itself
  - Filter can thrombose and obstruct the IVC
  - Does not prevent post-thrombotic disease
  - Patients with IVC filters still require chemical DVT prophylaxis as early as possible

Endocrine Dysfunction

- Serum Na$^+$ most commonly affected, but any pituitary or hypothalamic disorder may be seen
- Thought to be secondary to DAI and shearing damage of the hypothalamus and pituitary stalk
- Seen in 10% of TBI patients

Workup:
- Endocrinology consult
- Serum chemistry
- Serum cortisol—8 a.m.

- TSH, free T3 and T4
- FSH, LH, testosterone, prolactin
- IGF, IGF—II
- Vitamin D levels

Cerebral Salt Wasting (CSW)

Etiology:
- Direct neural effect on renal tubular function
- Leads to Na+ loss in urine, and hyponatremia
- Triggers ↑ ADH secretion (appropriate)

Risk Factors: SAH, TBI

Clinical:
- Polyuria, weight loss, dehydration
- Hypotension, orthostasis
- Hypovolemic hyponatremia

Treatment:
- Volume repletion (0.9% NS), follow BUN/Cr
- May need po NaCl, start 1 g bid and titrate with daily Na^+ levels

Syndrome of Inappropriate Anti-Diuretic Hormone Secretion (SIADH)

Etiology:
- Excessive anti-diuretic hormone (ADH) secretion (posterior pituitary)
- H_2O reabsorbed in the collecting ducts while Na^+ excreted

Risk Factors:
- CNS trauma, SAH
- Malignancy (small cell lung most common)
- Medications: Carbamazepine, SSRI, TCAs, cephalosporins, nicotine

Clinical:
- Altered mental status, lethargy, coma
- Anorexia, nausea/vomiting
- Seizure
- Hyponatremia and concentrated urine (>300 Osm)
- Euvolemic hyponatremia

Treatment:
- If presents with seizure or severe AMS, ICU transfer required, otherwise:
- Ensure euvolemic status (BUN/Cr ratio <20)
- Fluid restrict 1–1.5 L/day with strict Intake/Output records

- Replace Na$^+$ <15 mEq per 24 h (avoid central pontine myelinolysis)
  - NaCl 1 g po bid-tid and titrate by 1–2 g/day based on serum Na$^+$
  - 0.9% NS with loop diuretic (excretes more water than Na$^+$)
- If chronic, may start Demeclocycline 13–15 mg/kg/day divided q6–8 h

Diabetes Insipidus (DI)

Etiology:
- ADH deficiency/inability to reabsorb water in the collecting ducts

Risk Factors:
- Severe head injuries
- Skull fractures in or near the sella turcica may tear the stalk of the pituitary gland
- Hypoxia
- Pituitary surgery

Clinical:
- Polyuria
- Weakness, fever, psychic disturbances, prostration, death
- Hypovolemia with normal to increased Na+ level
- Urine Osm Na$^+$< Serum Osm Na$^+$

Treatment:
- Low Na+, low protein diet (reduce solutes to excrete)
- Desmopressin 0.05 mg po bid, increase as needed to total daily dose of 0.1–1.2 mg/day
- Increase PO H$_2$O, or hypotonic saline

Genitourinary Complications

Urethral Strictures/Erosions
- Minimize Foley catheter use

Urinary Tract Infections

Clinical:
- Change in behavior or mental status, fatigue
- Decreased participation/performance in therapy
- Increased spasticity

Treatment:
- Get a UA on admission and remove Foley, check trial of voids. If post-void residuals >400 mL, cath. If <250 mL for >24 h discontinue PVR
- Abx based on susceptibility (check hospital recommendations as they vary)
  - Fluoroquinolones may lower seizure threshold

Detrusor Hyperreflexia
Clinical:
- Most common bladder dysfunction after a brain injury secondary to impaired communication and mobility
- Neurogenic (spastic) bladder with uninhibited detrusor reflex (contraction)
  - Incontinent, small voids, normal residuals (<200 ml)
- Detrusor-sphincter dyssynergia may be seen with Pons lesions

Treatment:
- Timed-void program (provide urinal or commode at a regular scheduled intervals)
  - Void without instrumentation Q2 h during the day and QHS

- If unable to void or evacuate, intermittent straight catheterization may be necessary, q6–8 h with goal volume <500 ml
- Diapers and condom catheters may be needed
- Anticholinergic medication (to ↑ bladder capacity and decrease contractility)
  - Tolterodine 1–2 mg bid, titrate as needed up to 4 mg/day
  - Oxybutynin 5 mg bid-qid, titrate as needed up to 30 mg/day
    Side effects: sedation, dry mouth, mild memory impairment, confusion, agitation

Heterotopic Ossification

- Formation of mature lamellar bone in soft tissue
- Incidence: 11–76% in TBI, 10–20% are clinically significant [54]
- Greatest risk is during 3–4 months post-injury

Risk Factors:
- Prolonged coma (>2 weeks)
- Immobility

- Limb spasticity/tone (in the involved extremity)
- Associated long-bone fracture
- Pressure ulcers
- Edema

Clinical:
- Pain and ↓ ROM
- Local swelling, erythema, warm joint
- Muscle guarding, low-grade fever
- Joints most commonly involved: Hips > Elbows/Shoulders > Knees
- **Complications**: bony ankylosis, peripheral nerve compression, vascular compression, and lymphedema

Workup:
- Laboratory studies
  - Serum alkaline phosphatase (SAP)
    - Earliest and least expensive
    - Poor specificity (elevated with fractures)
  - Erythrocyte sedimentation rate (ESR)
    - Early inflammatory marker, nonspecific
- Plain X rays
  - Need 2–3 weeks for X-ray to demonstrate bone maturation
  - Soft tissue edema seen earlier
- Bone scan
  - Sensitive for early detection
  - Can be seen 2–4 weeks after TBI in Phase I (blood-flow phase)

Treatment:
- Bisphosphonates (Etidronate 20 mg/kg/day divided in two doses)
  - Inhibits growth but does not reverse or dissolve bone
- NSAIDs (indomethacin 25 mg tid)
- ROM to prevent ankylosis (gentle)
- Surgery—wedge resection
  - Must have clear goal: hygiene, positioning, ADLs, pain
  - Performed after 12–18 months to allow full maturation (controversial), indicated by decreased edema and normal labs
- Therapy
  - Controversial: Aggressive PROM may cause transverse microfractures. However, aggressive PROM and continued mobilization, once acute inflammatory signs have subsided, are indicated to help to maintain ROM.

References

1. Bullock MR, et al. Surgical management of acute epidural hematomas. Neurosurgery. 2006;58(3 Suppl):S7–15. discussion Si–iv.
2. Mayer S, Rowland L, Mayer S, Rowland L. Head injury. In: Rowland L, editor. Merritt's neurology. Philadelphia: Lippincott Williams & Wilkins; 2000. p. 401.
3. Besenski N. Traumatic injuries: imaging of head injuries. Eur Radiol. 2002;12(6):1237–52.
4. Victor M, Ropper A, Victor M, Ropper A. Craniocerebral trauma. In: Victor M, Ropper A, editors. Adams and victor's principles of neurology. 7th ed. New York: McGraw-Hill; 2001. p. 925.
5. Gennarelli T, Thibault L. Biomechanics of acute subdural hematoma. J Trauma. 1982;22(8):680.
6. Reymond M, et al. Aspirin as a risk factor for hemorrhage in patients with head injuries. Neurosurg Rev. 1992;15(1):21–5.
7. Singer RJ, Ogilvy CS, Rordorf G. Etiology, clinical manifestations, and diagnosis of aneurysmal subarachnoid hemorrhage, in Up To Date, D. Basow, Editor. 2012, Up To Date: Waltham, MA.
8. Hop JW, et al. Case-fatality rates and functional outcome after subarachnoid hemorrhage: a systematic review. Stroke. 1997;28(3):660–4.
9. Naidech AM, et al. Predictors and impact of aneurysm rebleeding after subarachnoid hemorrhage. Arch Neurol. 2005;62(3):410–6.
10. Latchaw RE, Silva P, Falcone SF. The role of CT following aneurysmal rupture. Neuroimaging Clin N Am. 1997;7(4):693–708.
11. Rordorf G, McDonald C. Spontaneous intracerebral hemorrhage: pathogenesis, clinical features, and diagnosis. In: Basow D, editor. UpToDate. Waltham, MA: UpToDate; 2011.
12. Ariesen MJ, et al. Risk factors for intracerebral hemorrhage in the general population: a systematic review. Stroke. 2003;34(8):2060–5.
13. Sturgeon JD, et al. Risk factors for intracerebral hemorrhage in a pooled prospective study. Stroke. 2007;38(10):2718–25.
14. Caplan LR. Etiology and classification of stroke. In: Basow D, editor. UpToDate. Waltham, MA: UpToDate; 2011.
15. Wardlaw JM, Mielke O. Early signs of brain infarction at CT: observer reliability and outcome after thrombolytic treatment – systematic review. Radiology. 2005;235(2):444–53.
16. Schellinger PD, et al. Evidence-based guideline: the role of diffusion and perfusion MRI for the diagnosis of acute ischemic stroke: report of the Therapeutics and Technology Assessment Subcommittee of the American Academy of Neurology. Neurology. 2010;75(2):177–85.
17. Davis PC, et al. Diagnosis of cerebral metastases: double-dose delayed CT vs. contrast-enhanced MR imaging. AJNR Am J Neuroradiol. 1991;12(2):293–300.
18. Brodd E, et al. Epidemiology and the nature of traumatic brain injuries. In: Vanderploeg R, editor. Traumatic brain injury. Washington, DC: Department of Veterans Affairs; 2004. p. 5.

19. Hunter JV, et al. Emerging imaging tools for use with traumatic brain injury research. J Neurotrauma. 2012;29(4):654–71.
20. Weinhouse GL, Young GB. Hypoxic-ischemic brain injury. In: Basow D, editor. UpToDate. Waltham, MA: UpToDate; 2011.
21. Rutland-Brown W, et al. Incidence of traumatic brain injury in the United States, 2003. J Head Trauma Rehabil. 2006;21(6):544–8.
22. Faul M, et al. Traumatic brain injury in the United States: emergency department visits, hospitalizations, and deaths. Atlanta: NCfIPaC Centers for Disease Control and Prevention; 2010.
23. Zaloshnja E, et al. Prevalence of long-term disability from traumatic brain injury in the civilian population of the United States, 2005. J Head Trauma Rehabil. 2008;23(6):394–400.
24. Teasdale G, Jennett B. Assessment of coma and impaired consciousness. A practical scale. Lancet. 1974;2(7872):81–4.
25. Bohannon RW, Smith MB. Interrater reliability of a modified Ashworth scale of muscle spasticity. Phys Ther. 1987;67(2):206–7.
26. Temkin NR, et al. A randomized, double-blind study of phenytoin for the prevention of post-traumatic seizures. N Engl J Med. 1990;323(8):497–502.
27. Elovic E, et al. Traumatic brain injury. In: Cuccurullo SJ, editor. Physical medicine and rehabilitation board review. New York: Demos Medical Publishing; 2010. p. 55.
28. Bontke CF, et al. Medical complications and associated injuries of persons treated in the traumatic brain injury model systems programs. J Head Trauma Rehabil. 1993;8(2):34–46.
29. Phuenpathom N, et al. Post-traumatic hydrocephalus: experience in 17 consecutive cases. J Med Assoc Thai. 1999;82(1):46–53.
30. Mazzini L, et al. Posttraumatic hydrocephalus: a clinical, neuroradiologic, and neuropsychologic assessment of long-term outcome. Arch Phys Med Rehabil. 2003;84(11):1637–41.
31. Annegers JF, et al. A population-based study of seizures after traumatic brain injuries. N Engl J Med. 1998;338(1):20–4.
32. Yablon SA. Posttraumatic seizures. Arch Phys Med Rehabil. 1993;74(9):983–1001.
33. van Hout B, et al. Relationship between seizure frequency and costs and quality of life of outpatients with partial epilepsy in France, Germany, and the United Kingdom. Epilepsia. 1997;38(11):1221–6.
34. Barlow KM, Spowart JJ, Minns RA. Early posttraumatic seizures in non-accidental head injury: relation to outcome. Dev Med Child Neurol. 2000;42(9):591–4.
35. Schwab K, et al. Residual impairments and work status 15 years after penetrating head injury: report from the Vietnam head injury study. Neurology. 1993;43(1):95–103.
36. Grafman J, Jonas B, Salazar A. Epilepsy following penetrating head injury to the frontal lobes. Effects on cognition. Adv Neurol. 1992;57:369–78.
37. Brooke MM, et al. The treatment of agitation during initial hospitalization after traumatic brain injury. Arch Phys Med Rehabil. 1992;73(10):917–21.
38. Deb S, Crownshaw T. The role of pharmacotherapy in the management of behaviour disorders in traumatic brain injury patients. Brain Inj. 2004;18(1):1–31.

39. Nickels JL, et al. Clinical use of amantadine in brain injury rehabilitation. Brain Inj. 1994;8(8):709–18.
40. Leone H, Polsonetti BW. Amantadine for traumatic brain injury: does it improve cognition and reduce agitation? J Clin Pharm Ther. 2005;30(2):101–4.
41. Zollman FS, Cyborski C, Duraski SA. Actigraphy for assessment of sleep in traumatic brain injury: case series, review of the literature and proposed criteria for use. Brain Inj. 2010;24(5):748–54.
42. Beetar JT, Guilmette TJ, Sparadeo FR. Sleep and pain complaints in symptomatic traumatic brain injury and neurologic populations. Arch Phys Med Rehabil. 1996;77(12):1298–302.
43. Clinchot DM, et al. Defining sleep disturbance after brain injury. Am J Phys Med Rehabil. 1998;77(4):291–5.
44. Mahmood O, et al. Neuropsychological performance and sleep disturbance following traumatic brain injury. J Head Trauma Rehabil. 2004;19(5):378–90.
45. Wilde MC, et al. Cognitive impairment in patients with traumatic brain injury and obstructive sleep apnea. Arch Phys Med Rehabil. 2007;88(10):1284–8.
46. Schott GD. From thalamic syndrome to central poststroke pain. J Neurol Neurosurg Psychiatry. 1996;61(6):560–4.
47. Bowsher D. Central post-stroke ("thalamic syndrome") and other central pains. Am J Hosp Palliat Care. 1999;16(4):593–7.
48. Patil VK, et al. Prevalence and treatment of headaches in veterans with mild traumatic brain injury. Headache. 2011;51(7):1112–21.
49. Chae J. Poststroke complex regional pain syndrome. Top Stroke Rehabil. 2010;17(3):151–62.
50. Baglin TP, Brush J, Streiff M. Guidelines on use of vena cava filters. Br J Haematol. 2006;134(6):590–5.
51. Becker DM, Philbrick JT, Selby JB. Inferior vena cava filters. Indications, safety, effectiveness. Arch Intern Med. 1992;152(10):1985–94.
52. Giannoudis PV, et al. Safety and efficacy of vena cava filters in trauma patients. Injury. 2007;38(1):7–18.
53. Ansell J, et al. Pharmacology and management of the vitamin K antagonists: American College of Chest Physicians Evidence-Based Clinical Practice Guidelines, 8th ed. Chest. 2008;133(6 Suppl):160S–98.
54. Melamed E, et al. Brain injury-related heterotopic bone formation: treatment strategy and results. Am J Phys Med Rehabil. 2002;81(9):670–4.

Chapter 2
Spinal Cord Injury

Jason W. Siefferman, Christopher Sahler, Donna G. D'Alessio,
Yolanda Scott, and Avniel Shetreat-Klein

Epidemiology of SCI [1]

Incidence: 12,000/year in the USA
Prevalence: ~265,000 in the USA
Age of Injury:
– Average age 40.7 years
– Bi-modal distribution between 16 and 30 years and 65+ years

Gender: 80.7% male
Race/Ethnicity:
– 66.5% Caucasian
– 26.8% African–American
– 8.3% Hispanic
– 0.9% Asian

Etiology:
– 40.4% Motor vehicle accidents
– 27.9% Falls

J.W. Siefferman, M.D. (✉)
Department of Anesthesiology, The Mount Sinai School of Medicine,
1 Gustave L. Levy Place, Box 1010, New York, NY 10029, USA
e-mail: jsiefferman@gmail.com

C. Sahler, M.D. • D.G. D'Alessio, M.D. •
Y. Scott, M.D. • A. Shetreat-Klein, M.D., Ph.D.
Department of Physical Medicine and Rehabilitation,
Mount Sinai Medical Center, New York, NY, USA
e-mail: christophersahler@gmail.com; dgdalessio@gmail.com;
  yscott80@gmail.com; avniel.shetreat-klein@mountsinai.org

K.A. Sackheim (ed.), *Rehab Clinical Pocket Guide:*
Rehabilitation Medicine, DOI 10.1007/978-1-4614-5419-9_2,
© Springer Science+Business Media, LLC 2013

- 15% Violence
- 8% Sports

Neurologic Level and Extent of Lesion:
- 39.5% incomplete tetraplegia
- 22.1% complete paraplegia
- 21.7% incomplete paraplegia
- 16.3% complete tetraplegia

Marital status:
51.9% of persons with spinal cord injury (SCI) are single at the time injury

Spinal Cord Injury Syndromes

Central Cord Syndrome

Cervical spinal cord injury affecting primarily the central tracts
Epidemiology: Most common, ~50% of incomplete injuries, 9% of traumatic SCI [2, 3]
Pathophysiology:
- Cord compression from anterior buckling of the ligamentum flavum during hyperextension in an already narrowed spinal canal [4]
- The affected tract carries fibers that mainly innervate distal upper limb musculature (functional deficits are more pronounced in the hands) [5]

Risk factors: Cervical stenosis and hyperextension injury
Clinical:
- Upper extremity weakness greater than lower extremity weakness
- Seen often in elderly patients with cervical spondylosis
- Usually results from a fall [4]

Prognosis:
- Favorable prognosis for functional recovery, especially in patients with initial classification of AIS D [6]
- Recovery typically occurs first in LEs, then bowel/bladder, then arms, then hands
- Better prognosis for younger than older patients [7]
  - Independent ambulation (87–97% vs. 31–41%)
  - Bladder function (83% vs. 29%)
  - Dressing (77% vs. 12%)

Brown-Sequard Syndrome (BSS)

Lateral hemisection of the spinal cord
Epidemiology: 2–4% of all traumatic SCI [8–10]
Etiology:
- Traditionally been associated with knife injuries
- May be a variety of etiologies, including closed spinal injuries with or without vertebral fractures [11, 12]

Clinical:
> At level: Loss of all sensory modalities and flaccid paralysis—Lower Motor Neuron (LMN) lesion
> Below level:
> - Ipsilateral loss of vibration, proprioception; spastic paralysis—Upper Motor Neuron (UMN) lesion
> - Contralateral loss of pain/temperature

Prognosis: [9, 11]
- Best prognosis for functional outcome of the incomplete SCI syndromes
- 75–90% of patients will ambulate independently upon discharge from rehabilitation
- 70% Independent for activities of daily living (ADL's)

Anterior Cord Syndrome

Injury to the anterior 2/3 of the spinal cord with preservation of the posterior columns
Epidemiology: 2.7% of all traumatic SCI [9]
Pathophysiology: [9, 13]
- Flexion injury, direct damage from bone fragment or disc compression
- Vascular insufficiency produced by occlusion of anterior spinal artery

Clinical:
- Bilateral loss of motor and pain/temperature
- Relative preservation of light touch, proprioception

Prognosis: 10–20% likelihood of motor recovery [14]

Posterior Cord Syndrome

Injury to the dorsal columns of the cord with relative sparing of the anterior 2/3
Epidemiology: Least common incomplete injury, incidence <1% [2, 9]
Etiology:
– Hyperextension injuries
– Posterior spinal artery occlusion
– Tumors
– Vitamin B_{12} deficiency

Clinical:
– Loss of proprioception and vibration sense
– Preservation of motor and pain/temperature

Prognosis: Poor for ambulation due to proprioceptive deficits

Conus Medullaris and Cauda Equina Syndromes

– *Conus medullaris* injuries affect the terminal spinal cord as well as lumbar nerve roots, resulting in UMN and LMN injury.
– *Cauda equina* injuries affect only the nerve roots (lumbar and/or sacral) and are therefore LMN injuries.

Epidemiology: [2]
– Cauda equina 5.2% of SCI
– Conus medullaris 1.7% of SCI

Etiology:
– Trauma, fracture, tumor, lumbar spondylosis, abscess, hematoma, spina bifida, ischemia

Clinical—Cauda equina:
– Loss of LE, anal, and bulbocavernosis reflexes
– Flaccid paralysis and atrophy of the LEs
– Flaccid bowel and bladder, impotence (may be spared if only lumbar roots are affected)
– Saddle anesthesia

Clinical—Conus medullaris:
– Combination of UMN and LMN depending on level
– Reflexes may be preserved or hyperactive

- Spasticity may develop in sacral muscles
- Bladder may be spastic
- Saddle anesthesia (loss of pain/temp)

Prognosis:
- Conus medullaris recovery is similar to other UMN spinal cord injuries
- Cauda equina injuries may represent a neuropraxia or axonotmesis, which may demonstrate progressive recovery
- Early diagnosis and surgical decompression predict better outcome [15]

SCI Assessment

Referring Physician: Name, hospital, and contact information
HPI:
- Clearly describe the mechanism of initial injury
- Determine if there was secondary trauma (TBI, fractures, blood loss, respiratory failure, etc.)
- Document if the patient was wearing a helmet or seatbelt, if applicable
- What did the patient feel immediately following the injury? Was there immediate loss of sensation and/or motor control, or did it develop progressively?
- Describe initial treatment course (i.e., intubation, use of steroids, emergent surgical interventions)
- Detail hospital course to date and any complications (skin breakdown, infection, DVT, significant laboratory or imaging findings)
- Document details including dates and names of surgeons if procedures performed (spinal stabilization, PEG tube, tracheostomy including type of trach and cuff versus uncuffed, IVC filter placement, and if it is removable)

Current Issues:
- Neuro—Subjective sensory and motor deficits
- Instability—Structural injury to spinal column requiring bracing or surgery for immobilization
- Pain—may be multiple types of pain. For each one, document location, quality, intensity, radiation, aggravating/alleviating factors. Document medications used for pain and their effectiveness.

- Bladder—voluntary voiding? incontinence? Sensation of genitals? on intermittent catheterization (IC), or Foley?
- Bowel—Sensation of rectum or bowel movements? voluntary bowel movements, or on a bowel program? incontinence?
- Spasticity—location, frequency, severity; causing pain, poor sleep, or interfering with function?
- Respiratory—comfortable? SOB? DOE? on vent or history of vent? secretion management requirement?
- Skin breakdown? Document location, stage, whether or not the patient was being turned regularly. Document type of mattress patient was on.
- Psych—symptoms of adjustment d/o or PTSD, flashbacks to event, nightmares, anxiety, disrupted sleep?
- Cardiovascular: symptoms of orthostasis (lightheadedness, syncopal episodes) or autonomic dysreflexia (headache, sweats, flushing)
- Diet—previous issues with dysphagia? Give special consideration if the patient underwent anterior cervical fixation which could cause vagal/recurrent laryngeal nerve damage. PEG tube?

PMH:
- **Include a Full Past Medical History**
- Any previous congenital or acquired spinal disorder (i.e., spina bifida, spinal stenosis)
- Any condition which may also limit function or which will need to be managed on the rehab unit (i.e., peripheral neuropathy, DJD, asthma/COPD)

PSH: Include dates of procedures
Medications:
- List home medications including herbal medicines and supplements.
- Medications used during previous hospital course.
- Make sure to list significant medicines (e.g., steroids, antibiotics) even if the patient is no longer taking them by the time of discharge to rehab.

Allergies: List drug and environmental allergies.
Social history:
- Type of housing and barriers to home access (single level house or third floor walk-up, narrow hallways, small bathrooms)
- With whom does the patient live?
- Support system (close family or friends)

- Employment history and education level
- Hobbies
- Substance abuse history

Prior Functional History:
- Ambulation: Independent or with assisted device?
- Exercise tolerance and reason for limitation (pain or SOB?)
- ADLs: Independent or require adaptive equipment or assistance?
- Did the patient have a home health aide?

Current (Admission) Level of Function:
- Function as documented on recent PT and OT notes
- Note any mobility restrictions/precautions or instructions for brace wear

ROS: Full review of systems

Physical examination: In addition to the standard medical physical examination, the SCI exam should emphasize the following elements:
- **Vitals:** Hypoxia, tachypnea, tachy- or bradycardia, hyper- or hypotension
- **Range-of-motion:** Active and passive
- **Muscle tone**: Passively range a joint at varying speeds and grade by modified ashworth scale (MAS) (Table 2.1) [16]
- **Strength:** Test key muscles (Table 2.2) and grade from 0 to 5 (Table 2.3)
- **Sensation:** Test light touch with cotton swab and pinprick in all dermatomes (Table 2.4), and grade from 0 to 2 (Table 2.5). Also check proprioception.

Table 2.1 Modified ashworth scale (MAS) [16]

Grade	Description
0	No increase in muscle tone
1	Slight increase in muscle tone, manifested by a catch and release or by minimal resistance at the end range of motion when the affected parts moved in flexion or extension
1+	Slight increase in muscle tone, manifested by a catch, followed by minimal resistance throughout the remainder (less than half) of the range or motion
2	More marked increase in muscle tone through most of the range of motion, but the affected part is easily moved
3	Considerable increase in muscle tone, passive movement is difficult
4	Affected part is rigid in flexion or extension

Table 2.2 Key muscles (myotomes)

Level	Muscle group
C5	Elbow flexors
C6	Wrist extensors
C7	Elbow flexors
C8	Flexor digit. Prof.
T1	Abd. Digit. Min.
L2	Hip flexors
L3	Knee extensors
L4	Ankle dorsiflexion
L5	Ext. Hall. Long.
S1	Ankle plantarflexion

Table 2.3 Manual muscle testing (MMT)

0	Total paralysis
1	Palpable or visible contraction
2	Active movement, full range of motion, gravity eliminated
3	Active movement, full range of motion, against gravity
4	Active movement, full range of motion, against gravity and provides some resistance
5	Active movement, full range of motion, against gravity and provides normal resistance
5*	Muscle able to exert, in examiner's judgment, sufficient resistance to be considered normal if identifiable inhibiting factors were not present
NT	Patient unable to reliably exert effort or muscle unavailable for testing due to factors such as immobilization, pain on effort or contracture.

Muscle strength is graded from 0 to 5 without +'s or −'s

– **Reflexes:** Biceps, Triceps, Patellar, Achilles; Babinski and Hoffmann
– **Skin:** Examine for breakdown (scapulae, ischia, sacrum, heels), infection; note tube/catheter/trach sites
– **Rectal:** Note *voluntary* and *involuntary* sphincter tone and whether stool is in the rectal vault.
– **Functional:** Bed mobility (rolling, bridging), supine → sit → stand, sitting and standing balance, and ambulation as able

Table 2.4 Key sensory points (dermatomes)

Level	Sensory point
C2	1 cm lateral to the occipital protuberance at the base of the skull
C3	In the supraclavicular fossa, at the midclavicular line
C4	Over the acromioclavicular joint
C5	On the lateral side of the antecubital fossa just proximal to the elbow
C6	On the dorsal surface of the proximal phalanx of the thumb
C7	On the dorsal surface of the proximal phalanx of the middle finger
C8	On the dorsal surface of the proximal phalanx of the little finger
T1	On the medial side of the antecubital fossa, just proximal to the medial epicondyle of the humerus
T2	At the apex of the axilla
T3	At the midclavicular line and the third intercostal space
T4	At the midclavicular line and the fourth intercostal space, located at the level of the nipples
T5	At the midclavicular line and the fifth intercostal space, located midway between the level of the nipples and the level of the xiphisternum
T6	At the midclavicular line, located at the level of the xiphisternum
T7	At the midclavicular line, one quarter the distance between the level of the xiphisternum and the level of the umbilicus
T8	At the midclavicular line, one half the distance between the level of the xiphisternum and the level of the umbilicus
T9	At the midclavicular line, three quarters of the distance between the level of the xiphisternum and the level of the umbilicus
T10	At the midclavicular line, located at the level of the umbilicus
T11	At the midclavicular line, midway between the level of the umbilicus and the inguinal ligament
T12	At the midclavicular line, over the midpoint of the inguinal ligament
L1	Midway between the key sensory points for T12 and L2
L2	On the anterior-medial thigh, at the midpoint drawn on an imaginary line connecting the midpoint of the inguinal ligament and the medial femoral condyle
L3	At the medial femoral condyle above the knee
L4	Over the medial malleolus
L5	On the dorsum of the foot at the third metatarsal phalangeal joint
S1	On the lateral aspect of the calcaneus
S2	At the midpoint of the popliteal fossa
S3	Over the ischial tuberosity or infragluteal fold
S4-5	In the perianal area, less than 1 cm lateral to the mucocutaneous junction

Table 2.5 Sensory grading

0	Absent
1	Impaired (either decreased or increased)
2	Normal
NT	Not testable

AISA Examination and Classification:
The ASIA Impairment Scale (AIS) allows for classification of the patient's injury according to the International Standards for Neurological Classification of Spinal Cord Injury, which facilitates research and communication between caregivers and has prognostic value.

- **Motor level**: Most caudal level that is graded 3/5 or greater with all segments cephalad graded normal (5/5) strength
- **Motor index score**: Calculated by adding the muscle scores of each key muscle group; a total score of 100 is possible.
- **Sensory level**: Most caudal dermatome to have normal sensation for both pin prick and light touch on both sides.
- **Sensory index score**: Calculated by adding the scores for each dermatome; a total score of 112 is possible for each pin prick and light touch.
- **Neurologic level of injury**: Most caudal level at which both motor and sensory modalities are intact.
- **Complete injury**: Absence of sensory and motor function in the lowest sacral segments (AIS A)
- **Incomplete injury**: Preservation of motor and/or sensory function below the neurologic level that includes the lowest sacral segments (AIS B, C, D, or E).
- **Skeletal level**: Level at which, by radiological examination, the greatest vertebral damage is found.
- **Zone of partial preservation (ZPP)**: Only applicable in complete injuries, refers to the levels caudal to the neurological level that remain partially innervated. Defined by the most caudal segment with some sensory and/or motor function.

Table 2.6 American spinal injury association impairment scale [17]

ASIA impairment scale	Description
A	No motor or sensory function is preserved in the lowest sacral segments
B	Sensory sparing in the S4-5 dermatome and/or deep anal sensation
	No voluntary muscle contraction more than three levels below the *motor* level
C	Sensory sparing in the S4-5 dermatome and/or deep anal sensation
	Voluntary muscle contraction more than three levels below the *motor* level
	More than half of the key muscles below the *neurologic* level are scored <3/5
D	Sensory sparing in the S4-5 dermatome and/or deep anal sensation
	Half or more of the key muscles below the *neurologic* level are scored ≥3/5
E	Normal neurologic function in all segments despite prior deficits

SCI Admission Orders

Admit to: Inpatient rehabilitation
Diagnosis: Type and level of spinal cord injury and etiology
Condition: Stable/fair
Allergies:
Vitals: Q Shift unless unstable (which would need more frequent vitals); include pulse oximetry for patients on ventilators, tracheostomies, or with respiratory impairment
Diagnosis: SCI—define by level and AIS classification
CV: SCI patients are likely to have new lower baseline BP, often relatively hypotensive (SBP 90-110); therefore prone to symptomatic orthostatic hypotension
- Compression stockings and abdominal binder OOB to prevent orthostasis
- Ensure appropriate fluid intake

Pulm on Ventilator: [18]
- Note ventilator settings from outside hospital; continue same settings on admission

- If unclear and there is no parenchymal lung injury, start CMV with tidal volume 10–15 cc/kg ideal body weight (about 1 L), rate 12, PEEP 5, titrate FiO_2 for SPO_2 to >92%
- Check ABG
- Daily Vital Capacity (VC) measurement
- See below and Respiratory section for further details

Pulm with Trach:

- Chest Physiotherapy every 6 h; use insufflator–exufflator with therapy
- CXR (evaluate for PNA or PTX)
- Check PFTs: (FEV_1, Vital capacity, Negative Inspiratory Force)
- Albuterol and Ipratropium nebs every 6 h standing and q4 prn
- Suctioning as needed
- Tracheostomy care orders - clean site with hydrogen peroxide then wash with NS
- Speech consultation for Passey-muir valve

Bladder with Foley: Remove Foley, wait 3 h, insert Foley, check U/A and Cx, and refer to Bladder section for further management
Bladder without Foley:

- Check U/A and Cx
- Check post-void residuals after each void for first 24 h using straight cath or bladder scan.
  - If volumes <200 cc AND patient is able to control voiding, allow patient to void
  - If volumes >200 cc OR patient is unable to control voiding, place a Foley and refer to Bladder section for further management

Bowel (UMN):

- Colace 100 mg po TID
- Senna 2 tabs po 8 h prior to bowel routine, this can be increased if needed to a max daily dose of (6 tabs/day)
- Bowel routine (digital stimulation) with mini enema or suppository 30 min after a meal
- If distended or having accidents, consider KUB to assess volume of stool in colon

Bowel (LMN):

- Requires manual disimpaction each morning after breakfast
- If possible, have patient seated in commode chair
- Bowel meds are adjusted for stool consistency to minimize accidents and allow for easy disimpaction

– If distended or having accidents, consider KUB to assess volume of stool in colon

Pain:
– MSK—Tylenol 650 mg q6h prn mild pain
– Oxycodone 5–10 mg po prn moderate–severe pain
– Neuropathic—gabapentin 300 mg tid–qid and/or nortriptyline 25 mg qhs

DVT prophylaxis: [19, 20]
Chemical prophylaxis may be contraindicated if recent surgery or hemorrhage
– Check LE duplex for undiagnosed DVT
  • If negative order sequential pneumatic compression devices (SCD)
– AIS D: Enoxaparin 40 mg SQ daily until D/C from Rehabilitation
– AIS C: Enoxaparin 40 mg SQ daily for 8 weeks
– AIS A or B: Enoxaparin 40 mg SQ daily for 8 weeks
  • If complicated (LE fracture, h/o thrombosis, cancer, heart failure, obesity, or age >70), needs to be continued for 12 weeks

Skin:
– Turn patient q2h while in bed to prevent skin breakdown
– Multipodis boots to prevent heel/calf skin breakdown and contractures
– If patient already has skin breakdown:
  • Document (photograph, measure, stage)
  • Initiate wound care plan (See Wound Care subsection)
– Pin care if HALO brace or external fixator present (instructions vary by surgeon)

Spasticity:
– Note level of current tone compared to discharge exam from prior hospital setting.
  • Acutely increased tone may indicate undiagnosed infection, fracture, or other pathology
  • Consider imaging, CBC, U/A & Cx, ESR, CRP, Alk Phos

Diet:
– Omeprazole 40 mg daily (for 2+ weeks post-injury to prevent GI stress ulcers)
– Tube feeding:
  • Convert calories/formula to 16- or 18-h overnight schedule

- Increase rate by 10 cc every 8 h to optimal target rate
- Nutrition consultation to optimize protein
- Oral feeding:
  - Speech and Swallow eval if dysphagia is suspected. Good idea for anyone in a C-collar.
  - Continue prior diet unless aspiration is suspected
- Weigh patient on admission and weekly

Activity:
- List precautions and restrictions, weight-bearing status of extremities
- Brace type(s) and instructions for wearing (at all times vs. OOB only)

Labs:
- CBC, BMP, LFTs, PT/PTT, U/A & Cx, TSH, Vit D 25, and 1,25
- Weekly CBC, and BMP unless otherwise indicated

Imaging:
- CXR if pulm or vent history
- KUB if bowel status unclear
- X-rays of orthopedic or surgical sites
- Consider LE duplex for DVT; required prior to pneumatic compression device use if no DVT prophylaxis for 72 h [19].

Consultations:
- **Speech:** Assess for aspiration and determine appropriate diet.
- Teach glossal-pharyngeal (frog) breathing if ventilator dependent
- Vocalization while on vent or with trach with speaking valve.

Nutrition: Optimize nutritional status and determine appropriate diet

Social work: Evaluate current living environment and social/financial support available for discharge planning

Psychology: Eval and continued therapy for adjustment disorder; Family counseling

Recreational and vocational therapy: For community reintegration, identifying outpatient services for returning to work, support groups

Therapy:
- **Dx**: Tetraplegia/paraplegia, medical diagnoses
- **Date of onset**

- **Precautions**: Mobility restrictions (i.e., Spine precautions, Cervical collar on at all times), cardiac (orthostasis), respiratory (RR 12–20), decreased sensation, Autonomic dysreflexia, skin breakdown, anticoagulation, hypoglycemia, etc
- **Weight-bearing status**: WBAT all extremities (unless there are any fractures)
- **Short-term goals**: Based on impairments, level of injury, and comorbidities, to be accomplished by discharge
- **Long-term goals**: Ideally maximized function based on level of injury and comorbidities

Physical Therapy Rx:
- Evaluate
- A/AA/PROM to LEs with stretching as indicated
- Tone-reducing techniques
- Strengthening to LEs
- Mat activities
- Transfers
- Sitting/standing balance
- Proprioceptive exercises
- Progressive ambulation with assistive device
- Stair negotiation as tolerated
- Home exercise program
- Trial of TENS, FES
- Ice ×20 min prn
- Splinting or bracing as indicated

Occupational Therapy Rx:
- Evaluation
- A/AA/PROM to UEs with stretching as indicated
- ADL training
- Fine motor coordination
- Neuromuscular reeducation
- Tone-reducing techniques
- Strengthening to UEs
- Splinting in neutral position or for tenodesis
- Functional transfers
- Work Simplification/Energy Conservation
- Adaptive device evaluation
- Durable Medical Equipment (DME) Evaluation
- Home evaluation to determine accessibility and need for equipment

- Trial of TENS, FES
- Ice or MHP ×20 min prn

Wheelchair Prescription:
- Power recline and/or tilt-in-space wheelchair with head, chin, or breath control
- Pressure relief cushion
- Postural support
- Safety belt

Adaptive Devices/Home Equipment that May Be Needed:
- Full electric hospital bed with side rails and Trendelenburg position
- Transfer board
- Power or mechanical "Hoyer" lift with U-sling
- Shampoo tray
- Handheld shower
- Padded reclining roll-in shower or commode chair with safety strap

Sequelae and Complications of SCI

Neurological Prognosis

Life expectancy:
Mortality rates are the highest during the first year after injury [1] (Table 2.7)
Life expectancy [1]
Causes of Death During First Year [21]
- 28% diseases of respiratory system
- 23% Ischemic/hypertensive heart disease

Table 2.7 Life expectancy (years) post-injury by severity of injury and age at injury, for those who survive the first 24 h [1]

Age at injury	Without SCI	Motor functional at any level	Para	Low tetra (C5–C8)	High tetra (C1–C4)	Ventilator dependent
20	58.6	52.6	45.2	40.0	35.7	17.1
40	39.4	34.1	27.6	23.3	19.9	7.3
60	22.4	17.7	12.8	9.9	7.7	1.5

- 9.7% PE
- 7.5% Sepsis

Functional Outcomes [22, 23]
(Dep = Dependent, A = Assist, Ind = Independent)
C1–C4:
- • **Respiratory**: Complete or partial phrenic nerve paralysis requiring ventilation initially
- • Dep for clearing secretions
- **ADLs and Transfers:** Dep
- **Pressure reliefs**: Ind with tilt-in-space power w/c
- **Mobility:** Ind in power w/c with head array or sip and puff

C5
- **Eating**: Mod Ind after setup with adaptive equipment such as wrist splint with utensil holder or universal cuff, bent fork or spoon, nonslip mat, plate guard, and possibly a mobile arm support
- **Grooming**: Min A after setup
- **Dressing**: A for upper body, Dep for lower body
- **Brushing teeth/grooming**: Min A after setup with wrist support and utensil holder
- **Bed mobility and transfers**: A
- **Bowel/bladder**: Dep
- **Driving**: Ind with adaptations

C6: Highest complete level that can live independently (if motivated)
- **Eating:** Ind or Mod Ind
- **Grooming:** A to Mod Ind
- **Dressing:** Ind for upper body, A for lower body
- **Bathing**: A to Mod Ind with wash mitt, handheld shower, U-shaped cuff, lever type faucet, grab bars, and shower chair
- **Bed mobility:** A to Ind
- **Transfers:** A to Mod Ind with transfer board for transfers on even surfaces. Uneven surfaces may require more assistance
- **Pressure reliefs:** Ind with power or manual w/c
- **Bladder:**
  - • Female: Continuous indwelling Foley most commonly used. May be Mod Ind for self-catheterization with a continent urinary diversion with an abdominal stoma for bladder access.
  - • Male: Potentially Mod Ind for intermittent catheterizations

- **Bowel:**
  - A for transfer and setup on recliner commode
  - Potentially Mod Ind for performance of bowel routine with rectal stimulation using suppository inserter and mirror guidance
  - A for cleanup

- **Mobility:**
  - Ind driving a van with w/c lift and hand controls from secured wheelchair
  - Ind with power w/c with standard arm controls
  - Potentially Ind with manual w/c indoors with modified hand rims. Power-assist wheels can be useful.

C7: Usual level of injury for functional independence
- **ADLs:** A to mod Ind
- **Bed mobility:** Min A to Ind
- **Transfers:** Mod Ind with transfer board
- **Bladder:**
  - Female: Ind with self-catheterization is possible, but technically difficult
  - Male: Mod Ind with intermittent catheterizations.
- **Bowel:** Mod Ind for performance of bowel routine with rectal stimulation using suppository inserter and mirror guidance
- **Mobility**:
  - Ind driving a car or van with hand controls
  - Ind with power w/c
  - Ind with ultra-lightweight manual w/c with modified hand rims, except over curbs and uneven terrain. Power assist wheels can be useful.
- **Typing:** Min A to Mod Ind (typing splint) for telephone and keyboard use

T2–T9
- **ADLs**: Ind
- **Transfers:** Ind for all including floor-to-chair transfers
- **Bowel/bladder:** Ind
- **Mobility:**
  - Ind with manual w/c including popping a wheelie and curbs
  - Mod Ind Ambulation for exercise with b/l KAFO and forearm crutches or walker

T10–Lumbar:
- **W/C**: Ind with manual w/c potentially including ↑/↓ stairs and escalators
- **Ambulation:** Mod Ind for ambulation with b/l KAFO and walker or crutches using swing-through gait—high energy expenditure. More for exercise than for functional mobility.

Neurologic Complications

Syringomyelia (posttraumatic cystic myelopathy)
- Cyst formation within the gray matter near the level of injury
- **Incidence:** 8% starting 2 months after injury [23]
- **Etiology:** unclear
  - Hematoma with enzymatic lysis?
  - Scarring with obstruction of CSF flow?
- **Clinical:**
  - Pain worse with valsalva
  - Ascending loss of reflexes
  - Ascending sensory loss in "cape" distribution
  - Change in spasticity
  - Postural changes
- **Workup:** MRI with contrast
- **Treatment:**
  - Avoid straining for bowel routine/urination
  - Neurosurgical consultation
  - Shunting
  - Cordectomy
- **Prognosis:** [23]
  - Pain reduction and motor recover>sensory recovery
  - Recurrence rate of ~50%

Peripheral Nerve Entrapment [3]
- Carpal tunnel and ulnar neuropathy most common
- **Incidence:** CTS 21–65%
- **Treatment:**
  - Relative rest
  - Splinting
  - Avoid direct pressure on nerves
  - Modify w/c propulsion and transfer techniques

- Padded gloves
- Surgical release/transposition
– See EMG chapter for further details

Respiratory [3, 18, 23]

Anatomy:
– Innervation:
  - Phrenic nerve (C3, 4, 5)—diaphragm
  - Vagus nerve—lung parasympathetics
– Inspiratory muscles: diaphragm (65–75% of volume), external intercostals, accessory muscles
– Expiratory muscles: abdominals, internal intercostals

Respiratory Changes After SCI:
– Increased residual volume
– Decreased vital capacity (VC) and tidal volume (TV)
  - Forced VC may initially be 50% of expected, but may improve to 60% [3]
– Paradoxical chest wall movement
  - Chest wall falls and abdomen protrudes during inspiration
– Diaphragm in biomechanically disadvantaged position
– Increased secretions from unopposed parasympathetics (Vagus n)

Impairment by level of injury: [3]
C2 or above:
– No respiratory muscle function (including diaphragm)
– Requires mechanical ventilation
– An intact phrenic nerve (EMG) may allow for diaphragmatic pacing

C3–4:
– Weak diaphragm, no active expiratory function
– Initially requires mechanical ventilation, many will wean

C4–C8:
– Intact diaphragm, but no active expiratory function
– Requires assistance for clearing secretion (insufflation–exsufflation, chest PT)
– Positioning to improve tidal volumes (supine>sitting by 15%)

T1–T5:
- No volitional intercostals or abdominal muscle function
- Requires assistance for clearing secretion (insulflator–exsulflator, chest PT)
- Positioning to improve tidal volumes (supine > sitting)

T5–T12:
- Weak intercostals and abdominals, weak cough
- Requires assistance for clearing secretion (insulflator–exsulflator, chest PT)

Respiratory Complications: [23]
- Occur in up to 67% of acute SCI patients
  - Pneumonia
  - Atelectasis
  - Respiratory failure
- Most common in high cervical (C1–C4) injuries
- Leading cause of death after SCI (21.7%) [24]
  - 72.3% due to pneumonia
- Risk increases with age, obesity, h/o asthma, COPD, or smoking
- Concomitant TBI may affect respiratory drive
- Sleep apnea (prevalence of 15–60%) [3, 24]

Prevention of Respiratory Complications: [23]
- Incentive spirometer
- Monitor VC and pCO_2
- Suctioning
- Chest PT
- Cough assist—manual or with insulflator–exsulflator (40 cm H_2O)
- Adequate hydration to thin secretions
- Teaching glossopharyngeal breathing
- Abdominal binder (increases VC 16–28% by prepositioning diaphragm)
- Medication
  - Inhaled bronchodilators (albuterol)
  - Oral mucolytics (guaifenesin, acetylcysteine)
  - Theophylline (decreases spasm, increases surfactant and diaphragmatic contractility)

Initial Workup:
- ABG
- Labs, including cardiac enzymes and toxicology

- CXR
- EKG
- Continuous Pulse Ox
- Pulmonary metrics:
  - Vital capacity (VC)
  - Forced expiratory volume in 1 s (FEV_1) or peak cough flow
  - Maximal Negative Inspiratory Force (NIF)
- Calculate Ideal Body Weight (IBW)
  - Males $= 50 + 2.3$(height in inches -60)
  - Females $= 45.5 + 2.3$(height in inches -60)

Mechanical Ventilation [18, 23, 24]
Indications:
- Respiratory failure
  - VC <15 cc/kg IBW, or <1L
  - NIF <20 cm H_2O
  - pO_2 <50
  - pCO_2 >50
  - Fatigue
- Intractable atelectasis
- Recurrent pneumonia related to atelectasis
- Tracheostomy if expect >5 days on vent

Mode:
- Continuous Mandatory Ventilation (CMV, formerly Assist Control) preferred
  - Fixed tidal volume, FiO_2, peak flow, and PEEP at set rate
  - Patient may trigger breath, and full tidal volume is delivered
  - Allows patient to speak if cuff partially deflated

Settings:
- Calculate Tidal Volume (TV) 10–20 cc/kg IBW [3]
- Increase TV 50–100 cc per day as tolerated to goal volume (>20 cc/kg IBW)
  - High tidal volumes is preferred for treating atelectasis
  - Reduces time to wean in SCI patients [25]
  - Stop increasing TV when
- Normal SPO_2 on room air (21%)
- No atelectasis
- Monitor pressures to avoid barotrauma
  - Peak pressure < 40 cm H_2O
  - Plateau pressure < 35 cm H_2O

- PEEP = 5 cm H_2O
  - May increase to improve pO_2 or decrease atelectasis
- Rate = 12
- FiO_2 = 21% (room air) unless underlying lung pathology
- Peak flow (rate of air delivery) = 60 L/min
- Sensitivity to trigger breath = −2 cm H_2O
- Do not allow the patient to override the ventilator settings [18]
- Set alarms
  - High pressure (peak inspiratory pressure + PEEP)
  - Low pressure (usually 10 cm H_2O + PEEP)
  - Low exhaled volume (TV—200 cc)

Alternative to traditional ventilator: [26, 27]
- Noninvasive Intermittent positive pressure ventilation (NIPPV) may be considered for patients with intact bulbar muscles and intact mental status
  - Apparatus similar to CPAP or BiPAP
  - Lower risk of pneumonia than with trach
  - Avoids complications of trach
  - More likely to be discharged home

Vent Weaning:
Indication: Vital capacity (VC) >10 cc/kg IBW
- VC of 15–20 cc/kg good predictor of successful weaning [28]
- Also consider CXR and ability to breathe on room air

Method: Progressive ventilator-free breathing (PVFB) [3, 24]
- Start by removing vent for 2–5 min TID
- Supine position with abdominal binder
- Increase time off vent as tolerated
- Provide humidified O_2 via trach collar
- More effective than SIMV in SCI [29]

Discontinue weaning if:
- VC drops by 50%
- Unable to maintain SPO_2 >92%
- RR >30
- HR >20 above baseline
- SBP change of 30 points
- Fatigue or altered mental status

Noninvasive ventilation may aide weaning [27]
- Intermittent positive pressure ventilation (IPPV)

- CPAP, BiPAP
- Intermittent abdominal pressure ventilator

Implanted devices: phrenic nerve stimulator, diaphragmatic pacing
- Require intact phrenic nerve
- May allow some patients to wean as well as improve speech and mobility

Bowel/GI

- **Anatomy/Physiology**Parasympathetic—pro-motility
  - Vagus nerve (CN X)—stomach through transverse colon
  - Pelvic splanchnic nerves (S2–4)—transverse colon to internal anal sphincter (IAS)
- Sympathetic—stasis
  - Celiac and Superior Mesenteric Ganglia (T4–12)—stomach through transverse colon
  - Inferior Mesenteric Ganglion (L1–3)—transverse and descending colon
- Somatic—External anal sphincter
  - Pudendal nerve (S2–4) motor and sensory to external anal sphincter (EAS)
- Reflexes
  - Gastrocolic
    - Trigger: Stomach/duodenal distention
    - Opens iliocecal valve
    - Increases colonic peristalsis
    - Timeframe: 15–60 min after meal
    - Mediated by cholecystokinin, serotonin, gastrin
  - Rectocolic and Recto-anal inhibition
    - Trigger: Rectal distention/stimulation
    - IAS relaxation and peristalsis
    - Mediated by pelvic nerve
    - Manual stretching/relaxation of EAS to allow stool evacuation

Acute SCI
- Atonic bowel/ileus
  - May last up to 7 days [3]
- **Treatment:**
  - NG tube to intermittent suction for decompression if vomiting or severe nausea

- IVF if unable to tolerate fluids
- TPN if >3 days
- PPI or H_2-blocker (unopposed vagal tone increases acid production)
- Abdominal massage, TENS
- May consider trial of metoclopramide 10 mg tid and/or erythromycin

Chronic SCI
- UMN Bowel (injury above conus medullaris)
- UMN Bowel (injury above conus medullaris)
  - EAS cannot be voluntarily relaxed, may be spastic
  - Intrinsic reflexes intact and may be hyperactive
  - May have spontaneous BMs (accidents)
- LMN Bowel (injury at or below conus medullaris)
- LMN Bowel (injury at or below conus medullaris)
  - EAS and colon flaccid
  - Intrinsic reflexes absent
  - Colonic dilation and storing of stool

Bowel Program Guidelines:
- **Goal:** to have planned, regular bowel evacuations to prevent complications such as constipation, diarrhea, pain, or unplanned bowel movements.
- Can be done in bed, but preferably, the patient should be sitting upright either in a padded commode chair or recliner commode
- Should be performed the same time every day
- Frequency and dosing of laxatives should coincide with established bowel routine
- During inpatient stay, bowel routine should be performed daily. It may change to an every other day as outpatient if the patient desires.

UMN Program
- Take advantage of reflexes
- Perform 1 h after a meal
- Use PR medication (suppository or mini-enema)±digital stimulation with lidocaine 2% jelly
  - Gently insert a gloved, lubricated finger into the rectum and slowly rotate the finger in a circular movement.
  - If tone persists, hold gentle pressure toward sacrum
  - Rotation is continued until relaxation of the bowel wall is felt, flatus passes, stool passes, or the internal sphincter contracts.

- • Digital stimulation is repeated every 5–10 min as necessary until stool evacuation is complete.
- – **Medications:** 3-2-1
  - • Docusate 100 mg po tid
  - • Senna 2–4 tabs 8 h prior to bowel routine
  - • 1 enema or suppository to initiate program

LMN Program

- – Manual stool evacuation required—no reflexes to assist removal of stool
- – Perform prior to bathing each morning to prevent accidents during day
  - • Insert one or two lubricated fingers into the rectum to break up or hook and remove stool.
  - • Performing on commode for gravity and valsalva assistance
- – Bulk stool for easy removal and to prevent accidents (psyllium, methylcellulose)
- – Perform 15–30 min after meal to take advantage of gastro-colic reflex

Bowel Medications

Bulking Agents

- – Allow stool to retain more water and produce gel to ease passage
- – **Onset of action:** 12–72 h
- – Examples:
  - • Psyllium (Metamucil)—1 Tablespoon daily—TID
  - • Methylcellulose (Citrucel)—1 Tablespoon daily—TID
  - • Dietary fiber—At least 15 g/day

Osmotics

- – Poorly absorbed polyvalent ions (Mag, Phos, Sulfate)
- – Increase intestinal H_2O and stimulate cholecystokinin
- – **Site of action:** All, mostly small bowel
- – **Onset:** ½–6 h
  - • Fleet's (sodium phosphate)—reduces K^+, may cause renal failure
  - • Mag citrate—300 mL = ~2 g elemental mag
  - • Mag hydroxide (MoM)
  - • Mag sulfate (Epsom salt)—most potent
  - • Mannitol (>20 g po)

Hyperosmotics
- Poorly absorbed carbohydrates or polymers
- Induce osmotic diarrhea—increased volume stimulates peristalsis
- **Site of action:** Colon
- **Onset:** ½–24 h
  - Glycerin supp—draws H_2O into rectum, stretching it to stim reflex
- Includes sodium stearate which irritates rectum
  - Miralax (polyethylene glycol)
- Avoid Lactulose and Sorbitol in SCI patients, as bacterial breakdown of these sugars can cause uncomfortable bloating

Stimulants (PO)
- Irritate bowel wall or stimulate plexus
- May also alter electrolyte secretion
- **Site of action:** Colon
- **Onset:** 6–10 h
  - Bisacodyl (Dulcolax)
  - Cascara
  - Casanthranol (anthraquinone stimulant, hydrolyzed by colonic bacteria)
  - Senna (Senokot)—stimulates Auerbach's plexus – peristalsis
- **Complications:** Melanosis coli (brownish discoloration of colon), Cathartic colon (atonic, redundant colon; associated w/ use >3×/week for >1 year.)
  - Aloin—an aloe derivative
  - Aloe and Rhubarb—converted by colonic bacteria into active agent.
- **Site of action:** Small intestine
- **Onset:** 2–6 h
  - Castor Oil—converted to ricinoleic acid

Stimulants (PR)
- **Onset:** ¼–1 h
  - Bisacodyl supp (in mineral oil)
  - Microlax 5 cc enema (contains sodium citrate, sodium lauryl sulfoacetate, sorbitol, glycerol, sorbic acid, and H_2O)
  - Glycerin supp
- Onset: 5–20 min
  - Bisacodyl enema (1.25 fl oz, 10 mg)
  - Magic Bullet supp (dulcolax in water base)
  - Docusate mini enema (Enemeez)

Enemas
- Large Volume (500–1,500 cc)
  - Soap Suds = Sodium lauryl sulfate
  - H_2O
  - SMOG (Saline, Mineral Oil, Glyercin)
- Standard
  - Fleet's (sodium phosphate), 133 cc—<u>Avoid in renal failure</u>
  - Mineral oil, 133 cc
  - Glycerin, 8 oz (or mix with H_2O for large volume)
- Mini/Micro
  - Docusate +/− Benzocaine (Enemeez)
  - Bisacodyl 10 mg, 1.25 oz (Dulcolax)
  - Microlax 5 cc

(Table 2.8) **Bowel Medications**

Bladder

Normal Bladder Anatomy/Physiology:
- Storage (Sympathetic)
  - Sympathetic (hypogastric nerve T11–L2)
    - Detrusor relaxation (β_3-adrenergic)
    - Internal sphincter contraction (α_1-adrenergic)
  - Somatic (pudendal nerve, S2–4)
    - External sphincter contraction
  - Parasympathetic (Pelvic splanchnic nerve, S2–4) motor fibers are inactive, sensory afferent fibers track detrusor stretching
  - Cerebral cortex inhibits the pontine micturition center
- Voiding (Parasympathetic)
  - Full bladder (>150 cc) activates parasympathetic sensory afferents
  - Pontine micturition center coordinates detrusor contraction and sphincter relaxation.
  - *Parasympathetic* (Pelvic splanchnic nerve, S2–4)
    - Detrusor contraction (cholinergic)
  - *Sympathetic* (hypogastric nerve, T11–L2) motor fibers are inactive
    - Internal sphincter relaxation
  - *Somatic* (pudendal nerve, S2–4)
    - External sphincter relaxation

Table 2.8 Bowel medications

Medication	Mechanism	Dosing	Side effects	Onset
Docusate	Emollient (increases stool fat content)	100 mg po TID	Soft stool	PO: 12–72 h
	Irritates rectal mucosa	Mini enema PR	Discomfort	PR: 10–20 min
Senna	Activates Auerbach's plexus—increases peristalsis	2–4 tabs (8.6 mg) po 8 h prior to bowel routine	Catatonic colon (with chronic use)	8 h
Bisacodyl	Irritates colonic mucosa → peristalsis and electrolyte secretion	10 mg po or pr daily or 20 mg po q8h ×3 for severe constipation	Discomfort	PO: 8 h PR: 15–30 min
Lactulose	Osmotic effect → colonic distention → peristalsis and H_2O secretion	15–30 ml po q6h prn (60 ml daily max)	Gas and bloating, accidents	2–6 h
Polyethylene glycol	Osmotic diuresis increases stool H_2O	17 g po daily-bid	Accidents	≤24 h
Magnesium citrate	Osmotic effect → colonic distention → peristalsis and H_2O secretion	150–300 ml po ×1	Increased serum Mg, accidents	2–6 h
Milk of magnesia	Osmotic diuresis	30–60 ml po q6h prn	Increased serum Mg, accidents	2–6 h

Neurogenic Bladder After SCI
Anatomy:
- Lack of continuity between the sacral nerves and the pontine micturition center results in detrusor-sphincter dyssynergia (DSD), or inability to coordinate contraction/relaxation of the detrusor and sphincter for voiding
- **UMN lesions** → spastic bladder, with preservation of sacral reflexes and higher voiding pressures due to DSD.
  - Bladder pressure >40 mmHg may cause hydronephrosis and eventual kidney failure
- **LMN lesions** (At or below S2) → flaccid bladder, with loss of sacral reflexes

Clinical: UMN and LMN may present as retention or incontinence
- Retention may result from:
  - Atonic detrusor (LMN bladder or acute SCI)
  - Sphincter contraction (persistent sympathetic tone, dyssynergia)
  - Other outlet obstruction (urethral stricture, prostate)
- Incontinence may result from:
  - Atonic detrusor with overflow (high volumes)
  - Detrusor Spasticity (low volumes)
  - Preexisting pelvic floor insufficiency

Treatment:
- The goal in bladder management is to maintaining low bladder pressures and continence while minimizing infections and the risk of upper tract deterioration [30]
- **Initial:** Indwelling Foley until spinal shock resolved and orthostasis controlled
- Trial of void (remove Foley—typically do this early in the AM for convenience)
  - Void with control
    - ° Check post-void residual (PVR)
      - If <200 cc, acute management complete
      - If >200 cc, may have DSD (UMN) or weak detrusor (LMN)
        - ▫ Intermittent catheterization (IC) prn PVR >200
        - ▫ If UMN, trial of tamsulosin 0.4 mg po qhs to relax sphincter
        - ▫ If LMN, trial of bethanechol 10 mg po tid to facilitate detrusor contraction, may titrate up to 100 mg qid
        - ▫ Consider urodynamic study if no improvement

- Spontaneous voiding (reflex voiding without control):
  - Check PVR
    - If <200 cc, may use condom catheter or diaper
    - If >200 cc, will require IC q6h or indwelling catheter
      - If UMN, trial of tamsulosin 0.4 mg po qhs to relax sphincter
      - If LMN, trial of bethanechol 10 mg po tid to facilitate detrusor contraction, may titrate up to 100 mg qid
  - May decrease spontaneous voiding, but <u>monitor PVRs</u>:
    - Anticholinergics to relax detrusor
      - Oxybutynin 5 mg po tid, titrate up to 15 mg
      - Tolterodine 2 mg bid
    - Adrenergics to increase sphincter tone (if on IC)
      - Pseudoephedrine 30–60mg bid (max 120mg/day)
    - Spasticity management (baclofen, tizanidine)
    - Botulinum toxin injected into the detrusor
  - May reduce voiding pressures:
    - Tamsulosin 0.4 mg po qhs to relax sphincter
    - Botulinum toxin injected into urinary sphincter
    - Transurethral sphincterotomy
  - Urodynamic study recommended to check voiding pressures [30]
    - No voiding after 8 h:
  - Check bladder volume (bladder scan or IC)
    - If <200 cc, hydrate and recheck
    - If >200 cc, start IC q6h
      - For LMN, trial of bethanecol 10 mg po tid, may titrate up to 100 mg qid
      - For UMN, trial of tamsulosin 0.4 mg po qhs + anticholinergic (oxybutynin, tolterodine)
- Catheterization programs
  - **Goal:** Maintain empty bladder to prevent hydronephrosis, UTI, and incontinence
  - **Methods:**
    - Intermittent catheterization (IC)
      - Start q6h and adjust frequency to maintain volumes 400–500 cc
      - May help train/strengthen bladder
      - Start patient training ASAP
      - Complications: UTI if poor technique

- Not recommended for patients with high urine output, AD, strictures, bladder capacity <200 cc, or who are unable to catheterize themselves and do not have a willing caregiver [30].
  ○ Indwelling urethral catheter
    - Appropriate for patients unable to perform self-IC or with high urine output
    - Complications: UTI, urethral erosion, stricture, bladder cancer, bladder/kidney stones
  ○ Suprapubic tube
    - Nongenital placement of indwelling catheter
    - Appropriate for patients with urethral abnormalities, recurrent obstruction, AD, skin breakdown
    - Complications: UTI, bladder cancer, bladder/kidney stones
  ○ Urinary diversion (i.e., Mitrofanoff)
    - Surgical procedure for a continent suprapubic conduit
    - May allow some patients to become independent with an IC program
    - May be performed with bladder augmentation

Workup: Urodynamic study helps to clarify voiding pattern by looking at:
– Sphincter and intravesicular (bladder) pressures
– Bladder emptying
– Timing, coordination, and strength of detrusor and sphincter contractions

Chronic SCI bladder management:
– Renal U/S yearly to check for hydronephrosis
– BMP checking renal function yearly
– Cystoscopy every 10 years if indwelling catheter to evaluate for bladder cancer

Urinary Tract Infection (UTI):
– Antibiotics only indicated for symptomatic bacteriuria or exacerbation of chronic UTI [31, 32]
  • Urinalysis with
    ○ Bacteria ($\geq 10^2$ cfu/mL for IC, $\geq 10^4$ cfu/mL for clean catch, or any amount with indwelling foley) [33]
    ○ 0–5 Squamous epithelial cells (marker for contamination)

- • Pyuria
- • Symptoms
  - ° Fever, dysuria, change in voiding, AD, increased spasticity
- – **Treatment course:** [31]
  - • Chronic SCI without fever—5 days
  - • Acute SCI without fever—7 days
  - • SCI with fever—14+ days
- – Antibiotic prophylaxis does not prevent UTI [31]

(Table 2.9) **Bladder Medications**

Spasticity

Tone: muscle resistance to passive stretch across a joint
Spasticity: velocity-dependent increase in tone due to hyperactive stretch reflex (UMN)
Rigidity: non-velocity-dependent increase in tone (basal ganglia)

Treatment Objectives:
- – Not all tone should be treated
  - • Lower extremity tone, for example, may facilitate standing transfers or ambulation without the need for bracing
- – Indications/Goals of treatment:
  - • Improve function: mobility, balance, ADLs, positioning, hygiene
  - • Decrease pain
  - • Prevent contractures
  - • Allow for uninterrupted sleep
- – Rule out pathological causes of increased spasticity
  - • Infection, pain, constipation, urinary retention, skin break-down, HO
- – Treatment varies by severity, location (generalized vs. focal), age, compliance, and comorbidities.
  - • Focal treatments for focal spasticity (i.e., botulinum, TENS, orthoses)
  - • Multiple muscles in multiple limbs, consider po medication ± focal treatments

Table 2.9 Bladder medications

Medication	Mechanism	Dosing	Side effects	Notes
Bethanecol	Muscarinic agonist (M2 and M3) → increases detrusor contractility	Start 10 mg po tid Increase 10 mg/dose Max 100 mg/dose	Hypotension, headache, GI cramping, lacrimation, sweating	Contraindicated in patients with asthma, CAD, gastric ulcers
Tamsulosin	α_{1A} adrenergic antagonist → relaxes smooth muscle of prostate and bladder neck	Start 0.4 mg po qhs May increase to 0.8 mg	Orthostasis	Do not use with nitro agents Contains sulfa
Doxazosin	α_1 adrenergic antagonist → relaxes smooth muscle of prostate and bladder neck	Start 1 mg po qhs Max dose 8 mg/day	Orthostasis, hypotension	
Tolterodine	Muscarinic antagonist (M1–M5) → relaxation of detrusor	Start 1–2 mg po bid Max 4 mg/day	Dizziness, dry mouth, constipation, confusion, drowsiness	Available in LA formulation
Oxybutynin	Muscarinic antagonist (M1, M3) → relaxation of detrusor	Start 5 mg po bid–tid Increase 5 mg/dose Max 30 mg/day	Dizziness, dry mouth, constipation, confusion, drowsiness	Available in XL and patch formulations
Pseudoephedrine	Norepinephrine release from presynaptic neurons → contraction of internal urethral sphincter and relaxation of detrusor	Start 30 mg po bid Max 120 mg/day	Tachycardia, palpitations, blurry vision, anorexia, vertigo	

Treatment—Therapy:
- Correct positioning, splinting, casting, tone-reducing orthoses
- Stretching, ROM exercises
- Modalities (TENS, FES)

Treatment—Oral Medication (See Table 2.10):
- **Baclofen**—GABA$_B$ agonist, pre- and post-synaptic
  - Start 10 mg po tid and titrate by 10 mg as needed, max 80 mg/day (theoretical)

  Side effects: sedation, seizure risk with sudden discontinuation

- **Tizanidine**—α_2 agonist, inhibits spinal interneurons
  - Start 2 mg tid–qid and titrate by 2 mg as needed, max 36 mg/day

  Side effects: sedation, dry mouth, orthostatic hypotension, elevated LFTs

- **Clonidine**—α_2 agonist
  - Use limited due to hypotensive effects, but may be used intrathecally in combination with baclofen for spasticity and pain
- **Dantrolene sodium**—blocks Ca^{2+} release from sarcoplasmic reticulum
  - Start 25 mg daily and titrate to 3–4 times a day as needed every 4–7 days, max 400 mg/day
  - Preferred for lack of cognitive and sedative side effects

  Side effects: Possible liver toxicity—Need to monitor LFTs frequently

- **Benzodiazepines**—GABA$_A$ agonists
  - Start clonazepam 0.5 mg po tid or qhs. May increase to 1 mg tid
  - Alternative is Valium 2–5 mg po qhs, may increase to 10 mg
  - Helpful for painful nocturnal spasms

  Side effects: tachyphylaxis, drowsiness, confusion

Treatment—Interventional:
- Chemical neurolysis with phenol or alcohol
  - Lasts 6–9 months, inexpensive

  Side effects: dysesthesias, weakness

- Botulinum toxin type A and type B
  - For spasticity in selected muscles
  - Onset 2–3 days, peak 2–3 weeks, duration of effect 3 months
  - May improve ambulation, positioning, and hygiene, and reduce pain [34]

Side effects: dysphagia, dyspnea, weakness, fatigue

- Intrathecal Baclofen Pump (ITB)
  - Consider for patients with ADL-limiting spasticity uncontrolled on oral medications (less sedating), including those with hemi-spasticity
  - Less effective for upper extremities

  Side effects: infection, pump may fail, risk of withdrawal seizures

- Spinal Cord Stimulator (SCS)
  - May improve motor control, but evidence is mixed; no recent studies

  Side effects: infection, spinal cord injury (Table 2.10)

Autonomic Dysreflexia (AD) [35]

Reflex sympathetic response to a noxious stimulus **below** the level of injury
- Associated with injuries at or above T6
- Considered a medical emergency
- Does not occur until out of spinal shock (first week); subsequently, patients remain at lifelong risk.

Pathophysiology:
- Noxious stimuli below the level of injury trigger a sympathetic reflex within the spinal cord
- Catecholamines are released, resulting in vasoconstriction
- The significance of the T6 level is that the sympathetic supply to the splanchnic vasculature originates from T6–L2.
  - Splanchnic vasoconstriction significantly decreases intravascular volume
  - Due to the SCI, the brain cannot inhibit the sympathetic outflow to the splanchnic circulation
- Combined with the LE vasoconstriction, systemic blood pressure rises
- The carotid baroreceptors trigger adjustment for hypertension
  - Increased vagal tone → bradycardia, vasodilation above level
  - Descending spinal inhibition of sympathetic outflow (blocked)

Table 2.10 Spasticity medications

Medication	Mechanism	Dosing	Side effects	Notes
Baclofen	$GABA_B$ agonist → pre- and post-synaptic inhibition	Start 10 mg po tid, increase by 5–10 mg/dose every 3–5 days	Sedation, confusion, constipation	Abrupt discontinuation may precipitate seizures
Dantrolene	Decrease release of calcium from sarcoplasmic reticulum	Start 25 mg daily, increase to TID, then increase dose by 25 mg every 3–5 days Max 400 mg/day	Weakness, fatigue, drowsiness, diarrhea, liver toxicity	Follow LFT's weekly
Diazepam	$GABA_A$ agonist → pre-synaptic inhibition	Start 2 mg po bid or qhs, may increase to 5 or 10 mg	Drowsiness, fatigue, confusion	Tachyphylaxis with tolerance and dependence
Clonazepam	$GABA_A$ agonist → pre-synaptic inhibition	Start 0.5 mg po tid or qhs, may increase to 1 mg	Drowsiness, fatigue, confusion	Tachyphylaxis with tolerance and dependence
Tizanidine	α_2 agonist → inhibits spinal interneurons	Start 2 mg tid–qid and titrate by 2 mg as needed Max 36 mg/day	Orthostasis, hallucination, sedation, dizziness, elevated LFTs	Follow LFT's *Tab* and *Cap* are not bioequivalent
OnabotulinumtoxinA	Cleaves SNAP-25, preventing exocytosis of presynaptic ACh vesicles at the neuromuscular junction	25–50 units/muscle Max 12–14 units/kg or 400 units in 3 months	Dysphagia, dyspnea, weakness, upper respiratory infection	Approved for elbow, wrist, and finger flexor spasticity only
RimabotulinumtoxinB	Cleaves synaptobrevin preventing exocytosis of presynaptic ACh vesicles	Start 2,500 units total Increase per muscle up to 50%	Dysphagia, dyspnea, weakness, upper respiratory infection	

Clinical:
- Systolic Blood Pressure >20 mmHg above baseline (>15 in kids)
- Anxiety
- Headache (HA)
- Blurred vision
- Nasal congestion
- Sweating/flushing/piloerection above level
- Bradycardia

Workup and Treatment:
1. Check blood pressure (BP) and pulse initially and after each adjustment
2. Elevate head/sit patient up to decrease intracranial pressure
3. Loosen restrictive clothing, remove socks, braces, or supports
4. Evaluate for bladder distension/tenderness
   (a) For indwelling catheter, ensure it is draining properly
      ° If blockage is suspected, irrigate with 10–15 mL of normal saline
      ° If the catheter does not start to properly drain after irrigation, then replace with new catheter
   (b) If no catheter, straight cath with lidocaine jelly
      ° If output >200 cc, start IC program (see Sect. 5.5)
      ° Collect U/A and culture
   (c) If no other cause is found, may consider flushing bladder with 5–10 cc lidocaine 1%
5. If SBP >150 or if HA, apply 1″ nitropaste to forehead
6. Check rectum for fecal impaction.(Use lidocaine jelly to prevent additional noxious stimulus)
7. Examine skin for breakdown and note BP response to position changes
8. If cause cannot be immediately identified, treat the pain triggering AD and continue workup with close monitoring of BP
   (a) Oxycodone 5 mg PO, or Morphine 4 mg IV
9. If BP continues to rise, treat with 2 in. of Nitropaste (can be wiped off if BP drops too much as AD resolves). This is usually applied to the forehead to ensure it is removed at appropriate time
10. If BP still continues to rise, use Nifedipine 10 mg capsule. Have patient bite capsule to speed effect. *Be prepared for possible hypotension when cause of AD is found and is resolved.*

Other Potential Causes of AD to Consider:
- Fracture, HO, DVT/PE, Infection
- GU: Bladder distention, kidney/bladder stone, blocked catheter, UTI
- GI: Appendicitis, impaction, gallstones, ulcers, hemorrhoids
- Skin: Constrictive clothing, burns, blisters, pressure ulcers, ingrown toenail, cuts
- Reproductive system: sexual intercourse, infection
  - Males: Ejaculation, epididymitis, scrotal compression
  - Females: Menstruation, pregnancy, vaginitis, ovarian torsion, fibroids

Preeclampsia Versus AD:
- Preeclampsia never occurs before 24 weeks gestation
  - Triad of HTN, Proteinuria, Edema
- AD may occur during labor. Resolves with epidural anesthesia

Pediatric population—threshold for pharmacologic intervention: [35]
- <5 years old: SBP >120
- 5–12 years old: SBP >130
- >13 years old: SBP >140

Heterotopic Ossification (HO)

Formation of mature lamellar bone in soft tissue
Epidemiology: [36, 37]
- Incidence: 10–78% in SCI
- Generally diagnosed 1–4 months post-injury, but can occur later
- Peak incidence at 2 months

Risk Factors:
- Complete > Incomplete (RR 2.0 ± 4.2) [37]
- Prolonged coma (> 2 weeks)
- Immobility
- Spasticity (in the involved extremity)
- Associated long-bone fracture
- Pressure ulcers
- Younger age

Clinical:
- Decreased ↓ ROM (20–30% of patients) [37]
- 3–8% develop ankylosed joints [37]
- Pain or AD
- Local swelling, erythema, warmth
- Low-grade fever
- Joints most commonly involved: Hips > Knee > Elbow > Shoulder > Hand > Spine [37]

Complications:
- Skin breakdown
- Nerve entrapment
- Loss of function

Workup:
- Laboratory Studies
  - Serum Alkaline Phosphatase (SAP) [38, 39]
    - ° May be elevated 7 weeks before the first clinical signs become apparent (but often elevated postoperatively without HO as well)
    - ° Peak levels occur 3 weeks after the appearance of clinical signs
    - ° Poor specificity (elevated with fractures)
  - CPK
  - Erythrocyte sedimentation rate (ESR)
    - ° Early inflammatory marker, nonspecific
- Plain X-rays
  - Only soft tissue edema seen early on
  - Need 2–3 weeks for bone maturation to be visible on X-ray
- Three phase 99m Technetium Bone Scan
  - Sensitive for early detection
  - Can be seen 2.5 weeks after SCI [37]
  - Will be normal in mature HO [23]

Treatment: [3]
- Bisphosphonates
  - Inhibits osteoclastic activity but does not reverse or dissolve bone
  - If CPK elevated
    - ° Etidronate 20 mg/kg/day divided in 2 doses ×6 months
  - If CPK normal
    - ° Etidronate 20 mg/kg/day divided in 2 doses ×3 months, then
    - ° 10 mg/kg/day ×3 months

- NSAIDs
  - Consider for inflammation if CRP >8 or CPK elevated
  - Indomethacin 25 mg tid ×2 weeks or until CRP <2 or CPK normal
- Therapy
  - Once acute inflammatory signs have subsided, gentle PROM is indicated to help maintain functional range
  - Avoid aggressive PROM as microtrauma may lead to further HO [40]
- Radiation therapy
- Surgery—Wedge resection
  - Must have clear goal: hygiene, positioning, ADLs, pain
  - Performed after 12–18 months to allow full bony maturation

Pressure Ulcers and Wound Care

Lesions resulting from unrelieved pressure which damages underlying tissue [41]

Pathophysiology [23, 41, 42]

- Prolonged or excessive tissue deformation (compression >70 mmHg, shear or tension) including possible ischemic distortion of the vasculature
- Muscle tissue is more sensitive than skin to pressure-induced ischemia
- Pressure ulcers develop in deep structures then progress superficially

Epidemiology [43, 44]

- 24% of Model Systems SCI patients developed at least one pressure ulcer during acute care or rehabilitation
- 15% had a pressure ulcer at their first annual examination, 20% at year 5, 23% at year 10
- Incidence in cervical complete > thoracic complete > incomplete
- Most frequent secondary medical complication of SCI in Model Systems [45]
- Second most common reason for rehospitalization in chronic SCI

Risk Factors [3, 45, 46]

Level and severity of the injury, violent injury, mobility status, gender, ethnicity, marital status, employment status, level of education, tobacco or alcohol use, prior pressure ulcer, nutritional status, anemia, incontinence, muscle atrophy, vascular insufficiency

Prevention: [47]
- Begin pressure relief techniques ASAP
- Avoid prolonged immobilization
- Daily visual and tactile skin inspection
- Turn or reposition patients every 2 h in bed
  - Eliminate stretching and folding of soft tissues and prevent shearing when individuals are repositioned.
  - Avoid side-lying directly on the trochanter.
- Prescribe pressure-relief regimen for w/c use (power or manual)
  - Weight shift every 15 min, reposition every hour [41]
- Apply pressure-reducing support surfaces preventively to protect soft tissues from injury
  - The support surface–skin interface should stay cool and dry
  - Use pillows or cushions to bridge contacting tissues and unload bony prominences (increase weight-bearing surface)
  - Avoid donut-type devices
  - Pressure mapping can help determine the best seating system and ensure pressure reliefs are effective [3]
- Therapy program should include muscle strengthening and cardio to prevent deconditioning
- Nutritional optimization and smoking cessation [3]
- Educate patient, family, and aide on ulcer prevention and treatment including skin examination

Clinical [3]
- Breakdown occurs over bony prominences
  - Seated: ischial tuberoscity, trochanters, elbows
  - Supine: Sacrum, heels, scapulae, occiput
- Daily physical exam should screen for early signs of potential breakdown
  - Check skin temperature (warmth or coolness)
  - Tissue consistency (firm or boggy feeling)
  - Sensation (pain, itching)

Complications [3]
Infection (cellulitis, osteomyelitis), pain, increased spasticity, AD, adjustment d/o
Staging of Pressure Ulcers [48]
- **Suspected Deep Tissue Injury**: Purple or maroon discoloration of intact skin or blood-filled blister due to underlying tissue damage

Stage I
- Non-blanching erythema of intact skin

Stage II
- Partial thickness loss of dermis with pink wound bed, no slough
- May also be intact or ruptured blister

Stage III
- Full thickness loss of dermis with exposed adipose.
- Slough may be present but should not prevent depth assessment
- Undermining and sinus tracts may be present

Stage IV
- Full thickness loss with exposed bone, muscle, or fascia
- Slough or eschar may be present but not cover wound bed
- Undermining and sinus tracts may be present

Unstageable
- Full thickness loss with depth assessment obscured by slough or eschar

Wound exam: [47]
- Location and appearance
- Size (length, width, and depth)
- Stage
- Exudate
- Odor
- Necrosis
- Undermining/Tunneling/Sinus tracts
- Healing (granulation, vascular supply, epithelialization)
- Margins and surrounding tissue integrity
  - Maceration (white discoloration and bogginess)

Treatment [47]
- Stage I
  - Monitor nutrition
  - Ensure turns q2h
  - Barrier films or lotions
- Stage II
  - Hydrocolloid gel (bid) or film dressing (leave on until it falls off)
- Stage III and IV
  - Surgical consultation
  - Debridement of eschar, necrotic tissue, and slough (unless on heel)

- ◦ Sharp with scalpel—stop when reach intact capillaries
- ◦ Enzymatic—collagenase bid
- • Cleanse at each dressing change with NS or wound cleanser
  - ◦ Irrigate with a pressure of 4–15 psi to reduce bacterial load [49]
- • Consider negative pressure therapy
- • Electrical stimulation
- • Maintain moist ulcer bed
- • Barrier cream to surrounding intact skin to prevent maceration and dressing to keep it dry
- • Check testosterone levels (men)
  - ◦ Men—testosterone 200 mg IM q2 weeks
  - ◦ Women—testosterone 50 mg IM q2 weeks
  - ◦ Follow serum levels 1 week after administration

Nutrition
- – Check labs, calorie count, serial weights to determine nutritional status
- – Low serum protein $\rightarrow$ interstitial edema $\rightarrow$ decreased O_2/nutrient delivery to skin, and increased tissue pressure $\rightarrow$ decreased blood flow [50]
  - • Total protein <6.4 g/dL [51]
  - • Albumin <3.5 mg/dL [52]
- – Diet:
  - • Total calories: 35–40 kcal/kg of body weight daily [53]
  - • Protein intake: [47]
    - ◦ Stage II—1.2–1.5 g/kg/day
    - ◦ Stage III or IV—1.5–2.0 g/kg/day
- – Micronutrients: [23]
  - • Multivitamin with minerals daily
  - • Vitamin C 1 g/day [23]
  - • Zinc does not affect the healing of pressure ulcers within 2–3 months [54] and may have harmful long-term effects [55]
  - • Arginine 7–15 mg/day [56]

Medical Complications

Orthostatic Hypotension

Definition: [57]
- Decrease in systolic blood pressure (SBP) by at least 20 mmHg, OR
- Decrease in diastolic blood pressure (DBP) by at least 10 mmHg
- Within 3 min of standing or being raised greater than 60° on a tilt table.

Clinical:
- Lightheadedness, blurry vision, nausea, dizziness, ringing of the ears, fatigue, palpitations, pallor, and syncope
- Found to limit 43% of therapy sessions in one study, with tetraplegic patients most affected [58]

Pathophysiology: [59]
- Carotid baroreceptors sense drop in BP, but due to the SCI, the signal cannot reach the sympathetic system (T1–L2) and trigger vasoconstriction
- Other factors:
  - Decreased plasma volume associated with prolonged supine position
  - Malnutrition/hypoalbuminemia
  - Cardiovascular deconditioning
  - Motor deficits leading to loss of skeletal muscle pumping activity

Treatment:
- Compression stockings and abdominal binder prior to sitting up
- Adequate hydration and nutrition
- Medication (if non-pharmacological methods insufficient):
  - NaCl tablets 1 g po BID-QID
    - Monitor BMP
    - Contraindicated in CHF
  - Midodrine 2.5–10 mg po TID
    - α_1 adrenergic agonist → vasoconstriction
    - **Side effects**: hypertension, urinary retention, headache, paresthesias
  - Fludrocortisone 0.1 mg daily
    - Aldosterone analog → Na^+ retention, K^+ excretion
    - **Side effects:** Hypertension, CHF exacerbation, dizziness, headache, weakness

Venous Thromboembolic Disease

Including Deep Vein Thrombosis (DVT) and Pulmonary Embolism (PE)

Epidemiology: [3, 23]
- DVT incidence in acute post-injury period: 47–100% (varies by study) [3]
- DVT incidence during Acute Rehab (Model Systems): 9.8% [60]
- PE incidence during Acute Rehab (Model Systems): 2.6% [60]
- 80% occur during the first 2 weeks
- PE #1 cause of death in acute SCI [23], #3 within first year [45]

Risk Factors: [23]
- Virchow's triad: [61]
  - Venous stasis
  - Vessel–wall (endothelial) damage
  - Hypercoagulable state
- Prior DVT
- Medical comorbidities: vascular disease, DM, cancer, obesity
- Older age

DVT Prophylaxis: [19]
- Sequential compression device (SCD) for first 2 weeks after injury
  - Lower extremity ultrasound if thromboprophylaxis delayed >72 h post-injury
- Consider IVC filter [62–64] if
  - Anticoagulant prophylaxis failed
  - Unable to anticoagulate (high risk of bleeding)
    - ° Anticoagulant prophylaxis still required once cleared
- Anticoagulant should be started within 72 h if not contraindicated
  - AIS D: Enoxaparin 40 mg SQ daily until D/C from Rehabilitation
  - AIS C: Enoxaparin 40 mg SQ daily for *up to* 8 weeks
  - AIS A or B: Enoxaparin 40 mg SQ daily for *at least* 8 weeks
    - ° If complicated (LE fracture, h/o thrombosis, cancer, heart failure, obesity or age >70), needs to be continued for 12 weeks
- Start PROM, mobilization ASAP

Clinical—DVT:
- Calf circumference asymmetry, edema, tenderness, low-grade fever, pain/tenderness (Homan's sign) [3]
- 10× more frequent in paretic leg [23]

Clinical—PE:
- Clinical signs and symptoms may be absent
- Dyspnea/desaturation, easy fatigability, tachycardia, EKG changes, flash pulmonary edema, chest pain, or hypoxic seizure
- Sudden death

Workup:
- Imaging
  - Venogram is gold standard [23]
  - Venous doppler
  - CT Angiogram (chest) + venogram (legs)
  - Ventilation/Perfusion (V/Q) scan if unable to have CTA
- ABG—$\downarrow PO_2$
- EKG [65, 66]
  - S1Q3T3—Prominent S in I, Q and inverted T in III
  - Right axis deviation
  - Right bundle branch block
  - ST elevation in VI and aVR
  - Tachycardia or AFib/flutter (Tachycardia may be only sign of PE in otherwise asymptomatic patient. Keep PE high on your list if other causes ruled out).

Treatment:
- Supplemental O_2, titrate SPO_2 >92%
- Medical consultation
- Hold PROM, mobilization for 48–72 h until anticoagulated [19]
  - Kirschblum et al. recommend 5–10 days of AC prior to mobilization [23]
- Discontinue pneumatic compression device
- IVC filter when anticoagulation is contraindicated
- Must start AC as soon as possible, even after filter placement [62]
  - Immediate-acting anticoagulant + warfarin, if not contraindicated
    - Heparin gtt (discuss goal with medicine and neurosurgery)
    - or LMWH, i.e., enoxaparin 1mg/kg q12h
  - Warfarin start 5 mg po daily, goal INR of 2–3
  - Treat for 6 months for proximal DVT

Hypercalcemia

Epidemiology: [23]
– 10–23% of patients with SCI
– More common in tetraplegia than paraplegia
– Peaks between 1 and 4 months post injury [67]
– More common in young men

Pathophysiology: [68]
– Loss of mechanical loading of the bone →increase in bone resorption
– In an acute SCI, loss of renal tubular reabsorption →decreased calcium excretion

Clinical:
– Constipation
– Abdominal pain
– Myalgia, arthralgia
– Lethargy and fatigue
– Confusion/psychosis
– Nausea/vomiting

Workup: [69]
    Serum calcium level (normal range 8.5–10.5 mg/dL)
    Correct for albumin concentration [2]
    Corrected Calcium=0.8× (normal albumin—patient's albumin)+patient's serum calcium

Treatment: [23, 69]
– Calcium level <12 mg/dL—immediate treatment not necessary
    • 0.9NS IV for adequate hydration (promote urinary excretion)
    • Avoid thiazides, lithium, and vitamin C
– Calcium 12–14 mg/dL
    • If chronic without symptoms, treat like mild hypercalcemia
    • If acute or with, then treat as severe hypercalcemia
– Calcium >14 mg/dL
    • 0.9NS IV @ 200–300 cc/h (decrease for CHF, etc.)
        ◦ Place Foley
        ◦ Urine output goal 100–150 cc/h
        ◦ Add loop diuretic for edema
        ◦ Stop when euvolemic

- Bisphosphonates [67, 69]
    - ° Pamidronate 60 mg IV over 4 h or 90 mg over 24 h
        - Inhibits osteoclast activity
        - Lowers Ca^{2+} over 3 days, nadir at 7
        - Side effects: Jaw osteonecrosis, fever, nausea, headache, myalgia, anemia
- Calcitonin 4 IU/kg IV or SQ q12h
    - ° May increase up to 6–8 IU/kg q6h
    - ° Increases renal excretion of Ca^{2+}, decreases bone resorption
    - ° May lower serum Ca^{2+} up to 1–2 mg/dL within 4–6 h
    - ° Peak effect within the first 48 h Nasal application not effective for hypercalcemia

Vitamin D Deficiency

Epidemiology
- Higher prevalence of vitamin D deficiency in SCI patients, 93% in one study [67, 70]
- Lower levels seen in African Americans [70, 71] and incomplete injuries [70]

Pathophysiology:
- Hypercalcemia $\rightarrow \downarrow$ PTH levels $\rightarrow$
    1. $\downarrow$ renal Ca^{2+} reabsorption
    2. $\downarrow 1,25(OH)_2 (D_3) \rightarrow \downarrow$ GI Ca^{2+} absorption
        - ° 30 ng/mL is needed for intestinal absorption [72]
- $\downarrow$ Sun exposure $\rightarrow \downarrow D_3$ levels [71]
    - Sunlight may provide up to 90% of our daily requirement

Workup:
- Serum 25-hydroxyvitamin D (D_2) and Ca^{2+}
    - Normal >30 ng/mL [72]

Treatment:
- Ergocalciferol (D2) or cholecalciferol (D3) [73]
    - 50,000 IU po weekly ×6–8 weeks, then
    - 800–1,000 IU po daily

Testosterone Deficiency (Hypogonadism)

Epidemiology:
– Prevalence
  • 83% in acute (<4 months) [74]
  • 43% in chronic [75]

Risk Factors:
– Testosterone levels drop with increasing time since injury [76, 77]
– Motor complete more commonly affected than incomplete [75]
– Lower levels associated with opiate use [75]
– Association with low albumin and hematocrit, and high AST levels [74]

Pathophysiology:
– SCI → ↓hGH, IGF-1, and testosterone [76]
– ↓Testosterone → ↓muscle mass and ↑fat mass [78]

Clinical:
– Muscle wasting
– Erectile dysfunction
– Decreased sex drive
– Fatigue
– Depression
– Increased cholesterol and lipid levels

Workup:
1. AM serum total testosterone level
   • Normal >325 ng/dL [75]
2. Serum FSH, LH and prolactin
   • In primary hypogonadism: ↑FSH, ↑LH, normal prolactin
   • In secondary hypogonadism: ↓FSH, ↓LH, possible ↑prolactin

Treatment:
– Testosterone enanthate or cypionate 200 mg monthly [78] or q2 weeks [79]
– Follow serum total testosterone halfway between dosages to ensure goal range (400–700 ng/dL) until steady, then q6–12 months [79]

Sexuality [80]

Men
Reflexogenic Erections
- Stimulation of somatic afferent fibers (pudendal nerve, S2–4)
- Efferent parasympathetic fibers (pelvic nerve, S2–4) trigger NO release

Psychogenic Erections
- Cortical modulation of above sacral reflex
- Mediated by sympathetic fibers from T11–L2

Ejaculation
- Sympathetic fibers from T11–L2 contribute to the hypogastric plexus

(Table 2.11) Prevalence of male sexual dysfunction after SCI: [81, 82]

Treatment:

Hypogonadism
- Check AM serum testosterone
- If low, may replace with 200 mg IM q2 weeks
- Recheck 1 week after injection to ensure dosing within therapeutic range

Phosphodiesterase-5 inhibitors
- Sildenafil 25 mg po daily prn
- Effective for UMN lesions only
- Avoid if taking nitrates
- Caution if prone to AD or hypotension

Intraurethral or intracorporeal prostaglandin E1 (alprostadil)
- May be effective for LMN lesions
- Caution if prone to AD (may be painful)
- **Side effects:** priapism, trauma

Table 2.11 Prevalence of male sexual dysfunction after SCI: [81, 82]

	Complete UMN (%)	Incomplete UMN (%)	Complete LMN (%)	Incomplete LMN (%)
Reflexogenic erection	>90	>90	12	
Psychogenic erection	<10	50	25	
Ejaculation	5	30	18	70

Vacuum pump
- Effective for LMN lesions
- **Side effects:** trauma, skin breakdown

Penile implants
- Complication rate 8–33% (erosion, infection)

Vibration
- Vibrator held along penile shaft
- Effective for UMN lesions only (96%)
- May trigger AD

Electroejaculation
- Rectal probe electrically stimulates the prostate
- 80–90% Success rates
- **Side effects:** AD, pain, rectal burns

Women
Vaginal Lubrication
- Reflexogenic and psychogenic by same pathways as ejaculation in men (see above)

Orgasm—achieved in <50% [83]
Menstruation [3]
- Acute SCI: 50–85% amenorrhea
- 50% menstruate at 6 months
- 90% menstruate at 1 year
- SCI does not affect female fertility once menstruation resumes

Pregnancy
- <10% of couples will have successful reproduction without assistance [84]
- 40% of men with SCI who have attempted to father children have done so

Infertility
- Erectile and ejaculatory dysfunction
- Poor semen quality (esp. motility)
  - Recurrent UTI or chronic inflammation
  - Testicular hyperthermia
  - Stasis of prostatic fluid
  - Sperm contact with urine (retrograde ejaculation)

Assisted Reproduction Success Rates
- Intrauterine insemination: 10–14%
- IVF: 30–40%

Complications of Pregnancy
- Preterm labor and low birth weight
- Autonomic dysreflexia
  - May be only manifestation of labor
    - Pre-eclampsia does not occur prior to 24 weeks
  - Treatment=epidural anesthesia
- Pressure ulcers
- Increased spasticity
- Recurrent UTIs
- Decreased pulmonary function
- Constipation
- Leg edema
- Thromboembolism
- May need to adjust wheelchair and transfer techniques

Pain

Epidemiology:
- 77–86% experience pain after SCI [85–88]
  - 20–33% report severe pain [3, 89]
- 66% have chronic pain [90]
- Type of pain varies with time post injury [91]
  - 2 weeks post injury—33% neuropathic, 67% musculoskeletal
  - 6 months post injury—60% neuropathic, 40% musculoskeletal

Classification:
(Table 2.12) The International Associate for the Study of Pain (IASP) Classification of pain after SCI [92, 93]

Upper extremity (UE) Pain:
- Most commonly reported pain after SCI [94]
- 30–50% patient report shoulder pain interferes with ADLs [95, 96]
- Acute: usually is related to SCI, more common with tetraplegia

Table 2.12 The international associate for the study of pain (IASP) classification of pain after SCI [92]

Broad type (tier 1)	Broad system (tier 2)	Specific structures/pathology (tier 3)
Nociceptive	MSK	Bone, joint, muscle trauma/inflammation
		Mechanical instability
		Overuse
	Visceral	Renal calculus, bowel, sphincter dysfunction
		AD headache
Neuropathic	Above level	Compressive mononeuropathy
		CRPS
	At level	Spinal root injury/compression
		Syringomyelia
		Dual level cord and root trauma
	Below level (>3 levels below NLI) [93]	Cord trauma/ischemia

- Chronic: more common in paraplegia, linked to overuse injury, poor seated posture, spasticity, subluxation, rotator cuff pathology [95, 97, 98]
- Common examples of shoulder pain: [99]
  - Bicipital tendonitis, subacromial bursitis, adhesive capsulitis, acromioclavicular sprain/strain, subluxation, cervical radiculopathy, spasticity, contractures, HO, or syrinx
  - Overuse injuries: [98]
    - ° 45% wrist or hand
      - CTS, ulnar nerve entrapment, DeQuervain's tenosynovitis, OA
    - ° 32% elbow injuries
      - Ulnar nerve entrapment, lateral epicondylitis, OA

Visceral Pain:
- **Clinical:** Abdominal pain or tenderness, nausea, vomiting, constipation, diarrhea, sweating, AD
- **Common causes:** Fecal impaction, bowel obstruction, bowel infarction, bowel perforation, cholecystitis, choledocholithiasis, pancreatitis, appendicitis, splenic rupture, bladder perforation, pyelonephritis, UTI, Renal calculus, dysreflexic headache, pressure sores

Neuropathic Pain:
- **Etiology:** Dysfunction in the peripheral and central nervous systems [100]
  - Neuronal hyperexcitability
  - Reduced inhibition
  - Neuronal reorganization/plasticity
- **Clinical:** tingling, burning, cramping, electric radiations, allodynia, hyperalgesia

Complications:
- Pain may present as general malaise, increased spasticity, or AD
- Patients with chronic SCI pain report their pain prevents them from performing ADLs and has contributed to a decrease in their quality of life [87, 101]

Workup:
- Determine the nature of the lesion, the neurological structures involved, and the changes in the surviving tissue [102]
- Physical exam
  - Determine the neurological level for neuropathic pain [103]
    ○ If there seems to be neuropathic pain above the known level of injury, have suspicion for secondary (higher) cord compression or ascending syrinx.
  - MSK and medical exam for identifying sources of nociceptive pain
- Additional testing with X-ray, CT, MRI, or electrodiagnostic studies may be indicated [103]
- For further information, refer to Siddall and Middleton, 2006 [104]

Treatment:
- Acute musculoskeletal pain and overuse injuries
  - Relative rest, ice, elevation, NSAIDs, device modifications, behavior modification, supportive orthoses, steroid injection
- Medication (See table 2.13)
  - If pain is not managed with medication after an adequate trial at maximum dose, then another drug with a different mechanism of action may be added [105]
    ○ Adequate trial lengths: [105]
      - Lidocaine—2 weeks
      - Gabapentin or TCA—6–7 weeks titration, then 1–2 weeks at max dose
      - Opiods and tramadol—4–6 weeks

- Therapy [95, 96, 99, 106]
  - ROM, strengthening, stretching, massage, splinting, modalities
  - Balanced shoulder exercise
    - ° Maintain proper sitting posture
    - ° Stretch anterior muscles
    - ° Strengthen posterior muscles
    - ° Rowing, backward wheeling
  - Proper wheelchair, positive seat angle, vertical and low backrest with adequate support for posture
  - Alternate techniques for transferring, weight shifting, mobility
- Psychological therapy [107]
  - Coping skills, cognitive behavioral therapy, exposure to social, sexual, and communication skill training
- Neuromodulation for *At Level* pain [100, 108]
  - Transcutaneous electric nerve stimulation (TENs)
  - Spinal cord stimulation
  - Deep brain stimulation
- Surgical interventions [100, 108]
  - Spine stabilization, decompression, synrinx cordotomy, cordectomy, myelotomy, doral root entry zone lesion (DREZ)
  - All surgical treatment options have limited support for effectiveness

Table 2.13 Pain medications

Medication	Mechanism	Dose	Side effects
Amitriptyline	Acts on $5HT_{2A}$ receptors increasing serotonin and norepinephrine concentrations in the central nervous system, inhibiting afferent pain signals [18, 19]	Start 25 mg po qhs Max: 150 mg/day	Drowsiness, dry mouth, dizziness, N/V, constipation, confusion, anxiety, insomnia, urinary retention, paresthesias, tremor, vision changes, QT prolongation, SIADH
Baclofen	$GABA_B$ agonist	5 mg po TID increase: 15 mg/day q3 days Max: 80 mg/day	Drowsiness, dizziness, weakness, confusion, hypotension, respiratory depression, withdrawal seizures
Duloxetine	Serotonin and norepinephrine reuptake inhibition → descending inhibition of pain	Start 30 mg po daily Increase after 1 week Max: 60 mg	Headache, somnolence, fatigue, nausea, dizziness, hyperhydrosis
Gabapentin	Interacts with $\alpha_2\delta$ subunit of voltage-gated N-type Ca^{2+} channels and indirectly with the NMDA receptor → inhibition of nociceptive signals [109, 110]	Start 100–300 mg po qhs Increase frequency to tid–qid Titrate by 200–300 mg/dose Max: 3,600 mg/day	Dizziness, drowsiness, ataxia, n/v, peripheral edema
Levetiracetam	Inhibits N-type voltage gated Ca^{2+} channels and acts as a $GABA_A$ agonist [111]	500 mg po q12h Increase by 1,000 mg/day q2 week Max: 3000 mg/day	Headache, N/V, diarrhea, anorexia, fatigue, dizziness, agitation, ataxia, withdrawal seizures Not effective for SCI pain [111]
Lidocaine topical	Inhibits Na^+ channels, stabilizing neuronal cell membranes and inhibiting nerve impulse initiation and conduction [112]	5% patch, 12 h on, 12 h off Max: 3 patches 5% ointment QID	Erythema, edema, burning, urticaria, arrhythmia

(continued)

Table 2.13 (continued)

Medication	Mechanism	Dose	Side effects
Methadone	μ-opioid agonist and NMDA antagonist	Start 1–2.5 mg po q8h–q12h Increase dose q10–14 days	Repiratory depression, hypotension, dizziness, sedation, N/V, constipation, QT prolongation
Milnacipran	Norepinephrine and serotonin (3:1) reuptake inhibition →descending inhibition of pain	Day 1: 12.5 mg Day 2–3: 12.5 mg bid Day 4–7: 25 mg bid Day 8: 50 mg bid Max: 100 mg bid	Nausea, constipation, headache, insomnia, hot flashes
Morphine	μ-opioid agonist [112]	Start 7.5 mg po or 2 mg IV Monitor for sedation, respiratory depression PO dose=3× IV dose	Repiratory depression, hypotension, drowsiness, constipation, pruritus, dry mouth, urinary retention
Pregabalin	Interacts with $\alpha_2\delta$ subunit of voltage-gated N-type Ca^{2+} channels and indirectly with the NMDA receptor → inhibition of nociceptive signals	Start 50 mg po TID Increase to 300 mg/day over 7 days Max: 600 mg/day	Dizziness, drowsiness, ataxia, tremor, n/v, peripheral edema, headache, blurry vision, weight gain
Tramadol	A low-affinity μ-opioid agonist and weak monoamine reuptake inhibitor [112]	50 mg po q6h prn Max: 400 mg/day	Dizziness, orthostatic hypotension, n/v, constipation, headache, pruritus, serotonin syndrome
Valproic acid	Blocks voltage-gated Na^+ channels suppressing high-frequency firing of neurons Indirect ↑GABA concentrations in CNS [113]	Start 250 mg po TID Increase by250 mg/dose Monitor serum levels (goal: 50–100 mg/L)	Headache, N/V, diarrhea, thrombocytopenia, dizziness, appetite changes, depression, insomnia, elevated AST/ALT, SIADH, vision changes

References

1. The National SCI Statistical Center. Spinal cord injury facts and figures at a glance. (2011). https://www.nscisc.uab.edu/PublicDocuments/reports/pdf/Facts%202011%20Feb%20Final.pdf. Accessed 3 Jul 2012.
2. McKinley W, et al. Incidence and outcomes of spinal cord injury clinical syndromes. J Spinal Cord Med. 2007;30(3):215–24.
3. Kirshblum S, Brooks M. Rehabilitation of spinal cord injury. In: Frontera WR, DeLisa JA, editors. Physical medicine and rehabilitation: principles and practice. Philadelphia: Lippincott Williams & Wilkins Health; 2010. p. 665–716.
4. Schneider RC, Cherry G, Pantek H. The syndrome of acute central cervical spinal cord injury; with special reference to the mechanisms involved in hyperextension injuries of cervical spine. J Neurosurg. 1954;11(6):546–77.
5. Levi AD, Tator CH, Bunge RP. Clinical syndromes associated with disproportionate weakness of the upper versus the lower extremities after cervical spinal cord injury. Neurosurgery. 1996;38(1):179–83. discussion 183-5.
6. Burns SP, et al. Recovery of ambulation in motor-incomplete tetraplegia. Arch Phys Med Rehabil. 1997;78(11):1169–72.
7. Penrod LE, Hegde SK, Ditunno Jr JF. Age effect on prognosis for functional recovery in acute, traumatic central cord syndrome. Arch Phys Med Rehabil. 1990;71(12):963–8.
8. Bohlman HH. Acute fractures and dislocations of the cervical spine. An analysis of three hundred hospitalized patients and review of the literature. J Bone Joint Surg Am. 1979;61(8):1119–42.
9. Bosch A, Stauffer ES, Nickel VL. Incomplete traumatic quadriplegia. A ten-year review. JAMA. 1971;216(3):473–8.
10. Brown-Séquard E. Course of lectures on the physiology & pathology of the central nervous system: illustrated by numerous engravings, representing the principal experiments and pathological cases. Lancet. 1858;72(1822): 109–12.
11. Roth EJ, et al. Traumatic cervical Brown-Sequard and Brown-Sequard-plus syndromes: the spectrum of presentations and outcomes. Paraplegia. 1991;29(9):582–9.
12. Tattersall R, Turner B. Brown-Sequard and his syndrome. Lancet. 2000;356(9223):61–3.
13. Cheshire WP, et al. Spinal cord infarction: etiology and outcome. Neurology. 1996;47(2):321–30.
14. Maynard Jr FM, et al. International standards for neurological and functional classification of spinal cord injury. American Spinal Injury Association. Spinal Cord. 1997;35(5):266–74.
15. Kennedy JG, et al. Predictors of outcome in cauda equina syndrome. Eur Spine J. 1999;8(4):317–22.
16. Bohannon RW, Smith MB. Interrater reliability of a modified Ashworth scale of muscle spasticity. Phys Ther. 1987;67(2):206–7.
17. Kirshblum SC, et al. International standards for neurological classification of spinal cord injury (revised 2011). J Spinal Cord Med. 2011;34(6): 535–46.

18. Consortium for Spinal Cord Medicine Clinical Practice Guidelines. Respiratory management following spinal cord injury: a clinical practice guideline for health-care professionals. J Spinal Cord Med. 2005;28(3): 259–93.

19. Consortium for Spinal Cord Medicine Clinical Practice Guidelines. Prevention of thromboembolism in spinal cord injury. 2nd ed. Washington, DC: Paralyzed Veterans of America; 1999.

20. Green D, et al. Prevention of thromboembolism after spinal cord injury using low-molecular-weight heparin. Ann Intern Med. 1990;113(8):571–4.

21. DeVivo MJ, Krause JS, Lammertse DP. Recent trends in mortality and causes of death among persons with spinal cord injury. Arch Phys Med Rehabil. 1999;80(11):1411–9.

22. Consortium for Spinal Cord Medicine Clinical Practice Guidelines. Outcomes following traumatic spinal cord injury: clinical practice guidelines for health-care professionals. J Spinal Cord Med. 2000;23(4):289–316.

23. Kirshblum S, et al. Spinal cord injuries. In: Cuccurullo SJ, editor. Physical medicine and rehabilitation board review. New York: Demos; 2010. p. 535–607.

24. Bryce TN, Ragnarsson KT, Stein AB. Spinal cord injury. In: Braddom RL, editor. Physical medicine and rehabilitation. Philadelphia: Saunders; 2007. p. 1285–350.

25. Peterson WP, et al. The effect of tidal volumes on the time to wean persons with high tetraplegia from ventilators. Spinal Cord. 1999;37(4):284–8.

26. Viroslav J, Rosenblatt R, Tomazevic SM. Respiratory management, survival, and quality of life for high-level traumatic tetraplegics. Respir Care Clin N Am. 1996;2(2):313–22.

27. Bach JR. Noninvasive respiratory management of high level spinal cord injury. J Spinal Cord Med. 2012;35(2):72–80.

28. Roth EJ, et al. Pulmonary function testing in spinal cord injury: correlation with vital capacity. Paraplegia. 1995;33(8):454–7.

29. Peterson W, et al. Two methods of weaning persons with quadriplegia from mechanical ventilators. Paraplegia. 1994;32(2):98–103.

30. Consortium for Spinal Cord Medicine Clinical Practice Guidelines. Bladder management for adults with spinal cord injury: a clinical practice guideline for health-care providers. J Spinal Cord Med. 2006;29(5):527–73.

31. Everaert K, et al. Urinary tract infections in spinal cord injury: prevention and treatment guidelines. Acta Clin Belg. 2009;64(4):335–40.

32. D'Hondt F, Everaert K. Urinary tract infections in patients with spinal cord injuries. Curr Infect Dis Rep. 2011;13(6):544–51.

33. National Institute on Disability and Rehabilitation Research Consensus Statement. The prevention and management of urinary tract infections among people with spinal cord injuries. J Am Paraplegia Soc. 1992;15(3):194–204.

34. Marciniak C, Rader L, Gagnon C. The use of botulinum toxin for spasticity after spinal cord injury. Am J Phys Med Rehabil. 2008;87(4):312–7. quiz 318-20, 329.

35. Consortium for Spinal Cord Medicine Clinical Practice Guidelines. Acute management of autonomic dysreflexia: individuals with spinal cord injury presenting to health-care facilities. J Spinal Cord Med. 2002;25 Suppl 1:S67–88.

36. Banovac K, et al. Prevention of heterotopic ossification after spinal cord injury with indomethacin. Spinal Cord. 2001;39(7):370–4.
37. van Kuijk AA, Geurts AC, van Kuppevelt HJ. Neurogenic heterotopic ossification in spinal cord injury. Spinal Cord. 2002;40(7):313–26.
38. Buschbacher R, et al. Warfarin in prevention of heterotopic ossification. Am J Phys Med Rehabil. 1992;71(2):86–91.
39. Orzel JA, Rudd TG. Heterotopic bone formation: clinical, laboratory, and imaging correlation. J Nucl Med. 1985;26(2):125–32.
40. Crawford CM, et al. Heterotopic ossification: are range of motion exercises contraindicated? J Burn Care Rehabil. 1986;7(4):323–7.
41. Bergstrom N, et al. Pressure ulcers in adults: prediction and prevention. Clinical Practice Guideline Number 3. Rockville: U.S. Department of Health and Human Services, Agency for Health Care Policy and Research; 1992. p. 101.
42. Daniel RK, Priest DL, Wheatley DC. Etiologic factors in pressure sores: an experimental model. Arch Phys Med Rehabil. 1981;62(10):492–8.
43. Yarkony GM, Heinemann AW. Pressure ulcers. In: Stover SL, DeLisa JA, Whiteneck GG, editors. Spinal cord injury: clinical outcomes from the model systems. Gaithersburg: Aspen Publications; 1995.
44. Richardson RR, Meyer Jr PR. Prevalence and incidence of pressure sores in acute spinal cord injuries. Paraplegia. 1981;19(4):235–47.
45. McKinley WO, et al. Long-term medical complications after traumatic spinal cord injury: a regional model systems analysis. Arch Phys Med Rehabil. 1999;80(11):1402–10.
46. Ho CH, Bogie K. Rehabilitation of spinal cord injury. In: Frontera WR, DeLisa JA, editors. Physical medicine and rehabilitation: principles and practice. Philadelphia: Lippincott Williams & Wilkins Health; 2010. p. 1393–409.
47. Consortium for Spinal Cord Medicine Clinical_Practice_Guidelines. Pressure ulcer prevention and treatment following spinal cord injury: a clinical practice guideline for health-care professionals. J Spinal Cord Med. 2001;24 Suppl 1:S40–S101.
48. National Pressure Ulcer Advisory Panel. (2007). Pressure ulcer stages revised by NPUAP. http://www.npuap.org/pr2.htm. Accessed 5 Aug 2012.
49. Rodeheaver GT, et al. Wound cleansing by high pressure irrigation. Surg Gynecol Obstet. 1975;141(3):357–62.
50. Krouskop T, et al. A synthesis of the factors that contribute to pressure sore formation. In: Ghista DN, Frankel HL, editors. Spinal cord injury medical engineering. Springfield: Thomas; 1986. p. 247–67.
51. Tourtual DM, et al. Predictors of hospital acquired heel pressure ulcers. Ostomy Wound Manage. 1997;43(9):24–8. 30, 32-4 passim.
52. Blaylock B. A study of risk factors in patients placed on specialty beds. J Wound Ostomy Continence Nurs. 1995;22(6):263–6.
53. Breslow RA, et al. The importance of dietary protein in healing pressure ulcers. J Am Geriatr Soc. 1993;41(4):357–62.
54. Brewer Jr RD, Mihaldzic N, Dietz A. The effect of oral zinc sulfate on the healing of decubitus ulcers in spinal cord injured patients. Proc Annu Clin Spinal Cord Inj Conf. 1967;16:70–2.
55. Eleazer GP, et al. Appropriate protocol for zinc therapy in long term care facilities. J Nutr Elder. 1995;14(4):31–8.

56. Stechmiller JK, Childress B, Cowan L. Arginine supplementation and wound healing. Nutr Clin Pract. 2005;20(1):52–61.

57. The Consensus Committee of the American Autonomic Society and the American Academy of Neurology. Consensus statement on the definition of orthostatic hypotension, pure autonomic failure, and multiple system atrophy. Neurology. 1996;46(5):1470.

58. Illman A, Stiller K, Williams M. The prevalence of orthostatic hypotension during physiotherapy treatment in patients with an acute spinal cord injury. Spinal Cord. 2000;38(12):741–7.

59. Claydon VE, Steeves JD, Krassioukov A. Orthostatic hypotension following spinal cord injury: understanding clinical pathophysiology. Spinal Cord. 2006;44(6):341–51.

60. Chen D, et al. Medical complications during acute rehabilitation following spinal cord injury–current experience of the Model Systems. Arch Phys Med Rehabil. 1999;80(11):1397–401.

61. Virchow R. Thrombosis and emboli (1846-1856). Canton: Science History Publications; 1998. p. 234.

62. Baglin TP, Brush J, Streiff M. Guidelines on use of vena cava filters. Br J Haematol. 2006;134(6):590–5.

63. Becker DM, Philbrick JT, Selby JB. Inferior vena cava filters. Indications, safety, effectiveness. Arch Intern Med. 1992;152(10):1985–94.

64. Giannoudis PV, et al. Safety and efficacy of vena cava filters in trauma patients. Injury. 2007;38(1):7–18.

65. Dubin D. Pulmonary embolism. In: Dubin D, editor. Rapid interpretation of EKG. Tampa: Cover Pub Co; 2000.

66. Conover MB. Acute pulmonary embolism. In: Conover MB, editor. Understanding electrocardiography. St. Louis: Mosby; 1996.

67. Maimoun L, Fattal C, Sultan C. Bone remodeling and calcium homeostasis in patients with spinal cord injury: a review. Metabolism. 2011;60(12): 1655–63.

68. Jiang SD, Jiang LS, Dai LY. Mechanisms of osteoporosis in spinal cord injury. Clin Endocrinol (Oxf). 2006;65(5):555–65.

69. Shane E, Berenson J. Treatment of hypercalcemia. In: Rosen CJ, editor. UpToDate. Waltham: UpToDate; 2012.

70. Nemunaitis GA, et al. A descriptive study on vitamin D levels in individuals with spinal cord injury in an acute inpatient rehabilitation setting. PM R. 2010;2(3):202–8. quiz 228.

71. Oleson CV, Patel PH, Wuermser LA. Influence of season, ethnicity, and chronicity on vitamin D deficiency in traumatic spinal cord injury. J Spinal Cord Med. 2010;33(3):202–13.

72. Heaney RP, et al. Peak bone mass. Osteoporos Int. 2000;11(12):985–1009.

73. Dawson-Hughes B, et al. Estimates of optimal vitamin D status. Osteoporos Int. 2005;16(7):713–6.

74. Schopp LH, et al. Testosterone levels among men with spinal cord injury admitted to inpatient rehabilitation. Am J Phys Med Rehabil. 2006;85(8):678–84. quiz 685-7.

75. Durga A, et al. Prevalence of testosterone deficiency after spinal cord injury. PM R. 2011;3(10):929–32.

76. Tsitouras PD, et al. Serum testosterone and growth hormone/insulin-like growth factor-I in adults with spinal cord injury. Horm Metab Res. 1995;27(6):287–92.

77. Celik B, et al. Sex hormone levels and functional outcomes: a controlled study of patients with spinal cord injury compared with healthy subjects. Am J Phys Med Rehabil. 2007;86(10):784–90.

78. Clark MJ, et al. Testosterone replacement therapy and motor function in men with spinal cord injury: a retrospective analysis. Am J Phys Med Rehabil. 2008;87(4):281–4.

79. Snyder PJ. Testosterone treatment of male hypogonadism. In: Matsumoto AM, editor. UpToDate. Waltham: UpToDate; 2012.

80. Consortium for Spinal Cord Medicine Clinical Practice Guidelines. Sexuality and reproductive health in adults with spinal cord injury: a clinical practice guideline for health-care professionals. J Spinal Cord Med. 2010; 33(3):281–336.

81. Linsenmeyer T. Sexual function and sexuality following spinal cord injury. In: Kirshblum S, Campagnolo DI, DeLisa JA, editors. Spinal cord medicine. Philadelphia: Lippincott Williams & Wilkins; 2002. p. 322–30.

82. Yarkony GM. Enhancement of sexual function and fertility in spinal cord-injured males. Am J Phys Med Rehabil. 1990;69(2):81–7.

83. Sipski ML, Alexander CJ, Rosen R. Sexual arousal and orgasm in women: effects of spinal cord injury. Ann Neurol. 2001;49(1):35–44.

84. Bennett CJ, et al. Sexual dysfunction and electroejaculation in men with spinal cord injury: review. J Urol. 1988;139(3):453–7.

85. Cardenas DD, et al. Gender and minority differences in the pain experience of people with spinal cord injury. Arch Phys Med Rehabil. 2004;85(11):1774–81.

86. Donnelly C, Eng JJ. Pain following spinal cord injury: the impact on community reintegration. Spinal Cord. 2005;43(5):278–82.

87. Ravenscroft A, Ahmed YS, Burnside IG. Chronic pain after SCI. A patient survey. Spinal Cord. 2000;38(10):611–4.

88. Siddall PJ, et al. A longitudinal study of the prevalence and characteristics of pain in the first 5 years following spinal cord injury. Pain. 2003;103(3): 249–57.

89. Bryce TN, Ragnarsson KT. Epidemiology and classification of pain after spinal cord injury. Top Spinal Cord Inj Rehabil. 2001;7(2):1–17.

90. Stormer S, et al. Chronic pain/dysaesthesiae in spinal cord injury patients: results of a multicentre study. Spinal Cord. 1997;35(7):446–55.

91. Siddall PJ, et al. Pain report and the relationship of pain to physical factors in the first 6 months following spinal cord injury. Pain. 1999;81(1–2): 187–97.

92. Siddall PJ, Yezierski RP, Loeser JD. Pain following spinal cord injury: clinical features, prevalence, and taxonomy. IASP Newsletter. 2000;3:3–7.

93. Siddall PJ, Yezierski RP, Loeser JD. Taxonomy and epidemiology of spinal cord injury pain. In: Yezierski RP, Burchiel KJ, editors. Taxonomy and epidemiology of spinal cord injury pain. Seattle: IASP Press; 2002. p. 9–24.

94. Dyson-Hudson TA, Kirshblum SC. Shoulder pain in chronic spinal cord injury, Part I: epidemiology, etiology, and pathomechanics. J Spinal Cord Med. 2004;27(1):4–17.

 95. Curtis KA, et al. Shoulder pain in wheelchair users with tetraplegia and paraplegia. Arch Phys Med Rehabil. 1999;80(4):453–7.
 96. Irwin R, Restrepo JA, Sherman A. Musculoskeletal pain in persons with spinal cord injury. Top Spinal Cord Inj Rehabil. 2007;13(2):43–57.
 97. Akbar M, et al. A cross-sectional study of demographic and morphologic features of rotator cuff disease in paraplegic patients. J Shoulder Elbow Surg. 2011;20(7):1108–13.
 98. Goldstein B. Musculoskeletal conditions after spinal cord injury. Phys Med Rehabil Clin N Am. 2000;11(1):91–108. viii-ix.
 99. Hastings J, Goldstein B. Paraplegia and the shoulder. Phys Med Rehabil Clin N Am. 2004;15(3):vii. 699-718.
100. Finnerup NB, Jensen TS. Spinal cord injury pain–mechanisms and treatment. Eur J Neurol. 2004;11(2):73–82.
101. Widerstrom-Noga EG, Turk DC. Exacerbation of chronic pain following spinal cord injury. J Neurotrauma. 2004;21(10):1384–95.
102. Yezierski RP. Pain following spinal cord injury: pathophysiology and central mechanisms. Prog Brain Res. 2000;129:429–49.
103. Haanpaa M, et al. NeuPSIG guidelines on neuropathic pain assessment. Pain. 2011;152(1):14–27.
104. Siddall PJ, Middleton JW. A proposed algorithm for the management of pain following spinal cord injury. Spinal Cord. 2006;44(2):67–77.
105. Dworkin RH, et al. Advances in neuropathic pain: diagnosis, mechanisms, and treatment recommendations. Arch Neurol. 2003;60(11):1524–34.
106. Dromerick AW. Evidence-based rehabilitation: the case for and against constraint-induced movement therapy. J Rehabil Res Dev. 2003;40(1): vii–ix.
107. Craig AR, et al. Long-term psychological outcomes in spinal cord injured persons: results of a controlled trial using cognitive behavior therapy. Arch Phys Med Rehabil. 1997;78(1):33–8.
108. Cioni B, et al. Spinal cord stimulation in the treatment of paraplegic pain. J Neurosurg. 1995;82(1):35–9.
109. Gu Y, Huang LY. Gabapentin actions on N-methyl-D-aspartate receptor channels are protein kinase C-dependent. Pain. 2001;93(1):85–92.
110. Hendrich J, et al. Pharmacological disruption of calcium channel trafficking by the alpha2delta ligand gabapentin. Proc Natl Acad Sci USA. 2008; 105(9):3628–33.
111. Finnerup NB, et al. Levetiracetam in spinal cord injury pain: a randomized controlled trial. Spinal Cord. 2009;47(12):861–7.
112. Teasell RW, et al. A systematic review of pharmacologic treatments of pain after spinal cord injury. Arch Phys Med Rehabil. 2010;91(5):816–31.
113. Johannessen CU. Mechanisms of action of valproate: a commentary. Neurochem Int. 2000;37(2–3):103–10.

Chapter 3
Neuromuscular Rehabilitation

Andres Deik, Paul Lee, and Daniel MacGowan

Basic Order Set for Neuromuscular Patients Being Admitted

Admit to: Inpatient or Outpatient Rehabilitation, depending on the reason for hospitalization
Referring Physician: Name, hospital, and contact information.
Vitals: Q shift change unless unstable
Nursing:

> **Secretion Management:** PRN suctioning. Anticholinergics can help secretion management but may exacerbate weakness. *Extreme caution is advised for their use in selected cases.*
>
> **Tracheostomy care orders:** clean with hydrogen peroxide and wash with NS at least once a day
>
> **Skin (especially in immobile patients):**
> ° Turn patient Q2 h
> ° Multipodis boots to prevent contractures and skin breakdown

A. Deik, M.D. (✉) • D. MacGowan, M.D., M.R.C.P.I.
Department of Neurology, Beth Israel Medical Center,
10 Union square east, Suite 5K, New York, NY 10003, USA
e-mail: amadiedo@chpnet.org

P. Lee, P.T.
Department of Physical Medicine & Rehabilitation,
Beth Israel Medical Center, New York, NY 10003, USA
e-mail: paullee@chpnet.org

K.A. Sackheim (ed.), *Rehab Clinical Pocket Guide:*
Rehabilitation Medicine, DOI 10.1007/978-1-4614-5419-9_3,
© Springer Science+Business Media, LLC 2013

IVF: NS or D_5NS at 50–75 cc/h if not taking PO, depending on hydration status. *Caution is advised with D_5 in Diabetics and with the volume infused if there is any concern for heart failure.*

Allergies: Including medication allergies, food and imaging contrast allergies.

Medications:

> **Fever/pain management:** Acetaminophen 650 mg PO Q4–6h prn pain or Temp > 100.4 (if no hepatic dysfunction). *AVOID opiates given the high risk of respiratory failure in some patients with neuromuscular conditions.*
>
> **Insomnia:** Trazodone 25–100 mg PO qhs or zolpidem 5–10 mg PO qhs. *Caution is advised when using these in patients at high risk of respiratory failure.*
>
> **Bronchospasm:** Albuterol and ipatropium nebulizations Q4–6h as needed for respiratory aide. *Caution is advised when concurrently using mucolytics as they may exacerbate bronchoconstriction.*
>
> **GI prophylaxis:** Esomeprazole 20–40 mg PO qd or pantoprazole 20–40 mg PO qd, 30 min prior to meals. Famotidine 20 mg IV Q12h is a reasonable IV alternative
>
> **Bowel regimen:**
> - ° Mild constipation: Docusate sodium 100 mg PO BID/TID and/or Sennosides 1–2 tabs PO QHS
> - ° Severe constipation: Miralax 1 capful/day dissolved in liquid
> - ° Fecal impaction: consider Fleet mineral oil enema.
>
> **DVT prophylaxis:** Heparin 5000 units SC q8–12h and/or intermittent pneumatic compression boots
>
> *Note: Medications that may potentially exacerbate muscle weakness and should be avoided include: anticholinergics, beta blockers, calcium channel blockers, muscle relaxants, antibiotics like aminoglycosides and fluoroquinolones, and botulinum toxin.*

Bladder regimen:
- If the patient has a foley catheter, a voiding trial may be attempted the morning after admission if the cause of bladder dysfunction has resolved. Otherwise, intermittent catheterization every 4–6 h may be required.
- Long-term goal: foley discontinuation within the first 2 days of hospitalization

- It is always important to rule out urinary tract infections or a medication side effect as the cause of urinary retention or incontinence.

Basic lab orders: CBC, CMP. Consider UA/UCx in patients with indwelling catheters

Special studies (in immobile patients):
- Chest X ray: If there is a concern for aspiration and atelectases.
- Chest CT with IV contrast: If there is a concern for PE, which may manifest as sudden dyspnea or unexplained tachycardia.

Motor Neuron Diseases

- Conditions leading to degeneration of the cortical pyramidal motor (the upper motor neuron) and/or the anterior horn motor neuron (the lower motor neuron) [1].
- Can rapidly lead to severe disability and death

Diagnosis: Distinguish between Progressive Muscular Atrophy (PMA, a purely lower motor neuron syndrome), Primary Lateral Sclerosis (PLS, a purely upper motor neuron syndrome) or Amyotrophic Lateral Sclerosis (ALS, a mixed upper and lower motor neuron syndrome)

Neurological:
- PMA: Hyporeflexia or areflexia with muscle atrophy are the dominant features [2]
- PLS: Spasticity, pseudobulbar affect and occasional disinhibition suggestive of frontal lobe dysfunction [3]
- ALS: Mixed atrophy and spasticity. There frequently is areflexia in the upper extremities while the legs are spastic and hyperreflexic [1]

Surgeries:
- Date and location of PEG insertion
- Date and location of Tracheostomy (know size and type of trach)
- Date and location of contracture release

Condition: Variable. ALS tends to progress rapidly over months, while PMA and PLS may remain stable for years [4]

Vitals: Patients with respiratory failure or assistive devices may require frequent checks

Diet:
- Start conservative. Speech and swallow assessment may be necessary

- Soft mechanical diet with thickened liquids in patients with dysphagia who are still able to eat may be appropriate.
- Advanced ALS patients may require exclusive PEG feeding. Eating for pleasure can be encouraged under the instructions of speech and swallow therapist.
- Ice chips are relatively safe and may provide comfort

Special Studies:
- As a part of the workup patients may undergo EMG/NCS testing

Respiratory Goal: Noninvasive positive pressure ventilation improves survival [5]. Bulbar-onset disease patients may need them earlier. Cough assistance devices and chest PT mobilize secretions and prevent lower respiratory infections [6].

Bladder Goal: Bladder function in motor neuron disease is generally spared until very late in the disease.

Physical Therapy
Early stage PT goals:
1. Restorative/preventive
  - Optimize independence with functional mobility and tasks
  - Strength training with progressive resistive exercises (PREs) using submaximal resistance on muscles that are strong or uninvolved [7]
  - Endurance training mild to moderate with no dyspnea
  - Stretching and ROM (all joints)
  - Home exercise program with general conditioning exercises, stretching
  - ROM (Assistive, active, and/or passive)
  - Caution: No PRE with muscles that are weakened by the disease. Avoid eccentric exercises, high-resistance exercises, exercising greater than three times a week, and inducing fasciculation and cramping. [8, 9]
2. **Compensatory:**
  - Energy conservation
  - Educate the patient in the importance of exercise, maintaining or increasing activity level, and refer to appropriate support groups
  - Assess need for appropriate assistive device (orthotics, cervical collars, slings, resting hand splints, volar wrist splints, adaptive equipment, rolling walker, or rollator)

Progressive Stage PT Goals:

1. **Compensatory**
   - Assess the need for home or work modifications (ramps, bathroom accessibility, and single level habitation)
   - Continue to assess the need for appropriate assistive device for safe ambulation and mobility
   - Wheelchair prescription (tilt in space, adjustable/removable leg rests, lateral trunk support, adjustable head rest, armrest, pressure relief cushion, i.e., Roho cushion)

2. **Preventive:**
   - pressure relieving devices (i.e., Pressure relieving mattress)
   - PROM, AAROM, AROM
   - continue submaximal exercises on muscles that are strong or uninvolved
   - continue mild to moderate endurance exercises
   - continue stretching, if limited with mobility or non-ambulatory, primarily focus on the following muscles: hamstring, iliopsoas, gastrocnemius/soleus, pectorals, latissimus dorsi, biceps, wrist flexors/extensors, pronators

Advanced Stage PT Goals:

1. Education: Caregiver education regarding transfers, positioning, pressure relief, and use of assistive devices
2. Preventive: contractures; PROM, stretching, and splinting (PRAFO, hand splints, cervical collars)
3. Position to assist with breathing

Bed Mobility: independent in early to mid-stage, train HHA and family in assisting patient with bed mobility in late stage

Transfers: independent in early to progressive stage, hydraulic patient lift and train HHA and family in assisting patient in late stage of disease

Pressure reliefs/positioning: hospital bed with pressure distributing mattress, pressure relief ankle foot orthotic (PRAFO), hand splints, cervical collars

Wheelchair propulsion:

Power→ refer to wheelchair clinic; tilt in space, postural support, and adjustable leg rest, head rest, seat height, arm rest, and interface depending on pts ability

Manual→ required with frontotemporal dementia

Standing: independent early to mid-stage, train HHA or primary care provider in guarding patient in standing

Ambulation: independent to modified independent in early stage, supervision or assistance usually required in middle stage, and typically non-ambulatory in late stage. Some PLS patients can walk in the late stages with assistance and the use of an assistive device if the strength of the limbs is preserved.

Occupational Therapy

Long-Term OT Goals:

Eating, grooming, dressing, and bathing:

1. **Early:**
   a. Assistive devices for bathroom: grab bar, tub bench, raised toilet seat
   b. Maintain independence for activities of daily living (ADLs)
   c. Assistive devices for dressing: dressing stick, reacher, long handled shoe horn, and button hook
   d. Assistive devices for eating: large diameter utensils, tray table, light weight "sippy cups," and plate guards

2. **Middle:**
   a. Recommend home visit from OT or Assistive technology professional (ATP)
   b. Assistive devices for bathroom: Three-in-one commode, shower chair, tub-transfer-bench, shower wheelchair, and long handled sponge

3. **Late:**
   a. Max to dependent assistance: hydraulic patient lift or track lift with U-shaped sling

Housekeeping/Meals: recommend home assessment for safety and activity level

Assistance required: max to dependent at late stage, moderate to minimum in middle stage, and minimum to no assistance required in early stage

Therapy Precautions: submaximal resistance for exercise and activity level, low to below moderate endurance training. Increased or prolonged weakness and fatigue is observed following overexertion.

HHA assistance that may be needed: 24 h is required at the late stage of disease

Speech: Severe dysarthria (caused by tongue atrophy and/or spasticity) is common in advanced disease or in bulbar onset motor neuron disease.

Assistive communication devices are useful [1]. Tablet technology is revolutionizing the market of assistive communication devices.

Nutrition: Soft mechanical diets and thickened liquids may be necessary if dysphagia is prominent, but may be insufficient to meet caloric needs. Early PEG tube insertion is a consideration.

Social Work: Needs change as the disease progresses. Social work may assist in the acquisition of adaptive devices, home equipment, and assessment of home safety.

Psychology: Rapid course of disease, depression, and pseudobulbar affect may need to be addressed. Support groups should be offered. Caregivers and family members may also benefit from counseling.

Wheelchair Prescription: power and manual: tilt-in-space, reclining, pressure relief cushion, postural support, and swing away adjustable leg rest, head rest, seat height, arm rest, and interface depending on pts ability

Adaptive Devices/Home Equipment that MAY be needed: hospital bed with pressure distributing mattress, ankle foot orthotics (AFO), pressure relief ankle foot orthotic (PRAFO), hand splints, cervical collars, commode, raised toilet seat, resting hand splints, enlarged grip/handles for utensils, pens, and other handheld devices, elastic shoelaces, rolling walker, rollator, single axis cane, lift chair, sliding board, seat up/down assist device

Inflammatory Demyelinating Polyneuropathies

- Immune-mediated disorders leading to demyelination of peripheral nerves with resultant lower motor neuron weakness [10].
- Proximal muscle weakness, areflexia, and ascending, length-dependent sensory loss without a clear sensory level may be present acutely [10]

Diagnosis: Acute Inflammatory Demyelinating Polyneuropathy (AIDP) or Chronic Inflammatory Demyelinating Polyneuropathy (CIDP)

Admit to: AIDP, also known as Guillain-Barre Syndrome (GBS) usually requires hospitalization and subsequent inpatient rehabilitation, whereas CIDP can usually be managed as an outpatient.

Neurological:
- When possible, it is important to distinguish between AIDP and acute exacerbations of CIDP.
- There are different variants of AIDP:
  ° GBS: Most common sensory-motor form [11]
  ° Miller-Fisher variant: Triad of ataxia (from severe deafferentation), areflexia and ophthalmoparesis without muscle weakness [12]

Surgeries: Date and location of Tracheostomy (know size and type of trach)

Condition: Mild AIDP cases may remain fully ambulatory, whereas severe cases can require mechanical ventilation

Vitals: As per the intensive care unit if on mechanical ventilation. In addition, patients on IVIG treatment are prone to autonomic instability and significant fluctuations in heart rate and blood pressure [13], so closer vital sign monitoring may be warranted.

Bowel regimen: Scheduled daily bowel regimen is crucial in immobile patients as it may prevent intestinal obstructions, a source of morbidity and mortality.

Diet: Patients with AIDP must remain NPO in case they require emergent intubation. When safe to eat, a high fiber diet and generous hydration are an important part of the bowel regimen.

IVF: IVIG has a potentially pro-coagulant effect [13] and dehydration should be avoided. Gentle hydration is advised in the elderly and others who may not adequately handle large fluid volumes.

Extremities: DVT prophylaxis is of utmost importance, especially while on IVIG

Skin: Turn Q2 if severely affected

Special Studies:
- Lumbar puncture and EMG/NCS testing [14]
- If intestinal obstruction is suspected, emergent abdominal imaging is warranted.

Respiratory Goal: Prolonged mechanical ventilation leading to Tracheostomy may be necessary. Goal is eventual respiratory independence.

Bladder Goal: Independent

Physical Therapy

Long-Term PT Goals:

Physical therapist evaluation will determine the need for an assistive device or a wheelchair for mobility upon D/C.

CIPD: Functional presentation may vary from nearly normal to requiring greater than 75% assistance to perform basic tasks and activities of daily living. The goals are to achieve all ADLs and mobility with independence or the least amount of assistance in a safe and effective manner.

AIDP—Guillain Barre syndrome:

- Bed Mobility: independent
- Transfers: independent
- Pressure reliefs/positioning:
  - During acute and disabled state electronic hospital bed with pressure distributing mattress, pressure relief ankle foot orthotic (PRAFO), and resting hand splints
  - Pressure relieving devices (PRDs) for insensitive areas
  - Daily skin inspections should be done, especially on bony prominences, weight bearing regions, and desensitized areas
  - Avoid having buttons, zippers, or seams in areas where they will be weight bearing
  - Position changes every 2 h in bed and every 15 min when sitting in a wheelchair
- Wheelchair propulsion:

  Power→ only in severe cases where recovery is impeded

  Manual→ light weight standard, independent
- Standing: independent
- **Ambulation:** independent to modified independent

Occupational therapy

Long-Term OT Goals:

Home evaluation for safety assessment and to determine the need for assistive devices.

  Eating, grooming, dressing, and bathing: independent

  Housekeeping/Meals: independent

  Assistance required: assistance required with heavy lifting and tasks requiring high level balance

Modalities Precautions: avoid modalities contraindicated for conditions with sensory loss

Therapy Precautions: submaximal resistance, mild to moderate cardio intensity

HHA assistance that may be needed: TBD by patient's need and functional level

Speech: Speech may be involved in cases of facial weakness

Nutrition: If patients are able to swallow, an anabolic diet will help recover any lost muscle mass.

Social Work: Social work may assist in the acquisition of adaptive devices, home equipment and assessment of home safety

Psychology: AIDP and CIDP are usually nonfatal diseases. Counseling may help coping with residual disability.

Wheelchair Prescription: refer to wheelchair clinic, AIDP: light weight folding standard, CIPD: depending on area and level of impairment and disability

Adaptive Devices/Home Equipment that MAY be needed: Tub transfer bench, grab bar, rolling walker, single axis cane, rollator, commode, PRAFO, resting hand splints, wheelchair, hospital bed (assist with respiration), slide board, seat up/down assist device

Acquired Myasthenic Syndromes

- Myasthenia Gravis (MG) and Lambert-Eaton Myasthenic Syndrome (LEMS) arise from dysfunction of neuromuscular transmission.
- In LEMS there is reduced pre-synaptic release of acetylcholine [15].
- In MG there is an antibody-mediated decrease in the concentration of the post-synaptic cholinergic receptor [16]

Diagnosis: Myasthenic crisis (typical cause of hospitalization)

Admit to: Once stable, patients are excellent candidates for inpatient rehabilitation.

Neurological:
- Proximal, bilateral muscle weakness [16]
- Reflexes tend to be spared [16]
- Bulbar symptoms may arise, leading to aspiration and respiratory failure. Head drop on admission [17] may predict respiratory failure. Tracheostomy and ventilatory support may be necessary.
- Autonomic dysfunction can be seen in LEMS but is not a feature of MG [15].

Surgeries:
- Date and location of thymectomy (if applicable)
- Date and location of PEG insertion (seldom needed)

- Date and location of Tracheostomy (know size and type of trach)

Condition: On occasion, patients will need intubation and ventilatory support.

Nursing: Patients with MG on an acetylcholine esterase inhibitor may develop copious secretions requiring suctioning, which, in the setting of an acute crisis, may predispose to respiratory failure. *If a myasthenic patient presents with an acute crisis, pyridostigmine must be discontinued immediately.*

Diet: NPO as they may require emergent intubation. If bulbar symptoms are present but the patient has been cleared to eat, soft mechanical diets and thick liquids may be preferable.

Medications: *Steroids exacerbate weakness in patients presenting with an acute crisis* [18].

Bladder regimen: Patients with LEMS and autonomic dysfunction may experience urinary retention or overflow incontinence [19].

IVF: If exposed to IVIG, dehydration must be avoided to diminish the risk of a procoagulant effect [13].

Extremities: Patients on IVIG are particularly prone to thrombotic events [13] and DVT prophylaxis is of utmost importance. Please see the basic order section for details.

Skin: Turn Q2 if immobile

Special Studies:
- EMG/NCS testing [20]
- Serum titers of anti Acetylcholine receptor binding [16]
- Serum titers of anti Voltage-Gated Calcium Channel (VGCC) antibodies [21]

Respiratory Goal: Severe cases may require mechanical ventilation and Tracheostomy. Goal is eventual respiratory independence.

Bladder Goal: Immune mediated incontinence may improve with immune therapy [19]

Physical Therapy
Long-Term PT Goals:
> **Bed Mobility:** Towards independence, depending on severity of disease
>
> **Transfers:** Independent (Class 1 through 3), towards independence or minimal assistance with Class 4a–5
>
> **Pressure reliefs/positioning:** cervical collar, electronic hospital bed to assist with breathing

Wheelchair propulsion:

Power→ Use for long distance or prolong out of house activity. If patient has compromised respiratory function patient may benefit from tilt in space, reclining, postural support, and adjustable head rest, swing away leg rest, and height.

Manual→ independent with short distances, difficulty managing manual wheelchair due to fatigue and proximal muscle weakness

Standing: Independent class 1–3, assistance or maximize physical ability with class 4a and 5.

Stairs: Independent to modified independent (require assistive device/handrail, increase time, and effort) for class 1–2, assistance required at level 3a and above.

Ambulation: Independent to modified independent (require assistive device, increase time and effort) with class 1–3, AFO required in some cases

Occupational Therapy
Long-Term OT Goals:

Eating, grooming, dressing, and bathing: Goal is to be independent or modified independent (use of assistive device, increase time, and effort). Activities that require keeping hands or arms above the shoulder or the head are more difficult for the patient to perform and may need assistance or frequent rests.

Housekeeping/Meals: light house duties are possible for patients who are ambulating without device. Independent with mild to moderate complex meal preparations.

Assistance required: assistance required for heavy lifting and moderate to high endurance tasks

Therapy Precautions: adjust the intensity of the rehabilitation program to the patient's presentation as they may have alternating "good" and "bad" days. Increased or prolonged weakness is observed after overexertion or reaching maximal capacity with exercises and activities on "good" days as well.

HHA assistance that may be needed: yes

Speech: Transient dysarthria is seen when facial weakness is prominent.

Nutrition: Patients at risk of aspiration may require liquid feeding via nasogastric tube or rarely PEG tube insertion. Speech and swallow evaluation will determine need for modified diet consistencies.

Social Work: Social work may assist in the acquisition of adaptive devices, home equipment, and assessment of home safety

Psychology: Some patients will require counseling in terms of coping with their diagnosis. Severe permanent disability from myasthenic syndromes is unusual, but possible.

Adaptive Devices/Home Equipment that MAY be needed:
Rollator, Rolling walker, single axis cane, electronic hospital bed, wheelchair, cervical collar, hand splints, elastic shoelaces, raised toilet seat, tub transfer bench, uplift seat assist device.

Muscular Dystrophies

- Congenital conditions were muscle tissue is replaced with fibrotic tissue [22].
- Myotonic dystrophy is the most common muscular dystrophy in adults [23].
- Duchenne's muscular dystrophy (or its milder version, Becker's muscular dystrophy) presents earlier in life and shortens life expectancy [24].
- Facioscapulohumeral muscular dystrophy (FSHMD) presents with weakness of facial muscles and scapular stabilization [25].
- Limb girdle muscular dystrophies (LGMD) are a broad group of disorders with different inheritance patterns [26].

Diagnosis: Muscular Dystrophy (specify what type, if known)
Neurological:
- Myotonic dystrophy: Patients have myotonia, which is the inability to relax quickly after sustained muscle contraction. Distal muscle weakness is the hallmark of type I, the most common form [23].
- Becker or Duchenne's muscular dystrophy: Patients present predominantly proximal muscle weakness. Hallmarks include the Gower's maneuver (where patients climb up their legs using their hands when attempting to stand) [27] and early bilateral calf hypertrophy [28].
- FSHMD: May involve the muscles of the trunk and the distal anterior compartment of the legs, causing great disability [25].
- LGMD cause proximal muscle weakness [26].

Surgeries:
- Date and location of muscle biopsy (if available)
- Date and location of Tracheostomy (know size and type of trach)

Condition: Disability will depend on stage of specific disease. Patients with Duchenne's usually succumb from complications of respiratory infections [29]. Patients with advanced Duchenne's muscular dystrophies may experience restrictive lung disease and require mechanical ventilation.

Diet: Regular diet unless there is an aspiration risk

IVF: *Patients with muscular dystrophies may have underlying and undiagnosed cardiomyopathies* [30]. A screening echocardiogram may guide safety of hydration.

Medications: *AVOID medications that are potentially myotoxic, including (but not limited to) statins, steroids, and HIV medications like AZT* [31].

Extremities: Patients with end-stage disease may be chronically immobile and at risk for DVT/PEs. Please see the basic order section for details.

Skin: Turn Q2 if immobile

Labs: TSH (given both hypo- or hyperthyroidism can lead to myopathy) [32, 33]

Special Studies:
- EMG/NCS testing
- Muscle biopsy
- Genetic testing may also be indicated [28]

Respiratory Goal: Advanced cases may require permanent mechanical ventilation [29]. Chest PT may aide in clearance of secretions.

Bladder Goal: Full bladder control

Physical therapy

Long-Term PT Goals:

Physical therapist goal is to maximize the patient's physical potential and capability.

1. **Restorative intervention**: improve or maximize functional capability for independence and self-care, submaximal resistive exercise to address disuse weakness and increase functional endurance in earlier stage of the disease.
2. **Maintenance:** promote quality of life, PROM, AROM, AAROM, stretches, and low to moderate exercises to all affected joints and muscles. Postural drainage, deep breathing, and secretion clearance to assist and maximize respiratory function.
3. **Preventive:** reduce or prevent significant deformity, bracing lower extremities to prevent contractures when weakness and immobility is present.

Bed Mobility: assistance required as weakness persists, treatment directed towards maximizing patient's ability to perform task independently and educating caregiver in assisting

Transfers: assistance required as weakness persists, treatment directed towards maximizing patient's ability to perform task independently and educating caregiver in assisting

Pressure reliefs/positioning: frequent turning when in bed, pressure relieving compensatory strategies, pressure relieving devices, promote ankle dorsiflexion, and trunk, hip, and knee extension posture and position to avoid contractures from prolonged sitting.

Wheelchair propulsion:

> Power→ wheelchair clinic referral, independent with hand-operated wheelchair
>
> Manual→ requires assistance

Standing: assistance required as weakness persists, treatment directed towards maximizing patient's ability to perform task independently and educating caregiver in assisting

Occupational Therapy
Long-Term OT Goals:

Assistance required: mechanical or electronic assisted arm support

Therapy Precautions: fatigue guidelines, overuse weakness especially with muscles grade less than 3 of 5, avoid heavy eccentric load or exercises

Speech: Facial weakness seen in FSHD may cause difficulties with phonation and chewing [34]. Severe dysarthria may require the use of assistive communication devices.

Nutrition: Severe dysphagia may lead to weight loss. PEG tube insertion may be considered if allowed by respiratory status.

Social Work: Needs change with disease progression. Social work may assist in the acquisition of adaptive devices, home equipment and assessment of home safety.

Psychology: Muscular dystrophies may be either fatal or lead to reduced life span with significant disability. Support groups should be offered. Caregivers and family members may also benefit from counseling.

Wheelchair Prescription: tilt in space, reclining, postural support, and adjustable head rest, swing away leg rest, and height.

Adaptive Devices/Home Equipment that MAY be needed:
Slide board, shower wheelchair, tub transfer bench, commode, strollers, hydraulic patient lift, mechanical or electronic assisted arm support, leg braces, PRAFO, AFO, resting hand splints, hospital bed with pressure distributing mattress

Acquired Myopathies

- Diverse group of muscle diseases secondary to:
  - ° Inflammation (as is the case of dermatomyositis and polymyositis)
  - ° Medications (statin- and steroid-induced myopathies)
  - ° Infections (like HIV)
  - ° Endocrinopathies (hyper- or hypothyroidism)
  - ° Idiopathic (as in the case of inclusion body myositis or IBM).
- Prognosis for these entities depends on the availability of disease modifying treatment, and thus varies depending on the specific cause.

Diagnosis: Acquired Myopathy (specify what type, if known)
Neurological:
- Presentation and manifestation depends on the myopathy type
- Inflammatory myopathies (and generally most myopathies) tend to be proximal
- IBM tends to affect the finger flexors [35] and the quadriceps
- Reflexes may be lost in advanced stages of disease

Surgeries:
- Date and location of Muscle biopsy (if available)
- Date and location of Tracheostomy, which may rarely be necessary (know size and type of trach)

Condition: Inclusion body myositis may evolve over years [36], while inflammatory myopathies may have a more rapid course [37].
Diet: Regular diet unless otherwise specified
IVF: *Caution is advised if there is a concern for cardiomyopathy.* When in doubt, obtain an echocardiogram, especially if aggressive hydration is required (in cases of rhabdomyolysis).
Medications: *It is important to avoid medications that are potentially myotoxic, including (but not limited to) statins, steroids, colchicine, and AZT* [31].
Extremities: Patients with end-stage disease may be chronically immobile and at risk for DVT/PEs. Please see the basic order section for details.
Skin: Turn Q2 if immobile
Labs: TSH (given both hypo- or hyperthyroidism can lead to myopathy) [31, 32]

Special Studies:
- EMG/NCS testing
- Muscle biopsy

Respiratory Goal: Respiratory compromise is rare. Goal should be respiratory independence.
Bladder Goal: Bladder involvement is not typical

Physical Therapy
Long-Term PT Goals:
Dermatomyositis: good functional recovery with early medical treatment.

Bed Mobility: independent, may require assistance if calcinosis is present
Transfers: independent, assistance if calcinosis is present
Pressure reliefs/positioning: contracture prevention
Wheelchair propulsion:

> Power: to be determined by PT/OT assessment if power wheelchair is needed
> Manual: to be determined by PT/O assessment if wheelchair is needed

Standing: independent, assistance required if calcinosis is present
Ambulation: independent to modified independent (uses assistive device, increase time and effort), assistance required if calcinosis is present

Occupational Therapy
Long-Term OT Goals:
Eating, grooming, dressing, and bathing: independent with basic ADLs and basic mobility skills, home assessment to determine the need for assistive device or modifications
Housekeeping/Meals: independent with simple tasks and meal preparation. Home assessment to determine the need of assistance or assistive devices.
Assistance required: depending on patient's cardiopulmonary status and if calcinosis is interrupting patients function
Therapy Precautions: exercise to be started only after inflammation is controlled
HHA assistance that may be needed: determined with a home assessment
Speech: Bulbar involvement is rare with acquired myopathies.
Nutrition: In patients experiencing rhabdomyolysis, a protein-restricted diet may be necessary if there is associated renal compromise.

Otherwise, an anabolic diet is preferred to aid in restitution of lost muscle mass.

Social Work: Social work may assist in the acquisition of adaptive devices, home equipment, and assessment of home safety.

Psychology: Some patients will require counseling in terms of coping with their diagnosis. Severe permanent disability is possible for some of these entities. Reversible myopathies may have a lower impact in a patient's quality of life.

Adaptive Devices/Home Equipment that MAY be needed:
Rolling walker, rollator, single axis cane, tub transfer bench, hospital bed, PRD

Polymyositis:
Physical therapist's goal is to maximize the patient's physical potential and capability. Variables associated with poor outcome of PM/DM were older age, pulmonary and esophageal involvement, and cancer.

Bed mobility: treatment directed towards maximizing patient's ability to perform task independently and educating caregiver in assisting the patient.

Transfers: treatment directed towards maximizing patient's ability to perform task independently and educating caregiver in assisting the patient.

Positioning/pressure relief:
- bedridden patients will require frequent turning or pressure distributing mattress. PRAFO with extremity rotation eliminating attachment.
- Pressure relieving devices (PRDs)
- Daily inspections should be done
- Avoid having buttons, zippers, or seams in areas where they will be weight bearing
- Position changes every 2 h in bed and every 15 min when sitting in a wheelchair

Ambulation: treatment directed towards maximizing patient's ability to perform task independently with an assistive device and educating caregiver in assisting the patient

Wheelchair details
Power: In some cases patient will require a power wheelchair, typically during an acute flare up of the disease. Independent with hand control.

Manual: OT/PT will need to assess if a patient is appropriate for a manual wheelchair due proximal weakness and potential respiratory and cardiac involvement.

Standing: treatment directed towards maximizing patient's ability to perform task independently and educating caregiver in assisting the patient

Eating/dressing/grooming: home assessment to determine the level of assistance and equipment the patient will require

Setup to modified independent typically needed upon discharge

Therapy Precautions: exercise can be started after the acute phase and when inflammation is controlled

Adaptive Devices/Home Equipment that MAY be needed:

Tub transfer bench, grab bar, rolling walker, single axis cane, rollator, commode, PRAFO, resting hand splints, wheelchair, hospital bed (assist with respiration), slide board, seat up/down assist device

Multiple Sclerosis

- Immune-mediated progressive demyelination of the central nervous system [38]
- Relapsing-remitting disease (the most common type) leads to accumulation of disability, while rarer forms may be more aggressive from onset [39]
- Signs and symptoms include numbness, tingling, ataxia, pyramidal weakness, and diplopia [40]
- Neuromyelitis optica (NMO) is a related condition causing longitudinally extensive myelitis [41]

Diagnosis: Multiple sclerosis (MS) exacerbation
Neurological:
- Pyramidal weakness
- Spasticity (sometimes even with sustained clonus)
- Impaired ambulation, hand dexterity, dysarthria
- Diplopia from extraocular movement abnormalities (often internuclear ophthalmoplegia) and/or decreased visual acuity from optic neuritis [39]

Surgeries (only in the most severe cases):
- Date and location of PEG insertion
- Date and location of Tracheostomy (know size and type of trach)
- Date and location of contracture release surgery

Condition: Stable/Fair. Disease modifying therapy has allowed pro- longation of time to disability, especially in relapsing-remitting disease

Vitals: Consider checking finger sticks at least twice daily if the patient is receiving steroid therapy and is obese or has a history of glucose intolerance.

Diet: Dysphagia may be prominent in very advanced disease, and the risk of aspiration should be considered. Caloric restriction may help prevent hyperglycemia in patients on steroid therapy.

IVF: Young MS patients are usually able to tolerate large fluid boluses. Dehydration may unmask underlying disability and must not be mistaken with an acute exacerbation.

Medications:

Percocet 1–2 tabs PO Q4–6h prn mod-severe pain

Can use Morphine for pain if increased LFTs or allergies to percocet

Neurontin 200 mg PO TID or Amitryptiline 25 mg PO QHS may help neuropathic pain

Consider oxybutinin starting at 5 mg PO BID for patients with spastic bladder.

Consider starting an insulin sliding scale should severe hyperglyce- mia from pulse steroids be encountered.

Bladder regimen: Many patients with MS develop spastic bladders and require intermittent catheterization [42] or permanent indwelling catheters that predispose them to recurrent urinary tract infections (UTIs). Acute UTIs may mimic acute MS exacerbations

Skin: Turn Q2 if immobile

Labs: UA, Ucx (always rule out a UTI in patients presenting with MS exacerbations)

Special Studies:
- Brain MRI
- Lumbar puncture

Respiratory Goal: Respiratory independence. Progressive forms of MS may require assistive devices, especially with significant lower brainstem or high cervical cord disease burden [43].

Bladder Goal: Some patients may become dependent on intermittent bladder catheterization to be able to void.

Physical Therapy
Long-Term PT Goals:
- Functional goals will vary depending on the course of the disease.

- Underlying goal for rehabilitation is to maximize the patient's general physical and functional capability.

Restorative intervention:
- Improving impairments, remediating functional limitations and disabilities to facilitate self-management skills
- Low to moderate intensity exercise, submaximal resistance, postural training, and functional endurance training

Preventive intervention:
- Minimize complications, impairments, and disabilities through course of the disease
- PROM, AAROM, AROM, stretching, weight bearing, splinting, and education

Compensatory intervention:
- Regaining or maintaining function with modifications to tasks, environment, and activity
- Using rolling walker, rollator, single axis cane, wheelchairs, home modifications, tub transfer bench, AFO, KAFO, and slide board

The following goals are set with a favorable disease course in mind.
Bed Mobility: independent
Transfers: independent or modified independent
Pressure reliefs/positioning:
- Patients with weakness and spasticity may have a difficult time shifting positions
- Spasticity and or spasms may create friction compromising the skin integrity
- Assess areas with superficial sensation deficits
- Pressure relieving devices (PRDs) for insensitive areas
- Daily inspections should be done
- Avoid having buttons, zippers, or seams in areas where they will be weight bearing
- Position changes every 2 h in bed and every 15 min when sitting in a wheelchair

Wheelchair propulsion:
> Power→ independent with hand controls
> Manual→ independent with short distance, recommend assistance with long distance due to weakness and fatigue

Standing: independent or modified independent

Ambulation:
- Maximize patient's ability towards independent or modified independent

Occupational Therapy
Long-Term OT Goals:
Eating, grooming, dressing, and bathing: home assessment to provide appropriate assistive devices and home modifications, typically require supervision or setup upon discharge from inpatient rehab, status may vary depending on severity of episode.
Teach energy conservation and activity pacing.
Housekeeping/Meals:
- Independent to modified independent with light housekeeping. Goal is to maximize function and reach independence.
- Assistance is typically required for meal preparations upon discharge

Assistance required: depending on patients functional capabilities
Modalities Precautions: avoid heat modalities
Therapy Precautions:
- Strict fatigue guidelines, require periodic rests during session, recommend morning session when body temperature is lowest, submaximal resistance less or equal to 70% MVC [44]
- Recommend to use performance measures: BP, HR, rating of perceived exertion (RPE), and expired gas analysis (VO2)
- Training intensity should be limited to 60–75% peak HR or 55–60% peak VO2 [45]
- Recommend 30 min/session or for patients more involved, three 10 min session/day
- Use handouts and pictures for patients with cognitive or memory deficits

HHA assistance that may be needed: yes, in advanced disease, or transiently after relapses causing severe motor impairment, particularly if the cervical cord is involved.
Speech: Patients may experience spastic speech, and thus require speech evaluation.
Nutrition: No dietary restrictions. Patients with severe dysphagia [46] may need PEG tube insertion, although this is rare.
Social Work: Needs change with disease progression, especially in the more aggressive variants. Social work may assist in the acquisition of adaptive devices, home equipment, and assessment of home safety.

Psychology: In the era of disease modifying therapy, MS is rarely a fatal condition. However, it can lead to significant accumulation of disability. Support groups should be offered. Caregivers and family members may also benefit from counseling.

Wheelchair prescription: Motorized wheelchair is preferred in advanced disease as patients may be unable to propel themselves.

Adaptive Devices/Home Equipment that MAY be needed:

Rolling walker, rollator, single axis cane, wheelchair, tub transfer bench, raised toilet seat, commode, AFO, KAFO, PRAFO, hydraulic patient lift.

References

1. Rowland LP. Diagnosis of amyotrophic lateral sclerosis. J Neurol Sci. 1998;160 Suppl 1:S6–24.
2. Rowland LP. Progressive muscular atrophy and other lower motor neuron syndromes of adults. Muscle Nerve. 2010;41(2):161–5.
3. Singer MA, Statland JM, Wolfe GI, Barohn RJ. Primary lateral sclerosis. Muscle Nerve. 2007;35(3):291–302.
4. Kim WK, Liu X, Sandner J, et al. Study of 962 patients indicates progressive muscular atrophy is a form of ALS. Neurology. 2009;73(20):1686–92.
5. Kleopa KA, Sherman M, Neal B, Romano GJ, Heiman-Patterson T. Bipap improves survival and rate of pulmonary function decline in patients with ALS. J Neurol Sci. 1999;164(1):82–8.
6. Wiebel M. [Non-invasive ventilation: possibilities and limitations in patients with reduced ability to cough]. Pneumologie. 2008;62 Suppl 1:S2–6.
7. Milner-Brown HS, Miller RG. Muscle Strengthening Through High-Resistive Weight Training in Patients with Neu- romuscular Disorders. Archives of Physical Medicine & Re- habilitation. 1988;69:14–19.
8. Kilmer DD. Response to resistive strengthening exercise training in humans with neuromuscular disease. American Journal of Physical Medicine & Rehabilitation. 2002;81:S121–S126.
9. Dal Bello-Haas V, Kloos AD, Mitsumoto H. Physical therapy for a patient through six stages of amyotrophic lateral sclerosis. see comment. Phys Ther . 1998;78:1312–1324.
10. Lunn MP, Willison HJ. Diagnosis and treatment in inflammatory neuropathies. J Neurol Neurosurg Psychiatry. 2009;80(3):249–58.
11. Ropper AH. The Guillain-Barre syndrome. N Engl J Med. 1992;326(17): 1130–6.
12. Fisher M. An unusual variant of acute idiopathic polyneuritis (syndrome of ophthalmoplegia, ataxia and areflexia). N Engl J Med. 1956;255(2):57–65.
13. Pierce LR, Jain N. Risks associated with the use of intravenous immunoglobulin. Transfus Med Rev. 2003;17(4):241–51.

14. Bahou YG, Biary N, al Deeb S. Guillain-Barre syndrome: a series observed at Riyadh Armed Forces Hospital January 1984–January 1994. J Neurol. 1996;243(2):147–52.

15. O'Neill JH, Murray NM, Newsom-Davis J. The Lambert-Eaton myasthenic syndrome. A review of 50 cases. Brain. 1988;111(Pt 3):577–96.

16. Drachman DB. Myasthenia gravis. N Engl J Med. 1994;330(25):1797–810.

17. Yaguchi H, Takei A, Honma S, Yamashita I, Doi S, Hamada T. Dropped head sign as the only symptom of myasthenia gravis. Intern Med. 2007;46(11): 743–5.

18. Miller RG, Milner-Brown HS, Mirka A. Prednisone-induced worsening of neuromuscular function in myasthenia gravis. Neurology. 1986;36(5):729–32.

19. Uemura M, Nishimura K, Nakagawa M, et al. [A case of Lambert-Eaton myasthnic syndrome associated with small cell lung carcinoma representing as urinary retention]. Hinyokika kiyo Acta urologica Japonica. 2003;49(9):535–8.

20. Meriggioli MN, Sanders DB. Myasthenia gravis: diagnosis. Semin Neurol. 2004;24(1):31–9.

21. Motomura M, Johnston I, Lang B, Vincent A, Newsom-Davis J. An improved diagnostic assay for Lambert-Eaton myasthenic syndrome. J Neurol Neurosurg Psychiatry. 1995;58(1):85–7.

22. Emery AE. The muscular dystrophies. Lancet. 2002;359(9307):687–95.

23. Bird TD. Myotonic Dystrophy Type 1. In: Pagon RA, Bird TD, Dolan CR, Stephens K, Adam MP, editors. GeneReviews™ [Internet]. Seattle (WA): University of Washington, Seattle; 1993–1999 Sep 17 [updated 2011 Feb 08].

24. Worton R. Muscular dystrophies: diseases of the dystrophin-glycoprotein complex. Science. 1995;270(5237):755–6.

25. Butz M, Koch MC, Muller-Felber W, Lemmers RJ, van der Maarel SM, Schreiber H. Facioscapulohumeral muscular dystrophy. Phenotype-genotype correlation in patients with borderline D4Z4 repeat numbers. J Neurol. 2003;250(8):932–7.

26. Bushby KM. Diagnostic criteria for the limb-girdle muscular dystrophies: report of the ENMC Consortium on Limb-Girdle Dystrophies. Neuromuscul Disord. 1995;5(1):71–4.

27. Sutherland DH, Olshen R, Cooper L, et al. The pathomechanics of gait in Duchenne muscular dystrophy. Dev Med Child Neurol. 1981;23(1):3–22.

28. Yiu EM, Kornberg AJ. Duchenne muscular dystrophy. Neurol India. 2008;56(3):236–47.

29. Matsumura T, Saito T, Fujimura H, Shinno S, Sakoda S. [A longitudinal cause-of-death analysis of patients with Duchenne muscular dystrophy]. Rinsho Shinkeigaku. 2011;51(10):743–50.

30. Sanyal SK, Johnson WW, Thapar MK, Pitner SE. An ultrastructural basis for electrocardiographic alterations associated with Duchenne's progressive muscular dystrophy. Circulation. 1978;57(6):1122–9.

31. Valiyil R, Christopher-Stine L. Drug-related myopathies of which the clinician should be aware. Curr Rheumatol Rep. 2010;12(3):213–20.

32. Mastaglia FL, Ojeda VJ, Sarnat HB, Kakulas BA. Myopathies associated with hypothyroidism: a review based upon 13 cases. Aust N Z J Med. 1988; 18(6):799–806.

33. Ramsay ID. Electromyography in thyrotoxicosis. Q J Med. 1965;34(135): 255–67.
34. Meyerson MD, Lewis E, Ill K. Facioscapulohumeral muscular dystrophy and accompanying hearing loss. Arch Otolaryngol. 1984;110(4):261–6.
35. Engel WK, Askanas V. Inclusion-body myositis: clinical, diagnostic, and pathologic aspects. Neurology. 2006;66(2 Suppl 1):S20–9.
36. Lotz BP, Engel AG, Nishino H, Stevens JC, Litchy WJ. Inclusion body myositis. Observations in 40 patients. Brain. 1989;112(Pt 3):727–47.
37. Tani K, Tomioka R, Sato K, et al. Comparison of clinical course of polymyositis and dermatomyositis: a follow-up study in Tokushima University Hospital. J Med Invest. 2007;54(3–4):295–302.
38. Compston A, Coles A. Multiple sclerosis. Lancet. 2008;372(9648): 1502–17.
39. Lublin FD, Reingold SC. Defining the clinical course of multiple sclerosis: results of an international survey. National Multiple Sclerosis Society (USA) Advisory Committee on Clinical Trials of New Agents in Multiple Sclerosis. Neurology. 1996;46(4):907–11.
40. Paty D, Studney D, Redekop K, Lublin F. MS COSTAR: a computerized patient record adapted for clinical research purposes. Ann Neurol. 1994;36(Suppl):S134–5.
41. Asgari N, Owens T, Frokiaer J, Stenager E, Lillevang ST, Kyvik KO. Neuromyelitis optica (NMO)—an autoimmune disease of the central nervous system (CNS). Acta Neurol Scand. 2011;123(6):369–84.
42. Lensch E, Jost WH. Autonomic disorders in multiple sclerosis. Autoimmune Dis. 2011;2011:803841.
43. Johansson KM, Nygren-Bonnier M, Schalling E. Effects of glossopharyngeal breathing on speech and respiration in multiple sclerosis: a case report. Mult Scler. 2011. doi:10.1177/1352458511430223.
44. White LJ, McCoy SC, Castellano V, et al. Resistance training improves strength and functional capacity in persons with multiple sclerosis. Mult Scler. 2004;10(6):668–74.
45. Dalgas U, Stenager E, Ingemann-Hansen T. Multiple sclerosis and physical exercise: recommendations for the application of resistance-, endurance- and combined training. Mult Scler. 2008;14(1):35–53.
46. Merson RM, Rolnick MI. Speech-language pathology and dysphagia in multiple sclerosis. Phys Med Rehabil Clin N Am. 1998;9(3):631–41.

Chapter 4
Orthopedic Rehabilitation

Joe Vongvorachoti and Crystal D. Thomas

Additional abbreviations

NWB   No weight allowed to be placed on affected limb
TTWB   (Toe Touch Weight Bearing) or TDWB (Touch Down Weight Bearing)=Affected limb may only touch for balance
PWB   (partial weight bearing)=Only a certain percentage of your body weight can be placed on affected limb. Percentage will be dependent on recommendations by MD
WBAT   (weight bearing as tolerated)=Place as much weight on affected limb as tolerated [90]

Disclaimer: The following is intended to be a general guideline. Every patient's rehabilitation course should be individualized based on various factors including, but not limited to, age, prior functioning, and other comorbidities. These guidelines can be overruled by clinical judgment or the surgeon's recommendations.

J. Vongvorachoti, M.D. (✉)
Sports Medicine and Spine, Hospital for Special Surgery,
New York, NY, USA
e-mail: vong2193@yahoo.com

C.D. Thomas, D.P.T.
30 Broad Street, 12th Floor, New York, NY 10004, USA

Outpatient Orthopedic Private Physical Therapy Practice,
Sports Physical Therapy of New York, NY, USA

K.A. Sackheim (ed.), *Rehab Clinical Pocket Guide:*   141
Rehabilitation Medicine, DOI 10.1007/978-1-4614-5419-9_4,
© Springer Science+Business Media, LLC 2013

Knee

S/P Total Knee Replacement

Knee OA (715.16)

- Usually secondary to severe osteoarthritis
- The knee is one of the most common joints affected by OA
- Most common age range—65–84 years of age
- Total knee replacement (TKR) is the definitive treatment for severe OA refractory to conservative treatments

Pathophysiology:
- Wear and tear
- Trauma
- Idiopathic

Symptoms:
- Preoperative—refractory knee pain and swelling especially with weight bearing activities, stiffness, deformity, instability
- Postoperative—swelling and inflammation of periarticular soft tissue, decrease in ROM due to swelling

Physical Exam:
- *Preoperative*
  - Inspection: Visible joint hypertrophy
    - ° Deformities: In OA one would find valgus deformities of the knee while in RA, one would typically see varus deformities.
    - ° Swelling: Possible degree of joint effusion and possibly concomitant pes anserine bursitis.
  - ROM: reduced passive range of motion, and crepitus
  - Palpation: Medial and/or lateral joint line tenderness [1]
  - **Provocative maneuvers**
    Clark test: superior compression of the patella supine while patient contracts quadriceps
- *Postoperative*
  - Inspection: staples or sutures in place
    - ° Potential for serosanguinous discharge
    - ° Residual effusion of knee joint after surgery
    - ° Warmth or erythema of surgical site

- ROM is guarded due to pain
- Strength: Muscle inhibition of quadriceps and hamstrings interferes with MMT

Imaging:
- **X-ray:** AP, Lateral, Merchants view (shows patellofemoral joint; patient supine with knees hanging down with 45° knee flexion) [2], Weighted PA view
  - Show narrowing of the joint space medially, laterally, or in patellofemoral joint
- **MRI**
  - Shows joint narrowing and cartilage loss
- *Postoperatively* non-weight-bearing AP and Lateral knee X-rays should be obtained in the immediate post-op period followed by weight bearing films by 6–8 weeks

Treatment:
- Deep venous thrombosis (DVT) prophylaxis
- Incision care with sterile gauze and frequent dressing changes
- Staples generally in place up to 2 weeks
  - May require a knee immobilizer
  - Postoperative pain relief
  - Analgesic or Nonsteroidal anti-inflammatory (NSAIDS) medications
    - ○ Tylenol 650 mg q4–6 h prn.
    - ○ Naproxen 500 mg BID prn, Motrin 600–800 mg TID, Mobic 7.5 mg BID prn with food, Celebrex 200 mg po bid prn with food. *Caution*: NSAIDS are controversial in the first few weeks because it may impair bone healing. Check with orthopedic surgeon first.
    - ○ Tramadol 50 mg 1 po q6 prn, vicodin 5/500 mg 1 po q6 prn, or Percocet 5/325 mg q4–6 h prn if pain refractory to above medications.
  - Minimize edema with frequent application of ice and elevation after PT

Rehabilitation Program:
Acute Phase **(Day 1 to 2 weeks; for most patients, this phase lasts until 5–7 days)**
Precautions: AVOID prolonged sitting, standing, or walking; AVOID pillow under the knee as this prevents full extension
Weight Bearing Status: WBAT

Goals: Minimize edema, reduce pain/inflammation, increase ROM to 90°, unassisted transfers, restore functional independence, perform independent home exercise program (HEP) [1]

Modalities:

- Cryotherapy to decrease swelling, improve ROM, function, and strength
- E-stim to the quadriceps for those who display inhibited recruitment [3]
- Neuromuscular Electrical Stimulation (NMES) combined with voluntary exercise may accelerate gains in quadriceps muscle strength and activation greater than voluntary exercise alone following total knee arthroplasty [4]

Program:

- Elevation to prevent edema
- Continuous Passive Motion (CPM) for 4–6 h daily—start at 40–60° flexion and progress as tolerated; increase approximately 5–10° per day but generally increase as tolerated by patient; discontinued after obtaining 90° pain free for 2 days. Discontinue Knee immobilizer if quad strength is above 3/5
- Chair transfers, Bed Mobility
- Activities of Daily Living (ADL) training—transfers, lower body dressing, etc.
- Strengthening: Isometric quadriceps, hamstrings, and hip exercises
  - Begin straight-leg-raise exercises, hip abduction, ankle pumps, quadriceps
  - Progress to closed-chain exercises as tolerated (bike)
  - Discontinue Knee immobilizer if quad strength is above 3/5
- Gait training: WBAT with bilateral upper extremity support (walker, axillary crutch) progress to single-hand support (cane)
- Stair Negotiations

Failure to attain proper ROM

- Adhesiolysis: lysis of adhesions using arthroscopy [5]
- Manipulation under anesthesia (MUA): gently applying a force to increase ROM [6]
- If ROM fails to meet goals, consider evaluation for adhesiolysis. Criteria are not well defined but generally include <80° knee flexion (time varies from day of discharge to 3 months) despite

aggressive PT. MUA is controversial because it may tear intra-articular tissue or cause Complex Regional Pain Syndrome (CRPS). Adhesiolysis may follow a trial of MUA [5–7].

Recovery Phase (2–8 weeks)
Precautions: AVOID prolonged sitting, standing, or walking; AVOID pillow under the knee as this prevents full extension; AVOID reciprocal stair climbing until good strength/control

Weight Bearing Status: WBAT

Goals: increase ROM to >105° and extension to 0°, decrease edema, ascend 4 step, normalize gait

Modalities: cryotherapy/elevation for edema, Electrical stimulation (E-stim) or biofeedback for quadriceps reeducation

Program:
- AROM flexion/extension
- Short crank ergometry (90 mm) for ROM > 90°
- Cycle ergometry (170 mm) for ROM >110°
- Patellar mobilization once staples/sutures removed and incision stable
- Straight-leg raises (SLR) progressive resistive exercises (PRE)
- Advance their dynamic and resistance exercise and freely pursue both open- and closed-chain kinetic exercises
- Balance and proprioceptive training (bilateral static balance activities progressing to unilateral static balance activities such as balance boards and machines such as Biodex)
- Transfers in/out of tub/shower and car
- Ambulation training advanced to single-handed or no device

Phase III (9–16 weeks)
Precautions: AVOID running and jumping

Weight Bearing Status: WBAT

Goals: increase ROM to >115°; independent in ADLs including putting on socks and shoes; reciprocal stair negotiation, maximize quadricep/hamstring strength for high-level activities; get up and go test <15 s (time it takes to stand up from an armchair, walk a 3 m, turn, walk back to the chair, and sit down.) [8]

Program:
- Patella mobilization/glides
- Quadricep/hamstring stretching
- Unilateral and eccentric leg press

- Up and down steps
- Ball/wall squats
- Balance/proprioception training with dynamic activities [1]

S/P Anterior Cruciate Ligament (ACL) Repair

ACL Disruption (717.83)

- Originates at the lateral intercondylar notch of femur and inserts lateral to medial tibial eminence
- Prevents anterior translation of the tibia with respect to the femur as well as hyperextension [9]

Pathophysiology:

- 78% due to noncontact mechanism [10]
- Rapid change of direction or cutting maneuvers combined with deceleration (soccer, basketball, lacrosse, football, skiing)
- Landing from a jump in or near full extension
- Pivoting with knee near full extension and a planted foot [11]

Physical exam:
- Inspection: may reveal swelling and erythema
- Provocative maneuvers
  - **Lachman:** with knee in 30° flexion, stabilize distal femur with top hand. Then translate the proximal tibia anteriorly with the bottom hand while translating the distal femur posteriorly. Test is positive when there is laxity or no end point compared to contralateral normal side [12].
  - **Pivot Shift test**
    ° With patient supine and knee extended, apply valgus and internal rotation force which anterolaterally subluxes the tibia
    ° Passively flex the knee and the iliotibial band (ITB) becomes a flexor and reduces the tibia at around 30°
    ° Most reliable under anesthesia [13]

Imaging:
- X-rays may show avulsion
- MRI without contrast shows tear on sagittal view (85–90% accurate)
- Arthroscopy is close to 100% accurate [9]

Treatment:
- Conservative with PT if no desire to have surgery or not involved in sports involving cutting
  - Rest, ice, compression, elevation
  - Knee immobilizer or hinged knee brace with crutches
  - Early knee ROM as tolerated
  - Gentle quadriceps strengthening
  - Hamstring strengthening [14]
- ACL repair or reconstruction with graft

Rehabilitation Program after ACL Surgery:
Phase I (Weeks 0–2)
Precautions: AVOID active knee extension 40–0°, ambulation without brace locked at 0°, heat, prolonged standing/walking.
Weight Bearing Status: Progress from PWB to WBAT.
Goals: full passive extension, decrease pain and swelling, ROM to 90° flexion, progressive weight bearing, prevent quadriceps inhibition, independent HEP [10].
Modalities: Cryotherapy: Ice 20 min out of every hour and elevate the leg with full knee extension to retard inflammation and reduce pain. Application of ice to the knee joint for 30 min is capable of completely reversing the Arthrogenic Muscle Inhibition (AMI) of the vastus medialis that resulted from induced knee joint effusion [4].
- NMES to reduce postsurgical muscle atrophy, increase muscle torque values, improve quadriceps femoris muscle strength and to improve functional recovery. NMES is more effective for strength training after ACL reconstruction when performed against isometric resistance [15].

Program:
- Passive knee extension with towel under heel
- Quadriceps reeducation
- Ambulation training with crutches
- Patellar mobilization
- Active flexion
- Hip PRE
- SLR with brace locked at 0°
- Upper body cardiovascular exercises
- HEP

Phase II (**Weeks 2–6**)
Precautions: AVOID reciprocal descending stairs until good alignment and quadricep control
Weight Bearing Status: Progress weight bearing status
Goals: ROM to 125°, minimize swelling, normal gait, ascend stairs without pain
Program:
- Wean off crutches when gait is non-antalgic
- Progress to CKC exercises—leg press, mini-squats
- Stair negotiation
- Proprioception training
- Active knee extension to 40°
- HEP

Phase III (**Weeks 6–14**)
Precautions: AVOID running or painful exercise
Weight Bearing Status: WBAT
Goals: full ROM, descend stairs reciprocally, LE flexibility
Program:
- Progress to deeper squats and lunges
- Isotonic knee extension 90–40° (CKC exercises preferred)
- Stair negotiation going down
- Retrograde treadmill
- Advanced proprioception training
- Quadriceps stretching
- Retrograde treadmill
- Agility exercises
- HEP

Phase IV (**Weeks 14–22**)
Precautions: AVOID sports until MD clearance
Weight Bearing Status: WBAT
Goals: run pain-free, maximize strength and flexibility
Program:
- Forward running if stepping down adequate
- Sports-specific training
- Plyometrics when near full strength
- Isotonic knee extension (CKC exercises preferred)
- HEP

Phase V (**>22 Weeks**)
Precautions: AVOID sports until MD clearance (full strength and ROM; able to perform sports-specific exercises/motions without limitations)
Weight Bearing Status: WBAT
Goals: build confidence in sport, maximize strength and flexibility
Program:
- Progress strengthening, flexibility, and agility
- Advanced plyometrics
- Brace for sport (surgeon's preference)
- Tailor program to limit pain/swelling
- HEP [10]

S/P Posterior Cruciate Ligament (PCL) Repair

PCL Disruption (717.84)

- Originates at the anterior medial intercondylar notch of femur and inserts lateral to posterior tibial plateau [9]
- Prevents posterior translation of the tibia with respect to the femur

Pathophysiology:
- 3% of all knee injuries
- Dashboard injury
- Severe posteriorly directed force to tibia with relatively fixed femur in knee flexion [16]

Physical Exam:
- Sag test—with knee flexed to 90° in supine position, observe for posteriorly displaced tibia
- Posterior drawer test—same position as above, but apply posterior force to tibia; positive if laxity or no end point

Imaging:
- X-rays may show avulsion
- MRI without contrast shows tear of PCL; less accurate than for ACL
- Arthroscopy is more accurate than MRI [9]

Treatment:
- Controversial whether requires surgery versus conservative treatment

Rehabilitation Program:
Acute Phase (Weeks 0–6)
Precautions: AVOID heat, ambulation without brace locked at 0°, excessive pain with therapy
Weight Bearing Status: Toe Touch Weight Bearing (TTWB) with crutches; progress at 2–6 weeks to 75%
Goals: Reduce pain and swelling, ROM to 90°, improve patellar mobility, independent HEP [16]
Modalities: Cryotherapy: ice and elevation 20 min out of every hour and elevate with knee in extension postoperative day (POD) #1. Taper off every day as tolerated.
- NMES 4 h for first 2 weeks. Then continue NMES to the Quadriceps: 60–0° of knee flexion for both isotonics and isometrics. Electrical stimulation is employed to facilitate and augment quadriceps contraction during specific exercises and is used in conjunction with voluntary quadriceps active contractions [17, 18].

Program:
- Passive extension (pillow under calf/ankle)
- Quadriceps reeducation with E-stim
- Patellar mobilization
- AAROM knee extension/passive flexion 0–70°; progress to 90° at week 4–6 as tolerated
- Hamstring and calf stretching
- SLR with brace locked at 0°
- Leg press from 60° to 0°
- Quadriceps sets at multiple angles (20–60°)
- Hip PRE
- Upper body cardiovascular exercise
- Learn HEP

Phase II (Weeks 6–12)
Precautions: AVOID resistive knee flexion exercises, prolonged sitting/ walking, NO active Open Kinetic Chain (OKC) hamstring exercises
Weight Bearing Status: PWB progress to WBAT when gait is non-antalgic
Goals: Increase ROM to 130°, restore normal gait, ascent 8 in. stairs and descend 6 in. stairs without pain, increase flexibility, protect patellofemoral joint

Program:
- Wean off crutches
- Brace change depending on surgeon
- Ergometry if ROM >115°
- AAROM
- Proprioception training
- Stair negotiation
- Pool gait training
- Knee Extension PRE with OKC

Phase III **(Weeks 12–20)**
Precautions: AVOID reciprocally descending stairs until patient has good quadriceps strength and control, resistive knee flexion exercises, prolonged standing/walking
Weight Bearing Status: WBAT
Goals: Full ROM, descend 8 in. stairs without pain, increase flexibility, protect patellofemoral joint.
Program:
- Leg press up to 80°
- AAROM and stretching
- Proprioception training on uneven surfaces
- Lunges
- Forward running
- Lower extremity PRE except NO active OKC hamstring exercises
  - Knee extension PRE to 80° with OKC exercises
- Descending stairs
- HEP [16]

S/P Knee Meniscal Repair

Meniscal Derangement (717.5)

- Medial meniscus is most common region torn

Pathophysiology:
- Degenerative
- Traumatic
  - Sudden acceleration or deceleration with change in direction
  - Common in football and skiing [9]

Symptoms:
- Pain, swelling, stiffness
- Pop

Physical Exam:
- Medial or lateral joint line tenderness
- **McMurray's test:** In supine position, hyperflex knee and apply internal rotation force to foot while extending the knee. Repeat with external rotation. Evaluates medial and lateral menisci respectively. Positive test includes click and pain.
- **Apley Grind test:** With patient prone and symptomatic knee flexed to 90°, apply axial load and external rotation; repeat with distraction of lower leg. Test is positive is axial load reproduces pain and distraction relieves pain [12].
- **Thessaly:** In single-leg stance, flex standing knee to 20°. Then rotate thigh and upper body externally and internally three times. Positive when it reproduces pain, locking, or catching [19].

Imaging:

- MRI without contrast of knee

Treatment:

- Total meniscectomy has been shown to cause degenerative changes in knee joint
- Partial meniscectomy still results in higher joint stresses than normal
- Attempts to repair meniscus are made when possible

Rehabilitation Program:
Acute Phase **(Weeks 0–6)**
Precautions: AVOID active knee flexion, ambulation without brace locked at 0°, prolonged standing/walking
Weight Bearing Status: TTWB for complex or radial tears
Goals: Full passive extension, decrease pain/swelling, ROM to 90°, quadriceps reeducation, HEP [20]
Modalities: Cryotherapy
- Transcutaneous Electrical Nerve Stimulation (TENS) [21]
Program:
- Quadriceps reeducation with E-stim
- Progressive weight bearing PWB to WBAT with brace locked at 0° and crutches
- Patellar mobilization
- AAROM to 90°

- SLR in all planes
- Hip PREs
- Pool ambulation (weeks 4–6)
- OKC quadriceps isometrics (submaximal at 60°) when ROM >85°
- Leg press to 60° when ROM >85°
- Upper body cardiovascular training
- HEP

Phase II (Weeks 6–14)

Precautions: AVOID descending stairs reciprocally until adequate quadriceps control
AVOID running and sports
Weight Bearing Status: Progressive weight bearing with crutches/cane (brace opened 0–60°)
Goals: Full ROM and normal gait, ascend and descend stairs without pain, HEP
Modalities: Cryotherapy
Program:
- Pool ambulation
- Wean off assistive device
- Brace changed by surgeon
- Patellar mobilization
- SLR in all planes with weights
- Neuromuscular training
- Balance training on uneven surfaces
- Leg press and modified squat
- OKC quadriceps isotonics (CKC preferred)
- Stair training, elliptical machine
- Upper body cardiovascular training
- HEP

Phase III (Weeks 14–22)

Precautions: AVOID sports until cleared by surgeon
Weight Bearing Status: WBAT
Goals: Running without pain, maximize strength and stability, confidence in sports movements, pass hop test, independence in gym program
Program:
- Squats <90° flexion
- Running backwards
- Forward running at 4 months if able to step down properly
- Lower extremity strengthening and flexibility

- Agility and sports-specific training
- Progress to lunges and plyometrics
- Isotonic and isokinetic training
- Hop test
- HEP [20]

Hip

Anatomy

1. *Capsule*
   - Covers the femoral head and most of its neck
   - Attached anteriorly at the intertrochanteric line; posteriorly, up to lateral half of the femoral neck
2. *Blood supply*
   - Crock described the arteries of the proximal end of the femur in three groups:
     1. Extracapsular arterial ring at the base of the femoral neck—formed by medial femoral circumflex artery and branches of the lateral femoral circumflex artery
     2. Ascending cervical branches of the extracapsular arterial ring on the surface of the femoral neck—penetrate the capsule of the hip joint at the intertrochanteric line, When they are close to the femoral head/neck junction, they are called retinacular arteries
        ○ Proximity to bone puts them at risk for injury in any fracture of femoral neck
     3. Arteries of the round ligament—a branch of the obturator or the medial femoral circumflex artery
        ○ Claffey reported that even if it is present, it is not capable of keeping the femoral head alive if all other sources of blood supply were compromised

- Femoral head becomes avascular by a displaced femoral neck fracture
- Excellent vascular supply to the metaphysis explains the absence of avascular changes in the femoral neck as opposed to the head
- Lateral group provides most of the blood supply to the femoral head and neck [22]

Hip Precautions

1. No flexion >90°
2. No adduction past midline
3. No internal rotation past neutral

S/P Total Hip Replacement

Hip OA (715.15)

- Most common reason for joint replacement is osteoarthritis, rheumatoid arthritis, avascular necrosis (AVN), posttraumatic, congenital hip disease, and infectious
- Indications: progressive pain and dysfunction, decline in mobility

Symptoms:
- *Pre-op*: groin pain that occasionally radiates to knee, gait disturbance (Trendelenberg gait), stiffness after sitting or lying down for a prolonged period of time. There should be no numbness/parasthesias.
- *Post-op*: swelling and pain is likely; however, patient should no longer have groin pain sensation

Physical Exam:
- *Pre-op*: antalgic gait pattern, weakness of hip abductors, positive FABER test.
- *Post-op*: Patients would have undergone either an anterior or a posterior approach to surgery. Posterior approach being more common. Patients will usually have staples in place. Make sure it is clean, dry, and intact.

Treatment:
- Post-op antibiotics given by surgical team
- Patients are often type and screened prior to surgery for potential post-op anemia. Blood transfusions may be necessary.
  - Generally speaking, patients with Hgb levels below 8 should be transfused but those who have Coronary Artery Disease should be kept at a Hgb level above 10.

- Pain regimen
- Elevation of limb to prevent edema accumulation.
- Wound Care: Dry sterile dressing once or twice a day until drainage has stopped. Then applying a thin layer of betadine with a dry gauze is recommended. Watch for symptoms of persistent drainage at which point antibiotics may be appropriate. Look for erythema around staples (if so, will need to remove staples sooner than 2 weeks post-op).

Rehabilitation Program:

Goal: Decrease pain and swelling, start exercise and ROM training (1 week), Guard against dislocation of the implant

- Abduction pillow while patient in bed
- Modalities: Ice per site to decrease swelling. TENS and Ultrasound contraindicated
- Avoid passive straight leg raises while in supine position
- ROM/Stretching—Will allow Thomas stretch of nonoperative extremity with post-op hip stretched gently into extension
- Patients are to be on Hip Precautions:
  - Posterior Hip Precautions—avoid hip flexion greater than 90°, adduction past midline, and internal rotation of the hip past neutral.
  - Anterior Hip Precautions—avoid hip extension, external rotation, adduction past midline
- Strengthening exercises to include quadriceps and gluteal isometrics, ankle pumps dorisflexion/plantarflexion, hip flexion only to below 45° in supine, sitting knee extension. Isometric hip abduction exercises in the initial week of therapy. Can progress to hip abduction exercises while lying supine and standing (gradual abduction and adduction) using available range. Side-lying hip abduction (against gravity) allowed 5 weeks post-op.
- Progressive Ambulation with assistive device (walker, crutches, or cane)
- Stair negotiations
- Transfer training
- Occupational Therapy can include Assistive device training with Reacher and Grabbers, Shoe horns, and Sock-Aids

After 6 weeks:
Goal: Advancement of strengthening exercises once hip precautions are over (after 6 weeks)
Program:
- Hip Abduction exercises with Theraband, sports-cords
- Prone-lying hip extensions allowed
- Treadmill and Retro treadmill exercises
- Concentric and Eccentric leg lift exercises
- Stationary Bike
- Closed Kinetic Chain exercises [23]

Subtrochanteric Fractures

Fracture; Closed; Unspecified Part of Femur, Thigh, Upper Leg (821.00)

- Fracture inferior to the greater and lesser trochanters
- Very high mechanical stresses and most difficult to stabilize [9]
- Rare compared to intertrochanteric fractures
- Unique pattern associated with bisphosphonate treatment: leads to transverse fractures [24]

Pathophysiology:
- Blood supply of hip: Transverse and descending branches of the lateral circumflex femoral artery [25]; poor blood supply [26]
- High-energy trauma: MVA or fall from high altitude
- Factors predisposing patients: osteoporosis

Physical Exam:
- Possible shortening of limb
- Limb external rotation [9]
- Check for upper limb injuries/fractures in elderly patients

Imaging:
- AP and lateral X-rays
- CT scan if extension into greater trochanter suspected [24]

Treatment:
- **Open reduction and internal fixation (ORIF) with a fixed-angle plate**

Rehabilitation Program:
Phase I (**Weeks 0–6**)
Precautions: AVOID weight bearing on affected leg; no isometrics first week
AVOID active adduction/abduction because of increased torque on fracture site [26]
Weight Bearing Status: TTWB
Goals: Ambulate with assistive device, transfer independently, increase ROM, decrease pain
Modalities: Cryotherapy
Program:
- Continuous Passive-motion Machine (CPM)
- PROM
- Touchdown weight bearing
- Transfers
- Gait training with assistive device
- Upper body strengthening for assistive device
- HEP

Phase II (**Weeks 6–12**)
Precautions: AVOID painful weight bearing
Weight Bearing Status: Advance weight bearing if X-rays show callus formation
Goals: Full weight bearing by 12 weeks
Program:
- PROM, AAROM, AROM
- PRE (resistance exercises starting with body weight, then progress to adding weights)
- Gait training; wean off assistive device by 12 weeks
- Stair negotiation
- HEP

Return to sports: 6 months [27]

Treatment:
Reconstruction nailing
- Second line option
- Osteoporotic and pathologic fractures

Rehabilitation Program:
Phase I (**Days 0–4**)
Precautions: AVOID painful ambulation

Weight Bearing Status: If cortical contact is good, WBAT with crutches or walker. If not, TTWB.

Goals: Ambulation with assistive device, increase ROM, decrease pain

Program:
- ROM
- Gait training
- Progress to SLR
- HEP, discharge in 3–4 days

Phase II **(Days 4–28)**

Precautions: AVOID painful ambulation

Weight Bearing Status: Progress weight bearing to WBAT when callus seen on X-ray

Goals: Progressive weight bearing if X-ray shows callus, strengthen hip abductors, improve ambulation.

Program:
- PRE especially hips
- Discontinue crutches/walker after able to stand on affected leg for 60 s and have equal hip abductor strength standing without Trendelenburg
- Swimming, stationary bike
- HEP

Phase III **(>4 weeks)**

Precautions: none

Weight Bearing Status: WBAT

Goals: FWB by 4–6 months, community ambulation by 6–8 weeks, begin driving motor vehicles at 8–16 weeks

Program:
- Ambulation training
- Driver training [28]

Femoral Neck Fractures

Fracture, Femur Neck; Closed; Intracapsular Section, Unspecified (820.00)

- Fracture medial to the intertrochanteric line

Pathophysiology:
- High-energy force in younger patients
- Low-energy force in elderly patients such as a fall
- 3–5% of femoral shaft fractures have associated femoral neck fracture
- Femoral neck fracture should be prioritized over most other closed fractures because femoral neck circulation can be compromised
- 15% associated with high-pressure intracapsular hematoma
- Blood supply and how affected by this type of fracture (see hip anatomy above)
- Factors predisposing patients: osteoporosis, poor balance, hyperparathyroidism, Parkinson Disease, Paget's Disease, spastic hemiplegia, postradiation of pelvis, metastatic disease [29]

Physical Exam:
- ROM is painful and should not be performed
- Assess neurovascular status

Imaging:
- AP and cross-table lateral X-rays
- CT scan may help with comminuted fractures

Treatment Preoperative:
- Immobilize leg with pillow under knee
- Traction has not been shown to be beneficial and can tighten anterior capsule
- If not sufficiently reduced, high risk of AVN
- Relative orthopedic emergency (controversial)
  - Surgery within 8 h, especially in patients <50 years old have better outcomes

Types of Surgical Treatment:
- ORIF if displaced and not able to be reduced in a closed manner
- Arthroplasty
  - Advanced rheumatoid arthritis or moderate osteoarthritis of the adjacent hip joint
  - Poor bone density, limited life expectancy
  - Pathologic fractures related to metastatic disease
  - Presence of severe psychiatric disease

Rehabilitation Program for ORIF:
Phase I **(0–7 days)**
Precautions: AVOID early excessive weight bearing

Weight Bearing Status: TTWB or PWB (depending on surgeon preference)
Goals: decrease pain, prevent DVT, ambulation and transfers
Program:
- Early mobilization in and out of bed, on and off toilet
- Transfers and gait training
- PWB with crutches in younger patient, walker in elderly patients
- Limit excessive ROM, especially PROM
- Quadriceps sets
- Upper body strengthening for assistive device
- Decubitus ulcer prevention
- ADLs

Phase II **(Weeks 2–6)**
Precautions: AVOID excessive weight bearing on affected side
Weight Bearing Status: PWB
Goals: progressively increase ambulation to 550 ft, improve balance, increase gait speed, improve "get up and go" test
Program:
- Increase weight bearing as tolerated (WBAT)
- Hip PROM for 6–8 weeks
- Stair negotiation nonreciprocally with upper extremity support
- Reciprocally if using a cane
- Outdoor ambulation on variable surfaces
- AROM hip in various positions (supine, standing, etc.)
- Strengthening exercises: isotonics and PRE
- Balance retraining

Phase III **(>6 Weeks)**
Precautions: AVOID excessive weight bearing on affected side
Weight Bearing Status: PWB; progress to WBAT after week 12
Goals: timed "up and go" test score of 16 s by 12 weeks, increase gait speed
Program:
- Gait training
- PRE
- Sports-specific training [30]

Rehabilitation Program for Arthroplasty (THA):
Phase I **(Weeks 0–2)**
Precautions: Hip precautions (no flexion >90°, adduction past midline, internal rotation) and abduction pillow for 6 weeks; Transfer out

of bed on surgical side (helps maintain precautions) [26]; AVOID lying on affected side

Weight Bearing Status: WBAT

Goals: prevent dislocation of hip joint, allow healing, early mobilization

Program:

- OOB day 1
- Cryotherapy
- Transfer and ambulation training
- WBAT
- Nonreciprocal stair negotiation
- ADLs

Phase II **(Weeks 2–8)**

Precautions: Hip precautions until week 6

Weight Bearing Status: WBAT

Goals: minimize pain and edema, normalize gait, independent ADLs

- AVOID heat, sitting >1 h
- Gait training
- Leg press
- Proprioception/balance training
- Pool therapy

Phase III **(>8 Weeks)**

Precautions: No running or jumping

Weight Bearing Status: WBAT

Goals: reciprocal stair climbing, return to normal activities

- Stationary bike
- Gait training
- Start forward step down program
- Leg press
- PRE lower extremities
- Advanced balance and proprioception training [30, 31]

Intertrochanteric Fractures

Fracture, Femur Neck; Pertrochanteric, Closed; Trochanteric Section, Unspecified (820.20)

- Between greater and lesser trochanters of femur
- Most common hip fracture [9]

Pathophysiology:
- low energy falls in osteoporotic patients
- F > M
- 90% occurs in patients >65 years old [32]

Symptoms:
- Hip pain

Physical Exam:
- Externally rotated and shortened limb [9]

Imaging:
- AP and lateral X-rays show fracture
- CT or MRI based on surgeon preference

Treatment:
- Sliding hip screw with two hole side plate for stable fractures
- Intramedullary (IM) hip screw for unstable fractures (significant disruption of posteromedial cortex)
  - Impending or pathologic fractures of proximal femur
- Hip arthroplasty (done less often due to higher perioperative mortality rate)
  - Pathologic fracture
  - Failed ORIF [32]

Rehabilitation for Patients with Screws:
Phase I (Weeks 0–6)
Precautions: AVOID adductor strengthening, PROM [25, 26]
Weight Bearing Status: WBAT
Goals: assisted transfers, ambulation, and lower body dressing; ambulation 100 ft with walker in 6 min
Program:
- OOB day 1
- Ambulation training with assistive device
- Begin stair training and outdoor ambulation after 2 weeks
- Balance training after 2 weeks
- Gentle isotonic strengthening
- Transfers
- A/AROM of hip and knee: limit adduction

Phase II (Weeks 6–12)
Precautions: None unless evidence of poor healing on X-ray
Weight Bearing Status: WBAT
Goals: maximize strength

Program:
- PROM
- Once there is radiographic evidence of fracture healing, start PRE
- Stair training
- Outdoor ambulation on variable surfaces
- Balance training

Phase III **(>12 Weeks)**
Precautions: None
Weight Bearing Status: WBAT
Goals: return to normal activities, stairs reciprocally, increase gait speed
Program:
- Stair training reciprocally
- Bicycling
- Isotonic and isokinetic machines
- Progressive gait training [32]

Rehabilitation for Patients with Arthroplasty:
- Individualized based on quality of intraoperative component-fixation and status of greater trochanter
- If trochanteric fixation used, AVOID hip abduction strengthening until trochanteric union
  - PWB for 6 weeks
  - Abduction orthosis
- see THA rehabilitation program [33]

Femoral Shaft Fracture

Fracture; Closed; Unspecified Part of Femur, Thigh, Upper Leg (821.00)

Pathophysiology:
- Trauma
- Pathologic fracture
- External iliac artery becomes the femoral artery after passing the inguinal ligament
- Profundus femoral artery branches off and gives rise to the medial and lateral femoral circumflex arteries

- It also gives off numerous perforating branches along the length of the femur that pass posteriorly
- Blood supply to the femur is from the primary nutrient vessel(s) and small periosteal vessels [34].

Symptoms:
- Thigh pain

Physical Exam:
- Check neurovascular status
- May have open wound if there is a break in the skin

Imaging:
- X-rays

Treatment:
Intramedullary Nail
Indications:
- Simple or comminuted fractures presenting below the lesser trochanter and extending distally to within 7 cm of the knee [35]

Rehabilitation Program:
Phase I (Weeks 0–8)
Precautions: AVOID painful ambulation
Weight Bearing Status: Progressive weight bearing in axially stable fractures (no or little comminution); usually delayed 6–10 weeks until callus formed in unstable fractures (moderate to severe comminution) [34]
Goals: early mobilization
Program:
- Early weight bearing (transverse or short oblique fracture)
- Partial weight bearing (PWB) 6–8 weeks (comminuted fracture) to permit callus formation
- AROM
- Gait training
- ADLs
- Pool therapy [35]

Phase II (>8 Weeks)
Precautions: AVOID painful ambulation
Weight Bearing Status: Progressive weight bearing in axially stable fractures (no or little comminution); usually delayed 6–10 weeks until callus formed in unstable fractures (moderate to severe comminution) [34]

Goals: maximize strength, return to normal activities
Program:
- AROM
- ADLs
- Gait training
- Stair negotiation

Most fractures unite in 3–5 months. [35]

Retrograde Nailing

Indications:
- Diaphyseal femoral-shaft fractures at least 5 cm below the bottom of the lesser trochanter down to the supracondylar femur including fractures with an intercondylar split.
- Fractures with associated musculoskeletal injuries

Rehabilitation Program:
Precautions: AVOID painful ambulation
Weight Bearing Status: Early weight bearing in axially stable fractures. Delayed 6–10 weeks until callus is apparent on postoperative radiographs in unstable fractures.
Goals: Full extension and flexion greater than 90° should be obtained between 6 and 8 weeks
Program:
- See above for rehab [36]

Pelvic Fractures

- 3–8% of ER fractures but 25% in patients with multiple fractures [37]

Pathophysiology:
- Trauma: falls and crush injuries

Symptoms:
- Pelvic pain
- Dizziness, lethargy (from blood loss)

Physical Exam:
- Palpate ASIS for integrity
- Compress the iliac wings together, then pull them apart (perform ONLY once as this may increase bleeding)
- Scrotal or labial hematomas indicate pelvic hemorrhage

- Rectal and vaginal exams for bony fragment lacerations
  - High riding prostate indicates urethral disruption
- Examine urethral meatus for bleeding

Imaging:
- AP and lateral X-rays
- Inlet X-ray (beam tilted 40° cephalad): sacral fractures, widening of SI or pubic symphisis
- Outlet X-ray (beam tilted 45° caudad): sacral, pubic rami, posterior iliac wing fractures [38]

Tile Classification
Tile A injuries—stable fractures, managed nonoperatively
Tile B injuries—rotationally unstable but vertically stable
Tile C injuries—both rotationally and vertically unstable

Diastasis of Symphysis Pubis

Fracture Closed; Specified Part of Pelvis; Other, Innominate Bone, Pelvic Rim (808.49)

- Arcuate ligament is main stabilizer between 2 pubic rami
- Seen in Tile B and C injuries
- "Open Book" injury: Diastasis of the symphysis pubis and external rotation of one innominate bone; posterior pelvic ligaments intact

Treatment:

ORIF if diastasis >2.5 cm

Rehabilitation Program:
Phase I (Weeks 0–8)
Precautions: AVOID painful ambulation
Weight Bearing Status: For Tile A and B, TTWB to PWB for 8 weeks
For Tile C, TTWB to PWB for 8–12 weeks
Goals: Ambulation with assistive device, transfers, ADLs
Program:
- Mobilized from bed to chair on the first or second day after surgery

- For isolated open-book injuries (Tile B), protected weight bearing on the injured side for 8 weeks
- For combined internal fixation of the anterior and posterior pelvic ring (Tile C), weight bearing should be delayed for 8–12 weeks
- Bed to chair transfers
- ADLs
- HEP

Phase II (>8–12 Weeks)
Precautions: AVOID painful ambulation
Weight Bearing Status: For Tile A and B, progress from PWB to WBAT
For Tile C, TTWB to PWB for 8–12 weeks
Goals: Restore normal gait, increase muscle strength and aerobic conditioning
Program:
- Strengthening directed at increasing hip abductor strength
- Aerobic conditioning
- Gait training
- Lower back-strengthening exercises and work-increasing programs for those who need to return to heavy labor [39]

Posterior Pelvic Ring Fractures

Fracture Closed; Specified Part of Pelvis; Other, Innominate Bone, Pelvic Rim (808.49)

Indications for surgery:

- Unstable posterior pelvic ring
- Sacroiliac (SI) joint dislocations; sacral fractures; certain, posterior, iliac "crescent" fracture-SI disruptions, and combinations of these

Treatment:
Conservative nonoperative treatment for stable fractures without displacement during hip ROM
- Frequent hip X-rays to ensure stability up to 6 weeks; may need X-rays at 8 and 12 weeks if still no signs of fracture healing

- Begin with TTWB as tolerated with walker/crutches then progress from PWB at 6 weeks

Iliosacral Screws (see above for indications)

Rehabilitation Program:
Dependent on associated injuries

Phase I **(Weeks 0–6)**
Precautions: AVOID painful ambulation
Weight Bearing Status: PWB
Goals: Ambulate with assistive device
Program:
- Protected weight bearing with crutches or walker
- Gait training
- Transfers
- ADLs

Phase II **(Weeks 6–12)**
Precautions: AVOID painful ambulation
Weight Bearing Status: Progress from PWB to WBAT
Goals: Ambulate without assistive device
Program:
- Advance weight bearing according to MD
- Wean off assistive device
- Advance ADLs
- HEP [40]

Acetabular Fractures (808.0)

- **Pathophysiology:**Trauma
- Axial load applied to femur
- Osteoporosis [41]

Symptoms:
- Hip pain
- Weak proximal thigh

Physical Exam:
- Check neurovascular status: especially femoral and obturator nerves (knee extension, hip abduction)
- Assess for any open wounds

Imaging:
- AP, internal oblique, external oblique X-rays
- CT scan for further details and preoperative planning

Treatment:
Kocher–Langenbeck Approach

Indications:
- Posterior wall, posterior column, posterior column and wall fractures

Rehabilitation Program:
Phase I **(Week 0–12)**
Precautions: Limit weight bearing
Weight Bearing Status: TTWB
Goals: early mobilization, increase strength and ROM
Program:
- Total hip arthroplasty precautions are not needed
- Partial, toe-touch weight bearing with crutches or a walker
- Out of bed on POD #1
- AROM
- Upper body strengthening for assistive device
- Stair negotiation
- Begin lower body strengthening later on

Phase II **(>12 Weeks)**
Precautions: AVOID painful ambulation
Weight Bearing Status: Progress from TTWB to WBAT
Goals: maximize strength and ROM, return to normal activities
Program:
- Progress to full weight bearing per MD
- AROM
- PRE
- Stair negotiation
- ADLs
- HEP [42]

Ilioinguinal Approach

Indications:
- Anterior wall and column fractures
- Most of both column fractures

Rehabilitation Program:
Phase I (Weeks 0–8)
Precautions: Limit weight bearing
Weight Bearing Status: PWB
Goals: ambulate with assistive device, increase ROM
Program:
- Partial-weight bearing up to 30 lb
- Gait training with assistive device
- Transfers
- ADLs
- Standing AROM of the hip
- HEP

Phase II (>8 Weeks)
Precautions: AVOID painful ambulation
Weight Bearing Status: Advance to WBAT
Goals: community ambulation without assistive device, strengthen hip muscles
Program:
- Full weight bearing
- Gait training; wean off assistive device
- AROM
- PRE with emphasis on hip flexors and abductors
- HEP [43]

Extended Iliofemoral Approach
- Indications:
- High transtectal transverse and T-type fracture patterns with involvement of the weight bearing dome
- Associated anterior column and posterior hemitransverse fractures
- Associated both-column fractures, with a posterior wall or a comminuted posterior-column lateral-dome involvement or extension into the sacroiliac joint
- Transverse or associated fractures where treatment has been delayed

Rehabilitation Program:
Phase I (Weeks 0–6)
Precautions: AVOID active abduction, any adduction, and flexion of the hip past 90°
Weight Bearing Status: TTWB

Goals: early mobilization, allow healing, ambulation with assistive device

Program:

- Sit at the edges of their beds with legs hanging off POD #1
- Transfer to chairs within the first 24–48 h
- CPM usually not necessary
- PROM
- After the removal of drains, toe-touch weight bearing up to 20 lb with crutches.
- Upper body strengthening exercises for crutch/walker use
- Gentle lower body strengthening toward end of phase (do NOT violate precautions)
- Gait training

Phase II (>6 Weeks)

Precautions: Slowly begin active abduction, adduction, and flexion of hip

Weight Bearing Status: Progress to full WBAT by 8–12 weeks

Goals: ambulation without assistive device, increase ROM

Program:

- Discontinue abduction/adduction/flexion precautions but AVOID excessive stretching
- AROM hips
- Gait training with cane; progress to independent ambulation
- PRE
- Stair negotiation
- HEP

Full activity: 6 months [44]

Tibial Fractures

Tibial Plateau Fracture

Fracture of Tibia and Fibula (823.00)

Pathophysiology:

- Common peroneal nerve courses around fibular neck and is at risk with severe displacement

- The trifurcation of the popliteal artery into the anterior tibial, posterior tibial, and peroneal arteries occurs posteromedially
- Majority due to high-speed motor vehicle accidents and falls from heights
- Direct axial compression usually with a valgus (more common) or varus (less common) moment
  - Anterior aspect of the femoral condyles is wedge-shaped
  - With the knee in full extension, the force drives the condyle into the tibial plateau
- Low-energy pedestrian accidents versus car fender accidents.
- When a single compartment is involved, it is usually the lateral plateau likely due to the normal 7° of valgus

Symptoms:
- Pain and swelling in knee
- Knee buckling
- Hemarthrosis unless joint capsule is disrupted

Physical Exam:
- Check neurovascular status: dorsalis pedis, posterior tibial, and popliteal arteries
- Assess knee ligaments
- Widening of the femoral-tibial articulation > 10° with stress exam indicates ligamentous disruption [45]

Imaging:
- AP and lateral X-rays

Treatment:
- If ankle-brachial index remains < 0.9 following a gentle manipulative reduction, obtain vascular consultation
- Nonsurgical if: <1 cm of shortening, 5° of valgus but no varus malalignment, 10° of malalignment in the anteroposterior plane, and 5–10° of external rotation but no internal rotation deformity, and low-energy trauma. However, there is no good evidence for nonsurgical reduction and many surgeons prefer surgical management.
- ORIF or Locked plating

ORIF of Tibia
Indications:
- Open plateau fractures, fractures with an associated compartment syndrome, and fractures with a vascular injury

- High-energy trauma with severe soft-tissue compromise in a young patient

Rehabilitation Program:
Phase I (Weeks 0–3)
Precautions: Limit ROM if there is swelling and tension on suture lines
Weight Bearing Status: Non-weight-bearing gait training with crutches or a walker
Goals: protect surgical site, increase strength, ambulate with assistive device
Program:
- Gentle ROM until bulky dressing is removed at 48 h
- If a meniscal tear was repaired, ROM is usually limited for the first 3 weeks with flexion stops at 60°
- Quadriceps strengthening

Phase II (Weeks 3–8)
Precautions: AVOID painful ambulation
Weight Bearing Status: Non-weight-bearing gait training with assistive device
Goals: 90° of flexion by 4 weeks, improve ambulation
Program:
- AROM and AAROM
- ADLs
- Stair negotiation

Phase III (>8 Weeks)
Precautions: AVOID painful ambulation
Weight Bearing Status: Weight bearing of up to 50% of body weight per MD, Progress weight bearing per MD (progression delayed to 10–12 weeks if surgeon determines intraoperatively that injury was extremely severe)
Goals: functional ROM, painless ambulation, normal alignment, resume normal activities
Program:
- Gait training
- PRE
- HEP

Resume most simple activities: 4–6 months
Running and vigorous athletic activities: delayed up to 1 year
However, patients rarely resume competitive athletics [46]

Locked Plating
Indications:
- Bicondylar tibial-plateau fractures, marked comminution, osteopenia or poor bone quality, and a bone gap secondary to loss of bone along one or both columns of the proximal tibia.

Rehabilitation:
Limited literature on rehabilitation in this type of surgery
Generally, TTWB for 4–6 weeks, then 50% weight bearing once callus forms
Can follow protocol for ORIF, which is more conservative [47]

Tibial Shaft Fractures (823.30)

Pathophysiology:
- Healing is slow in the tibia
- Postoperative knee pain is common and calms down over 4–6 months (Master)
- Five main causes: falls, sports injuries, direct blows or assaults, motor vehicle accidents, and gunshot injuries
  - Low-velocity injuries associated with a muzzle velocity of <2,000 ft/s are more commonly seen in civilian practice
  - High-velocity injuries are produced by military weapons
- Court-Brown and McBirnie's epidemiologic study of 523 fractures found 76.5% were closed and 23.5% were open fractures.
  - Average age of the patients with closed fractures was 35.6 years, and 42.4 years for the open fractures [48].

Symptoms:
- Lower leg pain and swelling
- Possible open wound

Physical Exam:
- Check neurovascular status: tibial and peroneal nerves, capillary refill
- Assess for any open wounds: may be only a small puncture wound
- Assess all knee ligaments: high incidence of ligament injuries [49]

Imaging:
- AP and lateral X-rays

Treatment:
- Chem 7 and urinalysis: myoglobinuria can cause renal failure

Intramedullary Nailing
Indications:
- Ipsilateral fracture of the femur, ankle, or foot
- Vascular injury
- Compartment syndrome
- Bilateral fractures

Rehabilitation Program:
Phase I (Weeks 0–4)
Precautions: AVOID resisted knee flexion/extension
Weight Bearing Status: PWB. In an unstable pattern (severe comminution) or an unreliable patient, weight bearing is not recommended for at least 6–8 weeks
Goals: prevent deformities and contractures, decrease swelling
Program:
- Posterior splint with the ankle neutral or in slight dorsiflexion to prevent an equinus deformity
- The patient remains in a splint until the swelling decreases (1–6 weeks)
- PWB in reliable patient
- Cryotherapy
- Gentle ROM per MD

Phase II (Weeks 4–8)
Precautions: AVOID resisted knee flexion/extension
Weight Bearing Status: In an unstable pattern (severe comminution) or an unreliable patient, weight bearing is not recommended for at least 6–8 weeks.
Goals: reduce unnecessary patellofemoral stress, decrease swelling
Program:
- Progress weight bearing per MD
- Thick elastic stocking for mild swelling
- Quad sets with SLR
- AROM especially of ankle
- Crutch training and upper body strengthening

Phase III (Weeks 8–16)
Precautions: AVOID painful ambulation

Weight Bearing Status: Progress weight bearing to WBAT. In unstable pattern, begin with PWB
Goals: start to walk without assistive device
Program:
- PRE hips
- Gait training

Phase IV (>16 Weeks)
Precautions: Return to sports gradually
Weight Bearing Status: WBAT
Goals: return to normal activities and possibly competitive sports
Program:
- Bicycling and swimming
- Sports-specific exercises
- Off-balance training
- Slow return to running

Return to running: 6–12 months
Full recovery: 1.5–2 years [49]

ORIF Tibial Shaft
- Alternative surgical option

Rehabilitation Program:
Precautions: AVOID painful ambulation
Weight Bearing Status: Weight bearing will be advanced to partial (50 kg) by 6–8 weeks and to full by 8–12 weeks
Goals:
Program:
- POD #1, PWB (20 kg) on the affected side
- Drain is usually removed after 2–4 days, then surgical dressing next day
- Then begin AAROM and AROM for ankle, hip, and knee
- See rehab protocol above [50]

Pilon Fracture (823.80)

- Pilon is synonymous with Plafond
- Distal tibia fracture
- 3–9% of tibia fractures
- More likely due to axial loading

Pathophysiology:

Two Types
- Rotational type
  - Relatively low-energy injury such as during recreational skiing; spiral in nature and are generally associated with little articular comminution and limited surrounding soft-tissue injury
- Axial compression type
  - High-energy motor-vehicle crashes, falls from a considerable height, and crush injuries; articular and metaphyseal comminution and significant soft-tissue injury

Symptoms:
- Ankle pain and swelling

Physical Exam:
- Check neurovascular status
- Assess for other fractures and soft-tissue injury [51]

Imaging:
- AP, lateral and mortise X-ray views: may need to extend X-rays proximally to assess entire tibia/fibula
- CT scan to assess for articular fractures [52]

Treatment:

Indications for surgery:
- Articular fracture displacement of ≥2 mm
- Unstable fractures of the tibial metaphysic
- Open pilon fractures

Rehabilitation Program:
Phase I (**Weeks 0–6**)
Precautions: limit weight bearing
Weight Bearing Status: TTWB
Goals: healing of surgical site, learn HEP
Program:
- Discharged to home in 24–48 h
- Postoperative splint and maintaining toe-touch weight bearing.
- Splint is removed and the incisions are inspected POD #8–12
- Ankle is immobilized again in a short-leg splint.
- When the sutures are removed, placed in a removable boot
- Then initiate AAROM ankle, subtalar joint, and foot/toes
  - Four times per day for 20 min each
- HEP

Phase II (**Weeks 6–12**)
Precautions: limit painful ambulation
Weight Bearing Status: PWB if alignment and fixation maintained on X-ray; otherwise maintain TTWB
Goals: improve ambulation, increase strength and ROM
Program:
- Aggressive AAROM of ankle
- AAROM and PROM of subtalar joint and foot
- Muscle strengthening
- Proprioception training
- HEP

Phase III (**>12 Weeks**)
Precautions: limit painful ambulation
Weight Bearing Status: Advance to full weight bearing
Goals: independent ambulation, maximize ROM, return to work
- Wean from boot and crutches
- PRE
- AROM and stretching of ankle, subtalar, and foot
- Laborers require a period of work hardening [51]

Ankle Fractures (824.8)

Pathophysiology:
- Increased body mass and history of smoking
- Highest incidence of ankle fractures occurs in elderly women
- Most ankle fractures are isolated malleolar fractures (66% of fractures)
- Bimalleolar fractures occur in 25%
- Trimalleolar (medial, lateral, and posterior malleoli) fractures occur in 7%
- Open fractures are rare (2%)
- Described by the likely mechanism: Predominantly rotational or predominantly axial-loading injuries
    - Rotational malleolar fractures are less-severe injuries
- Four major fracture types were described: supination-adduction, supination-external rotation (SER), pronation-abduction, and pronation-external rotation (PER) fractures [53]

Symptoms:
- Ankle pain and swelling

Physical Exam:
- Check neurovascular status
- Assess open wound if present

Treatment:
ORIF of ankle
- Mortise widening and talar shift especially if fibular displaced >2 mm
- Bimalleolar fractures

Rehabilitation Program:
Phase I (**Weeks 0–2**)
Precautions: AVOID weight bearing; wear splint to prevent equinus contracture
Weight Bearing Status: Non-Weight Bearing (NWB)
Goals: decrease swelling, allow surgical site to heal
Program:
- Short-leg, posterior, stirrup splint until good dorsiflexion of ankle
- Cryotherapy
- Leg elevation

Phase II (**Weeks 2–6**)
Precautions: AVOID weight bearing
Weight Bearing Status: NWB
Goals: ambulation with assistive device, decrease edema, increase ROM
Program:
- Reliable patients are instructed in AROM ankle and subtalar joint
- Removable short-leg orthotic
- Gait training with assistive device
- ADLs

Phase III (**Weeks 6–12**)
Precautions: AVOID painful ambulation
Weight Bearing Status: progress to WBAT
Goals: improve ambulation, decrease edema
Program:
- Progress weight bearing per MD
- AAROM, AROM, PROM

- Proprioception training
- Gait training
- HEP

Phase IV (**>12 Weeks**)
Precautions: AVOID sports until full strength, ROM, and agility
Weight Bearing Status: WBAT
Goals: return to normal activities and sports
Program:
- PRE
- Agility and sports-specific training

Persistent dependent swelling may persist for many months
- Compression stockings or elastic wraps.

Return to driving: patient's judgment
- However, simulated braking time returned to normal at 9 weeks [54]

Talus Fractures (825.21)

Pathophysiology:
- Uncommon: 2% of lower extremity injuries
- 2/3 of talus is covered in articular cartilage
- All fractures are articular injuries
- Trauma
- Talar neck fracture: Hyperdorsiflexion
- Other parts of talus: Inversion and eversion forces such as in sports
- Fractures of neck and body commonly occur together

Symptoms:
- Foot pain and swelling

Physical Exam:
- Neurovascular exam especially with posteriormedial displacement (risk of osteonecrosis) [55]
- Check integrity of medial and lateral ankle ligaments: apply inversion and eversion stress

Imaging:
- AP, lateral, and oblique X-rays
- CT scan for occult fractures and showing fracture pattern

Treatment:
ORIF
Indications:
- Disruption of articular congruity and/or loss of talar length, alignment, and rotation
- Talar neck and body fractures displaced more than 1–2 mm

Rehabilitation Program:
Precautions: AVOID weight bearing on affected side
Weight Bearing Status: NWB for 10–12 weeks
Goals:
Program:
- Bulky dressing with a posterior splint at first
- AROM of ankle, subtalar, and midfoot joints when placed into removable boot
- Physical therapy (PT) is started on a case by case basis depending upon the patient's ability to comply and progress with a HEP [56]

Lisfranc (825.25)

- In most displaced injuries, metatarsals displace dorsally and laterally on the tarsal bones

  - **Pathophysiology:**

- Trauma: Fall from height or MVA
- Sports: Hyperplantarflexion
  - Cuneiforms, cuboid, and or metatarsals fractures are commonly associated
- Crush injury [57]

Symptoms:
- Midfoot pain
- Swelling

Physical Exam:
- Check neurovascular status: including dorsalis pedis and posterior tibial arteries
- Fixed position of toes indicates tendon entrapment

Imaging:
- AP, lateral, and oblique X-rays
- CT scan not usually ordered: difficult to interpret

Treatment:
- Closed reduction if only bony injury

ORIF of Tarsometatarsal Joint

Indications:
- Displaced injuries and subtle injuries that have instability in two planes
  - Will result in loss of arch and/or deformity

Rehabilitation Program:

Phase I (Weeks 0–2)
Precautions: Placed in short-leg posterior plaster splint
Weight Bearing Status: NWB
Goals: decrease pain, ambulation with assistive device
Program:
- Short-leg, posterior, plaster splint at the end of the operation
- Gait training with crutches or walker.
- ADLs.

Phase II (Weeks 2–6)
Precautions: Limit weight bearing on affected leg
Weight Bearing Status: If the injury was isolated, the patient reliable, and fixation secure, the splint is replaced with a removable brace. If not, short leg NWB cast for another 4 weeks.
Goals: protect surgical site, allow healing
Program:
- If the injury was isolated, the patient reliable, and fixation secure, the splint is replaced with a removable brace.
- If any of these three factors is absent, a short-leg non-weight-bearing cast is recommended for an additional 4 weeks.
- Gait training with crutches or walker
- ADLs

Phase III (Weeks 6–10)
Precautions: AVOID painful ambulation
Weight Bearing Status: PWB with removable protective boot
Goals: increase ROM and strength, independent HEP

Program:
- Self-directed PT: ROM, PRE
- Swimming and bicycling
- Gradually advance weight bearing by end of phase per MD
- If mild swelling, start wearing regular shoe
- Compression stockings

Phase IV **(>10 Weeks)**
Precautions: AVOID running and jumping for 9–12 months
Weight Bearing Status: Progress to WBAT. Begin to wear regular shoe.
Goals: return to work and sports
Program:
- Advance to standard work shoe
- Custom-molded full-length insole of a nonrigid material such as cork or pelite
- Return to heavy labor in 3–4 months

Most patients have some symptoms in the foot for up to 2 years
Many will have lifelong symptoms [58]

Upper Extremity Fractures/Surgical Repair

Proximal Humerus Fractures (812.00)

- 5% of all fractures
- Axillary artery gives rise to anterior humeral circumflex artery at the inferior border of the subscapularis muscle
- It anastomoses with the posterior humeral circumflex artery (accompanies the axillary nerve through the quadrilateral space)
- Ascending branch of the anterior humeral circumflex artery comes lateral to the bicipital groove and supplies articular segment of humerus
- This vessel then becomes the arcuate artery and supplies the humeral head [59]

Four-Part Classification (Snider 1997)
Four parts of the humerus:
1. Greater tuberosity
2. Lesser tuberosity

3. Head
4. Shaft

Fragment = portion angulated >45° or displaced at least 1 cm

One part: Nondisplaced, impacted fractures
Two part: One fragment is displaced in reference to others
Three part: Two fragments are displaced
Four part: All fragments are displaced

Common locations
- Surgical neck (most common): can injure axillary nerve with anterior fracture-dislocation
- Anatomical neck: can injure axillary nerve with anterior fracture-dislocation
- Greater tuberosity: can injure rotator cuff muscles as they attach here
- Lesser tuberosity: can injure subscapularis as it attaches here

Symptoms:
- Severe pain, swelling, and ecchymosis
- Numbness/tingling, weakness

Physical Exam:
- Inspection can show swelling, ecchymosis, painful ROM [60]
- Check neurovascular system for compromise which can lead to AVN
- Medial or lateral deformity depending on the pull of the rotator cuffs on the fractured part
  - Deformities not usually seen due to swelling [59]
- Surgical neck fractures can be involve Axillary nerve
  - Can see weakness of teres minor and deltoid (Shoulder ER and abduction)
  - Decreased sensation at lateral shoulder
- Radial and ulnar nerves more involved than median nerve

Imaging:
- AP and lateral X-rays of shoulder
- Axillary X-ray is best for glenoid articular fractures but may be difficult due to pain
- CT is helpful for articular involvement, degree of fracture displacement, impression fractures, and glenoid rim fractures
- MRI is generally not indicated unless concerned about RTC integrity [60]

Treatment:
- Loss of consciousness and posterior fracture/dislocation indicates seizure: perform appropriate workup [59]
- One part fracture: see above
  - Conservative treatment with early ROM and sling immobilization for 6 weeks
  - AROM, pendulum exercises as tolerated
- Two, Three, and Four Part fractures:
  - Surgical intervention—arthroplasty or ORIF

Arthroplasty
Indications:
- Four-part fractures and fracture dislocations
- Head-splitting fractures
- Impression fractures involving more than 40% of articular surface
- Selected three-part fractures in older patients with osteoporotic bone

ORIF
Indications:
- All other fractures requiring surgery

Rehabilitation Program for ORIF:
Phase I (Weeks 0–4)
Precautions:
- If greater tuberosity repaired, wait for soft tissue to heal before active abduction or external rotation
- If lesser tuberosity repaired, AVOID active internal rotation or passive external rotation
- NWB
- AVOID ROM outside of surgeon preference

Weight Bearing Status:
Goals: early mobilization, protect surgical site
Modalities: Cryotherapy
Program:
- Pendulum exercises immediately
- Gentle AAROM once wound is healed around 2 weeks

Phase II (Weeks 4–8)
Precautions: AVOID leaning on affected arm
Weight Bearing Status: PWB per surgeon if X-rays show fracture healing around 6–8 weeks

Goals: increase ROM
Program:
- When wound is healed, begin gentle AAROM (see precautions in phase I)
- ADLs within specified ROM

Phase III (>8 Weeks)
Precautions: AVOID excessive weight bearing on affected side early in phase
Weight Bearing Status: Advance to WBAT per surgeon
Goals: increase strength, maximize ROM, return to normal activities [61]
Program:
- PROM, AROM
- Begin PRE
- Functional activities with affected arm [62]

Rehabilitation Program for Arthroplasty:
Phase I (Weeks 0–6)
Precautions: AVOID ROM outside of surgeon preference
Weight Bearing Status: NWB
Goals: prevent contracture, reduce pain
Program:
- Early PROM with abduction in scapular plane to 90° POD #1
- Start pendulum exercises POD #2
- Cryotherapy
- PROM forward elevation and supine external rotation with a stick

Phase II (Weeks 7–12)
Precautions: AVOID excessive weight bearing
Weight Bearing Status: Advance to WBAT
Goals: increase ROM, strengthen shoulder
Program:
- AAROM with pulley
- Isometrics for rotator cuff and deltoid
- Start PRE after 2–3 weeks
- ADLs [63]

Phase III (>12 Weeks)
Precautions: AVOID heavy lifting and painful ADLs
Weight Bearing Status: WBAT
Goals: return to normal activities

Program:
- AROM and stretching
- PRE
- Functional activities
- Sports-specific training [61]

Humeral Shaft Fractures (812.20)

- Relatively common fracture; up to 5% of all fractures

Pathophysiology:
- Fall on outstretched hand (FOOSH)
- MVA

Symptoms:
- Upper arm pain and swelling

Physical Exam:
- Swelling and deformity
- Assess radial nerve

Imaging:
- AP and lateral X-rays

Treatment:
- Minor fractures can be treated with splinting for 2 weeks
- Severe displacement and radial nerve injury require surgery [9]
- ORIF versus IM nailing based on surgeon preference

Rehabilitation Program for ORIF:
Phase I (**Weeks 0–6**)
Precautions: AVOID painful ROM
Weight Bearing Status: NWB
Goals: FROM in elbow and shoulder by 6 weeks
Modalities: Cryotherapy
Program:
- Sling for first 1–2 days
- Then AROM
- ROM of other joints
- PROM and stretching later in phase

Phase II **(Weeks 6–12)**
Precautions: limit weight bearing on affected side
Weight Bearing Status: PWB if X-rays show healing; otherwise NWB
Goals: increase strength
Program:
- Light weights at 6 weeks
- Regular weights at 12 weeks
- PROM, AROM
- ADLs

Phase III **(>12 Weeks)**
Precautions: limit painful weight bearing
Weight Bearing Status: progress to WBAT
Goals: return to normal activities
Program:
- Heavy work can start at 16 weeks
- Sports-specific training
- Ease into sports at 16 weeks [64]

Rehabilitation Program for IM Nail:
Precautions: AVOID painful ROM
Weight Bearing Status: NWB until surgeon feels fracture is stable
Goals: regain full ROM and strength
Program:
- Sling for 4–6 weeks
- Pendulum exercises and gentle PROM of elbow after POD#2
- No formal PT required
- HEP tailored based on method of nailing, fracture stability, and patient health [65]

Distal Radial Fractures (813.41)

- Most common fractures of the forearm

Pathophysiology:
- FOOSH
- Other Trauma
- In ages 35–64, incidence is greater in women.

Physical Exam:
- Pain and swelling at distal radius
- Check pulse and sensation
- Palpate for deformity

Symptoms:
- Wrist pain and swelling

Imaging:
- AP and lateral X-rays of forearm
- Consider hand, clavicle, and other parts of ipsilateral arm depending on pain
- Colles' Fracture: dorsal angulation of distal fragment
- Smith (Reverse Colles') Fracture: ventral angulation of distal fragment [9]

Treatment:
- Orthopedic referral for closed reduction with casting
- Closed reduction with external fixation
- Percutaneous pinning
- Open Reduction with Internal Fixation (ORIF)

Rehabilitation Program:
Protective Phase **(Weeks 0–6)**
Precautions: report early signs of CRPS to MD (unresolved joint stiffness, swelling, hypersensitivity, allodynia, shiny skin)
Weight Bearing Status: NWB
Goals: maintain immobilization, decreased edema and pain, FROM of other joints
Program:
- Early shoulder ROM to prevent adhesive capsulitis
- Elbow ROM
- Gentle, pain-free forearm rotation with MD approval
- Gentle wrist ROM in all planes
- Tendon gliding
- Hand intrinsic exercises
- Wrist splint in 0–20° wrist extension: open thenar and distal palmar crease to prevent stiffness

Stability Phase **(Weeks 6–8)**
Precautions: limit painful weight bearing
Weight Bearing Status: PWB if evidence of healing on X-rays; otherwise NWB

Goals: increase ROM of wrist and forearm, decrease edema, light use of involved arm
Modalities: Cryotherapy
Program:
- Wean off splint based on surgeon (when callus seen on X-ray)
- External fixator removed if present
- Scar friction massage
- Retrograde massage, gentle heat or contrast baths for edema
- Light, compressive garment (Coban, Tubigrip)
- Gentle AAROM and AROM of wrist and forearm
- Isolated wrist extension exercises to prevent use of finger extensors as primary wrist extension mechanism
- Gentle mobilization if fracture stable
- Fine motor coordination
- ADLs

Phase III (**>8 Weeks**)
Precautions: AVOID pain and compensations
Weight Bearing Status: progress to WBAT
Goals: Maximize strength, return to previous activities
Program:
- PROM and stretching
- Joint mobilization
- Serial static progressive splinting
- Isometric and dynamic gripping and pinching
- Wrist and forearm PRE
- Activity-specific activities and return to sport [66]

Scaphoid Fracture (814.01)

- More common in younger, active patients
- Four parts: proximal pole, waist, distal pole, and tuberosity
- 70% occurs at the waist, 20% at proximal pole
- 5–10% nonunion with immobilization
- Distal pole has rich blood supply
- Proximal pole has poor blood supply and require prolonged immobilization
- Fracture at waist can cause AVN, delayed union, or nonunion

Pathophysiology:
• FOOSH with wrist hyperextended and radially deviated

Symptoms:
• Wrist pain and swelling

Physical Exam:
• Tenderness of scaphoid and anatomic snuffbox [67]
• Neurovascular exam checking for integrity of median, ulnar, and radial nerves; capillary refill
• May have gross deformity from displacement of carpus to prominence of individual carpal bones

Imaging:
• AP, lateral, oblique, and "scaphoid" views show fracture and/or dislocation

Treatment:
Closed reduction with Percutaneous Pinning (CRPP)
• Minimally displaced fractures

ORIF
• Displaced fractures

Rehabilitation Program:
Protective Phase (**Weeks 0–4**)
Precautions: early motion in shoulder to prevent adhesive capsulitis
Weight Bearing Status: NWB
Goals: prevent adhesive capsulitis, minimize pain and edema
Modalities: Cryotherapy
Program:
• Volar or bivalve forearm thumb spica splint: 0–20° wrist extension; thumb immobilized with IP joint free
• Rest, compression garment
• Tendon gliding
• Interossei exercises
• ROM in other joints of ipsilateral arm

Phase II (**Week 4–16**)
Precautions: limit painful weight bearing
Weight Bearing Status: PWB if evidence of healing on X-rays; otherwise NWB
Goals: increase ROM, light functional use of wrist/hand
Modalities: Cryotherapy

Program:
- Continue splint; use static progressive splints later on
- Scar massage once wound is fully healed
- Thumb, wrist, and forearm ROM
- Progress to AAROM and PROM
- Isolated wrist extension exercises
- Fine motor coordination
- ADLs

Phase III (>16 Weeks)
Precautions: progress strengthening slowly, AVOID pain
Weight Bearing Status: progress to WBAT
Goals: maximize ROM and strength, return to work
Program:
- PROM, stretching
- Isometrics
- Grip and pinch strengthening
- PRE for wrist and forearm
- Work conditioning [68]

Finger Fractures (816.00)

- Distal phalangeal fractures are the most common
- Metacarpal neck fractures occur mostly at ring and small fingers (Boxer's fracture)
- Thumb proximal phalanx fracture is more common than metacarpal shaft fracture
- Bennett's fracture: fracture subluxation of thumb metacarpal base

Pathophysiology:
- Axial load or "jamming" injuries
- Diaphyseal fractures and joint dislocations occurs when hand is trapped resulting in a bending component
- Digits caught in furniture or equipment can cause a torsional stress leading to spiral fractures
- Crushing mechanisms in industrial work environments

Symptoms:
- Pain, swelling

Physical Exam:
- Capillary refill should be <2 s
- Two point discrimination at 6 mm
- Strength testing: finger flexors/extensors at DIP, PIP, and MCP
- ROM
- Rotation and angular deformity

Imaging:
- AP, lateral, and oblique X-rays show fracture and displacement
- Individual digits should be viewed separately to minimize overlap [69]

Treatment:
ORIF or Percutaneous Pinning
- Displaced, transverse fractures
- Fractures into joint line
- Flexor digitorium profundus avulsion injuries
- Angulated, malrotated, open, or multiple metacarpal fractures
- Thumb Ulnar Collateral Ligament (UCL) tear

Rehabilitation Program:
Phase I (Week 1)
Precautions: protect surgical site; no motion of joints adjacent to fracture until clinical union
Weight Bearing Status: NWB
Goals: reduce edema and pain, protective immobilization
Modalities: Cryotherapy
Program:
- Custom Thermoplastic Splint: hand/forearm-based gutter versus volar-based splint
- elevation
- ROM of uninvolved joints of ipsilateral arm

Phase II (Weeks 2–6)
Precautions: AVOID resistive exercises, excessive passive stress to injury
Weight Bearing Status: PWB if evidence of healing on X-rays; otherwise NWB
Goals: free gliding tendons, nonadherent scar
Program:
- Continue splint
- Scar management
- Heat modalities

- AAROM and AROM
- Tendon gliding
- Light functional use of hand in splint

Phase III **(>7 Weeks)**
Precautions: AVOID resistive exercises or static progressive splints until fracture healed
Weight Bearing Status: progress to WBAT
Goals: maximize ROM, increase strength and endurance, independent in ADLs
Program:
- Wean from splint
- Scar management
- AROM, PROM, stretching
- Eventually start PRE to hand and wrist
- Functional activities [70]

S/P CTS Release (354)

Indications:
- Atrophy of abductor pollicus brevis
- Severe and nearly constant numbness and/or pain
- Failure of conservative treatment [71]

Rehabilitation Program:
Phase I **(Weeks 0–4)**
Precautions: AVOID unnecessary elbow flexion because it may irritate the nerve
Weight Bearing Status: NWB
Goals: prevent contractures, maintain ROM
Program:
- Tendon and nerve gliding
- Bulky dressing is used to restrict wrist range of motion in the first 2 days
- ROM for fingers, wrist, and arm
- Wrist splint in neutral position for 3 weeks

Phase II **(>4 Weeks)**
Precautions: AVOID painful activities; Return to work with a 2-lb weight restriction

Weight Bearing Status: WBAT
Goals: return to work and normal activities
Program:
- AROM
- Strengthening of hand intrinsics
- HEP
- At 6–8 weeks, full activity without restrictions [72]

S/P Ulnar Nerve Decompression (354.2)

Indications:
- No improvement after 4–6 weeks of conservative treatment (night splinting, NSAIDS)
- Electromyography (EMG) shows compression at elbow

Pathophysiology:
- Repetitive/prolonged compression of ulnar nerve at elbow

Symptoms:
- Numbness/tingling in medial 1½ digits

Physical Exam:
- Decreased sensation in ulnar distribution
- Positive Tinel at elbow
- Symptoms with ulnar stretch: elbow flexion, wrist extension

Imaging:
- MRI

Treatment:
Ligament release (in situ decompression)
Anterior transposition of ulnar nerve (subcutaneous or submuscular)
Medial Epicondylectomy

Rehabilitation Program:
Phase I (Weeks 0–2)
Precautions: AVOID painful exercises, elbow extension > 90°, sensory
Weight Bearing Status: NWB
Goals: reduce edema and pain, prevent contractures in other joints, independent HEP

Modalities: Cryotherapy
Program:
- If flexor-pronator muscles are reattached, AVOID active wrist flexion/extension or forearm pronation
- Elbow in sling or splint: 90° with forearm and wrist in neutral
- Compression wrapping, elevation
- AROM elbow flexion, forearm pronation, and supination guided by pain
- Gentle PROM elbow flexion
- AROM to other joints
- HEP

Phase II **(Weeks 3–7)**
Precautions: same as Phase I; AVOID excessive elbow flexion/extension
Weight Bearing Status: NWB
Goals: scar management, increase ROM, free nerve adhesions, task modification
Program:
- Same precautions as phase I
- Wean splint
- Scar massage
- Elbow/forearm AROM progressing to PROM
- Progress elbow extension
- Ulnar nerve gliding
- Hand and pinch strengthening
- Isometric elbow exercises ~70° at 4 weeks
- ADLs

Phase III **(>8 Weeks)**
Precautions: slowly introduce and progress PRE
Weight Bearing Status: progress to WBAT
Goals: maximize ROM, increase strength and endurance, increase grip/pinch, return to normal activities
Program:
- Scar mobilization
- Ulnar nerve gliding
- Stretching
- Grip and pinch strengthening
- Begin PRE to elbow
- Forearm and wrist strengthening

- Dexterity exercises
- Progress to sports-specific training [73]

S/P Rotator Cuff Repair

Partial Tear of Rotator Cuff (726.13)

- Most commonly affects supraspinatus [9]
- Supraspinatus: shoulder external rotator, keeps humerus in glenoid fossa with shoulder movement, assists deltoid in abduction, depresses humeral head
- Infraspinatus: shoulder external rotator, stabilizes glenohumeral joint, depresses humeral head
- Teres minor: shoulder external rotator, stabilizes glenohumeral joint, depresses humeral head
- Subscapularis: shoulder internal rotator, depresses humeral head [74]

Pathophysiology:
- Degeneration of tendon
- Poor potential for healing
- Vascular insufficiency
- Repetitive trauma
- Extrinsic mechanical pressure from surrounding coracoacromial arch [75]

Symptoms:
- Pain in lateral shoulder

Physical Exam:
- Drop arm test: Passively abduct arm to 90° and instruct patient to lower arm slowly. Positive if patient cannot perform indicating RTC tear.
- Empty can test: Arm abducted in scapular plane to 90° with thumbs down. Apply downward pressure to resist. Positive if weak or causes pain [76].

Imaging:
- MRI shoulder: highest quality image of shoulder, shows muscle atrophy or fatty infiltration, high cost, claustrophobia

- Arthrography: easily interpretable, limited to detecting full-thickness tears, invasive, involves contrast dye, rarely gives info about quality of tendon or precise location
- Ultrasonography: useful for full-thickness tears; difficulty revealing small tears; small, partial tears and degenerative and scarred tissue may look similar [75]

Treatment:
- Since 1980, trend toward arthroscopic surgery rather than open surgery
- Preserves deltoid; decreased post-op pain and stiffness
- Arthroscopic-assisted mini-open repair versus all-arthroscopic repair

Phase I (Weeks 0–3)
Precautions: AVOID active movements, pain with ROM, and isometrics; Sling immobilization when resting
Weight Bearing Status: NWB
Goals: protect RTC repair, decrease pain and inflammation, increase shoulder external/internal rotation to 45° and forward flexion to 120°
Modalities: Cryotherapy [77]
- TENS for pain management. High Volt for increased localized circulation. NMES to prevent rotator cuff inhibition/disuse atrophy and to assist with isometric and isotonic exercises and for scapular stabilization [78].
Program:
- Patient education on sleeping and activities
- Pendulum exercises
- AAROM forward flexion in supine
- PROM by therapist
- AROM of other joints in ipsilateral arm
- Scapula stabilization exercises
- Submaximal deltoid isometrics in neutral later in phase
- HEP

Phase II (Weeks 3–7)
Precautions: AVOID active elevation of arm, maximal RTC exercises
Weight Bearing Status: slowly progress to PWB
Goals: protect RTC repair, decrease pain and inflammation, increase forward flexion and external rotation ROM to almost 100% normal

Program:
- Discontinue sling per MD
- AAROM
- Pool therapy
- Physio ball scapular stabilization below 90°
- Isometrics: submaximal ER/IR, progress deltoid
- Isotonic exercises for scapula and elbow
- Humeral head stabilization exercises
- HEP

Phase III (**Weeks 7–13**)
Precautions: AVOID shoulder "hiking," heavy lifting, jerking movements; limit overhead activity
Weight Bearing Status: progress to WBAT
Goals: minimize pain and inflammation, FROM, increase strength, normal scapulothoracic rhythm, light ADL <90°
Program:
- Limit overhead activities
- Cryotherapy PRN
- Functional ROM: towel exercises
- Periscapular strengthening
- RTC isotonic exercises when scapular strength established
- Scapular rhythm exercises
- Upper body ergometer

Phase IV (**Weeks 14–19**)
Precautions: overhead activity only when achieved good shoulder stability
Weight Bearing Status: WBAT
Goals: strength 5/5, neuromuscular control, normal scapulothoracic rhythm throughout FROM
Program:
- Progress to overhead activity: latissimus pull down
- Isotonics for periscapular and RTC
- Stretching
- Scapular stabilization
- Plyometrics <90° per MD

Phase V (**Weeks 20–24**)
Precautions: AVOID painful activities
Weight Bearing Status: WBAT

Goals: maximize ROM, strength, and neuromuscular control for work, sports, and daily activities

Program:
- MD clearance for sports: Usually when patient has full ROM and strength without pain. It also depends on type of surgery, level of athlete, type of sport.
- Progress isotonics for periscapular and RTC
- Stretching
- Sports-specific exercises
- Plyometrics >90° per MD
- Interval training for pitchers and overhead athletes [77]

S/P Total Shoulder Arthroscopy

Shoulder OA (715.11) [79]

Pathophysiology:
- Degenerative
- Idiopathic

Symptoms:
- Shoulder pain

Physical Exam:
- Restricted ROM especially forward elevation, external rotation, and internal rotation
- Grinding on passive ROM
- Posterior joint line tenderness compared to contralateral normal side
- Ratcheting sensation felt when resisting ER, but normal strength

Imaging:
- AP, scapular lateral, and axillary view X-rays show joint space narrowing, osteophytes, sclerosis or cystic changes in humeral head; may see subluxation of humeral head posteriorly [9]
- MRI needed if RTC or other injury suspected

Treatment:
- PT
- Shoulder arthroplasty

Phase I **(0–6 weeks)**
Precautions: wearing sling when not in therapy [80]
Weight Bearing Status: NWB
Goals: Relieve pain, reduce edema, protect joint, and restore function [61], return to sedentary work by 2–3 weeks [80]
Modalities: Cryotherapy
– TENS for pain management. High Volt for increased localized circulation. NMES to prevent rotator cuff inhibition/disuse atrophy and to assist with isometric and isotonic exercises and for scapular stabilization [78]
Program:
• No active ROM, NWB, sling immobilization
• Pendulum exercises, progressive isometrics, gentle passive ROM
• Toward end of stage, progress to gentle active ROM such as wall-walking
• Elbow, wrist, and hand ROM and exercises
• Scapulothoracic mobilization
• Scapular strengthening

Phase II **(6–12 weeks)**
Precautions: AVOID painful activities
Weight Bearing Status: Begin weight bearing at 8 weeks [80]
Goals: Abduction to 150°, pain control, external rotation to 45°
Program:
• ROM based on MD
• Discontinue sling, start light weights
• PROM
• AAROM, progressive AROM
• Humeral head control exercises
• Isometrics: deltoid in neutral
• Internal rotation at 6 weeks
• Pool therapy
• Begin light upper body ergometry
• Scapular retraction with elastic bands
• HEP

Phase III **(12–16 weeks)**
Precautions: AVOID scapular hiking
Weight Bearing Status: progress to WBAT
Goals: no pain with ADLs, abduction to 160°, internal rotation to T12, normal scapulothoracic rhythm >90°, maximize strength

Program:
- Progress ROM, stretching
- PRE for scapula, elbow
- Isometrics: deltoid away from neutral
- Scapular stabilization
- Pool therapy
- Upper body ergometry
- Row and chest press
- HEP

Phase IV (**>16 weeks**)
Precautions: AVOID heavy lifting
Weight Bearing Status: WBAT
Goals: maximize ROM and strength, normal scapulothoracic rhythm >100°
Program:
- A/AROM, PROM
- Posterior capsule stretching, towel stretch
- PRE
- Scapular rhythm exercises
- Proprioceptive neuromuscular facilitation
- Sports-specific training [61]

POSTOPERATIVE COMPLICATIONS

Specifics on work up and treatments may be found in the Medical Complications and Emergencies In Rehabilitation Chapter.

Postoperative Fever

- Normal temperature is 37 °C. Fever is >38 °C
- *Fever workup*: chest X-ray, urinalysis, urine culture, blood cultures—from two separate sites, wound culture swab, CBC with differential
- Low grade fever may be due to cytokine release following tissue trauma and can be treated with Tylenol. Physician must ensure no underlying infection

- *Other noninfectious causes*: transfusion, postoperative atelectasis, hematoma, venous thromboembolism (VTE), acute myocardial infarct, intracranial pathology, pancreatitis, alcohol withdrawal, and medications
- *Infectious causes*: urinary tract infection (UTI), respiratory infection, wound infection, intravascular cathether-associated infection, gram negative septicemia, abdominal sepsis, Clostridium difficile colitis, and fungal infection
  - Infectious causes usually occur around POD #5 [81]

Atelectasis

- Occurs POD #1–5
- *Risk factors*: secretions, decreased alertness, aspiration, mechanical obstruction, smoking history, surgery >3 h, COPD, poor general health, use of pancuronium as neuromuscular blocker, BMI >25 kg/m^2

Symptoms: shortness of breath
Diagnosis: Chest X-ray
Treatment
  - Keep patient upright rather than supine in bed
    - ° Oxygen by nasal canula
    - ° Incentive spirometry
    - ° Early mobilization
  - Treat underlying cause (Pulmonary Complications) [82]

Urinary Tract Infection

- Most common cause of post op fever
- UTI accounts for 40% of infectious causes of postoperative fever

Diagnosis: Fever, suprapubic tenderness on physical exam and urine labs

Treatment
- Remove catheter as soon as possible
- Antibiotics: Bactrim or fluoroquinolone depending on susceptibility [83]

Pneumonia

- Second most common cause of postoperative fever
- *Risk factors*: age >65, immunocompromised, thoracoabdominal trauma or surgery, serious comorbidities, decreased alertness, malnutrition, ventilator.

Diagnosis
- Sputum culture, tracheal aspirate (in addition to general workup)

Treatment
- Antibiotics according to hospital guidelines [82]

Wound Dehiscence

- Separation of the layers of a surgical wound
- *Risk factors*: overweight, older age, poor nutrition, Diabetes Mellitus, smoking, malignant growth, presence of prior scar or radiation at site, noncompliance with post-op instructions, surgical error, increased abdominal pressure, long-term use of steroids, kidney disease, immune problems
- Symptoms: bleeding, pain, swelling, redness, fever, broken sutures, open wound
- Diagnosis: wound and tissue cultures, CBC
  - Consider X-ray or ultrasound to assess extent of wound
- Treatment:
  - Antibiotics
  - Frequent changes in wound dressing
  - Resuturing
  - May need surgical removal of contaminated dead tissue [84]

Wound Infection

- Fever on POD # 5–7
- Open fracture should be treated with prophylactic antibiotics starting before surgery. Duration of antibiotics is poorly studied.

Antibiotics should be continued 1–3 days after surgery unless otherwise needed.

Physical exam: Erythema, induration, swelling, warmth, wound dehiscence

- Must differentiate from contact dermatitis associated with local irritation from the wound dressing/tape. This also causes erythema. Contact dermatitis is usually accompanied by pruritis and vesicles, and has the shape of the dressing [81].
- If there is erythema but no swelling or fluid collection, treat with antibiotic based on surgeon preference.

Treatment
- Cover for Staph aureus with Cefazolin 1 g IV q6–8 h [85]
- If infection is more serious and there is concern for osteomyelitis, consider Oxacillin 2 g q6 h IV (methicillin-sensitive) or Vancomycin 1 g q12 h IV (MRSA). Consult Infectious Disease to ensure proper coverage [81]
- If fluid collection, copious drainage, and fever are present, patient may need wound opening and likely debridement. Consult Infectious Diseases [85, 86].

    Wound dressings: prevent infection, absorb exudates, hypoallergenic, and occlude
    - Semi-impermeable films: OpSite, Tegaderm, Bio-Occlusive
    - Occlusive hydrocolloids (Duoderm) are permeable to water vapor and oxygen
    - No concensus on superiority of a specific type of dressing [81]

Seroma

- Collection of serum in tissue spaces
- *Risk factors*: Diabetes Mellitus, obesity, poor vascular status, smoking, chemotherapy, radiation therapy, and use of steroids
- Complications: infection, slower healing, need for surgical interventions [87]
- Normal dressing after surgery: Dry sterile dressing with gauze [88]
  Symptoms
  - Discomfort around wound, pain, redness

Treatment
– Most seromas resolve in 4 weeks
– Slings or special wraps have been proposed but have the risk of limiting ROM
– Aspiration is well-tolerated if patient experiences significant discomfort [89]
– Limited evidence that negative pressure wound therapy prevents seroma formation after THA [88]

Venous Thromboembolism

- <u>Virchow's triad:</u> hypercoaguable state, venous stasis, and endothelial injury
- Incidence between 6 and 60%
- *Risk factors*: orthopedic trauma with femur or tibia fracture, advanced age, recent blood transfusion, surgery

Deep venous thrombosis (DVT)
- *Symptoms*: calf pain and swelling, unilateral pitting edema
- Diagnosed with Ultrasound doppler

Pulmonary embolism (PE)
- *Symptoms*: dyspnea, chest pain, hemoptysis, syncope, hypotension, right sided heart failure if embolism is large
- Work up:
    – EKG—shows sinus tachycardia but nonspecific
    – Labs—Fibrin D-Dimer but very nonspecific especially after trauma or postoperatively
    – Pulmonary angiography—gold standard
        ○ CT angiography is less invasive with a specificity of 96% and sensitivity of 83%
- PE can be fatal in 2/3 of patients

Treatment: DVT and PE are usually *treated* with warfarin or Low Molecular Weight Heparin (LMWH). Treatment will depend on hospital protocol and/or vascular consult.

<u>Thromboembolic Prevention/Prophylaxis</u>
- Early mobilization, adequate hydration to prevent hemoconcentration and physical prophylaxis

- Addition of compression stockings have not been shown to reduce DVT and compliance is poor
- Chemical prophylaxis
  - DVT prophylaxis is usually dictated by the surgeon when patient is postoperative
  - LMWH and Fondaparinux are shown to be effective and are the most common agents used.
- One large study showed that Aspirin significantly reduced VTE, but a major criticism is that some patients may have also received other means of chemoprophylaxis.
- Duration of prophylaxis is also controversial. Some evidence suggests that there is increased risk up to 3 months after surgery and that there may be rebound thrombophilia after cessation of prophylaxis after discharge. Many patients are discharged after 7–10 days. Therefore, the duration of prophylaxis will be dependent on the extent of injuries, risk of bleeding, patient mobility and balance, and ultimately the surgeon's preference.
- *Inferior vena cava filters* do not fully eliminate the risk of PE and may increase risk of DVT. Generally used if chemoprophylaxis is contraindicated (intracranial bleeding, abdominal injury) [83].

References

1. Cahill JB, Kosman LM. Total knee arthroplasty. In: Cioppa-Mosca J, Cahill JB, Cavanaugh JT, et al., editors. Postsurgical rehabilitation guidelines for the orthopedic clinician. St. Louis, MO: Mosby Elsevier; 2006. p. 21–7.
2. Merchants View. http://eorif.com/KneeLeg/Xray%20knee.html. Accessed 7 Nov 2011.
3. Brosseau L, et al. Thermotherapy for treatment of osteoarthritis. Cochrane Database Syst Rev 2003;4:CD004522.
4. Placzek JD, Boyce DA. Orthopaedic physical therapy secrets. 2nd ed. St. Louis, MO: Mosby Elsevier; 2006.
5. Jerosch J, Aldawoudy AM. Arthroscopic treatment of patients with moderate arthrofibrosis of after total knee replacement. Knee Surg Sports Traumatol Arthrosc. 2007;1:71–7.
6. Baydar ML, Gur E, Kirdemir V, Engin AS. The role of arthroscopic adhesiolysis in the treatment of the arthrofibrosis and the partial ankylosis of the knee. Acta Orthop Traumatol Turc. 1994;28(5):379–83.
7. Fitzsimmons SE, Vazquez BS, Bronson MJ. How to treat the stiff total knee arthroplasty? A systematic review. Clin Orthop Relat Res. 2010;468:1096–106.

8. Okumiya K. The timed "up & go" test is a useful predictor of falls in community-dwelling older people. J Am Geriatr Soc. 1998;46(7):928–30.

9. Brown DP, Freeman ED, Cuccurullo S. Musculoskeletal medicine. In: Cuccurullo S, editor. Physical medicine and rehabilitation board review. New York, NY: Demos Medical Publishing; 2004. p. 191–255.

10. Cavanaugh JT. Anterior cruciate ligament reconstruction. In: Cioppa-Mosca J, Cahill JB, Cavanaugh JT, et al., editors. Postsurgical rehabilitation guidelines for the orthopedic clinician. St. Louis, MO: Mosby Elsevier; 2006. p. 426–37.

11. Alentorn-Geli E, Myer GD, Silvers HJ, et al. Prevention of noncontact anterior cruciate ligament injuries in soccer players. Part 1: Mechanisms of injury and underlying risk factors. Knee Surg Sports Traumatol Arthrosc. 2009;17(7):705–29.

12. Andrus S, Malanga GA, Stuart M. Physical examination of the knee. In: Malanga GA, Nadler SF, editors. Musculoskeletal physical examination: an evidence-based approach. Philadelphia, PA: Mosby Elsevier; 2006. p. 279–94.

13. Sports Medicine Institute: University of Minnesota Orthopaedics. Pivot Shift. http://www.sportsdoc.umn.edu/Clinical_Folder/Knee_Folder/Knee_Exam/pivot%20shift.htm. Accessed 7 Nov 2011.

14. Kaufman MS. Knee injuries and conditions. In: Harrast MA, Finnoff JT, editors. Sports medicine: study guide and review for boards. New York, NY: Demos Medical Publishing; 2012. p. 277–89.

15. Feil S, Nevell J, Minogue C, Paessler HH. The effectiveness of supplementing a standard rehabilitation program with superimposed neuromuscular electrical stimulation after anterior cruciate ligament reconstruction. Am J Sports Med. 2011;39(6):1238–47.

16. Cavanaugh J. Posterior cruciate ligament reconstruction. In: Cioppa-Mosca J, Cahill JB, Cavanaugh JT, et al., editors. Postsurgical rehabilitation guidelines for the orthopedic clinician. St. Louis, MO: Mosby Elsevier; 2006. p. 440–50.

17. Ittivej K, Prompaet S, Rojanasthien S. Factors influencing the treatment of posterior cruciate ligament injury. J Med Assoc Thai. 2005;88:S84–8.

18. Wilk KE. Rehabilitation of isolated and combined posterior cruciate ligament injuries. Clin Sports Med. 1994;13(3):649–77.

19. Karachalios T, et al. Diagnostic accuracy of a new clinical test (the Thessaly test) for early detection of meniscal tears. J Bone Joint Surg Am. 2005;87:955–62.

20. Cavanaugh JT, Gately CT. Meniscal repair and transplantation. In: Cioppa-Mosca J, Cahill JB, Cavanaugh JT, et al., editors. Postsurgical rehabilitation guidelines for the orthopedic clinician. St. Louis, MO: Mosby Elsevier; 2006. p. 454–64.

21. Jarit GJ, Mohr KJ, Waller R, Glousman RE. The effects of home interferential therapy on post operative pain, edema, and range of motion of the knee. Clin J Sports Med. 2003;13(1):16–20.

22. Tornetta P. Hip dislocations and fractures of the femoral head. In: Bucholz RW, Heckman JD, Court-Brown CM, editors. Rockwood & Green's fractures in adults. Philadelphia, PA: Lippincott Williams and Wilkins; 2006. p. 1715–50.

23. Tucker CY, Diamond A. Total hip arthroplasty. In: Cioppa-Mosca J, Cahill JB, Cavanaugh JT, et al., editors. Postsurgical rehabilitation guidelines for the orthopedic clinician. St. Louis, MO: Mosby Elsevier; 2006. p. 3–15.

24. Leung K. Subtrochanteric fractures. In: Bucholz RW, Heckman JD, Court-Brown CM, editors. Rockwood & Green's fractures in adults. Philadelphia, PA: Lippincott Williams and Wilkins; 2006. p. 1827–44.

25. Netter FH. Lower Limb. In: Netter FH, editor. Atlas of human anatomy. 3rd ed. Teterboro, NJ: Icon Learning Systems; 2003. p. 467–528.

26. Ganz SB. Hip fracture. In: Cioppa-Mosca J, Cahill JB, Cavanaugh JT, et al., editors. Postsurgical rehabilitation guidelines for the orthopedic clinician. St. Louis, MO: Mosby Elsevier; 2006. p. 59–72.

27. Gardner MJ, Johnson EE, Lorch DG. Subtrochanteric femur fractures: plate fixation. In: Wiss DA, Anglen JO, Bak SF, et al., editors. Master techniques in orthopaedic surgery: fractures. Philadelphia, PA: Lippincott Williams & Wilkins; 2006. p. 276–87.

28. Russell T. Subtrochanteric femur fractures: reconstruction nailing. In: Wiss DA, Anglen JO, Bak SF, et al., editors. Master techniques in orthopaedic surgery: fractures. Philadelphia, PA: Lippincott Williams & Wilkins; 2006. p. 292–315.

29. Leighton RK. Fractures of the neck of the femur. In: Bucholz RW, Heckman JD, Court-Brown CM, editors. Rockwood & Green's fractures in adults. Philadelphia, PA: Lippincott Williams and Wilkins; 2006. p. 1753–88.

30. Santos ERG, Swiontkowski MF. Femoral neck fractures: open reduction internal fixation. In: Wiss DA, Anglen JO, Bak SF, et al., editors. Master techniques in orthopaedic surgery: fractures. Philadelphia, PA: Lippincott Williams & Wilkins; 2006. p. 208–14.

31. Anglen JO. Femoral neck fractures: arthroplasty. In: Wiss DA, Anglen JO, Bak SF, et al., editors. Master techniques in orthopaedic surgery: fractures. Philadelphia, PA: Lippincott Williams & Wilkins; 2006. p. 217–27.

32. Baumgaertner MR, Taksali S. Intertrochanteric hip fractures: intramedullary hip screws. In: Wiss DA, Anglen JO, Bak SF, et al., editors. Master techniques in orthopaedic surgery: fractures. Philadelphia, PA: Lippincott Williams & Wilkins; 2006. p. 249–62.

33. Haidukewych GJ. Hip arthroplasty for intertrochanteric hip fractures. In: Wiss DA, Anglen JO, Bak SF, et al., editors. Master techniques in orthopaedic surgery: fractures. Philadelphia, PA: Lippincott Williams & Wilkins; 2006. p. 265–73.

34. Nork SE. Fractures of the shaft of the femur. In: Bucholz RW, Heckman JD, Court-Brown CM, editors. Rockwood & Green's fractures in adults. Philadelphia, PA: Lippincott Williams and Wilkins; 2006. p. 1845–910.

35. Browner BD, Caputo AE, Mazzocca AD, Wiss DA. Femur fractures: antegrade intramedullary nailing. In: Wiss DA, Anglen JO, Bak SF, et al., editors. Master techniques in orthopaedic surgery: fractures. Philadelphia, PA: Lippincott Williams & Wilkins; 2006. p. 324–48.

36. Ostrum RF, Farrell ED. Femoral shaft fractures: retrograde nailing. In: Wiss DA, Anglen JO, Bak SF, et al., editors. Master techniques in orthopaedic surgery: fractures. Philadelphia, PA: Lippincott Williams & Wilkins; 2006. p. 352–9.

37. Kanlic EM, Pacheco HO. Pelvic fractures: external fixation and C-clamp. In: Wiss DA, Anglen JO, Bak SF, et al., editors. Master techniques in orthopaedic surgery: fractures. Philadelphia, PA: Lippincott Williams & Wilkins; 2006. p. 621–2.

38. Starr AJ, Malekzadeh AS. Fractures of the pelvic ring. In: Bucholz RW, Heckman JD, Court-Brown CM, editors. Rockwood & Green's fractures in adults. Philadelphia, PA: Lippincott Williams and Wilkins; 2006. p. 1584–662.

39. Temple DC, Schmidt AH, Sems SA. Diastasis of the symphysis pubis: open reduction internal fixation. In: Wiss DA, Anglen JO, Bak SF, et al., editors. Master techniques in orthopaedic surgery: fractures. Philadelphia, PA: Lippincott Williams & Wilkins; 2006. p. 640–8.

40. Routt MLC. Posterior pelvic-ring disruptions: iliosacral screws. In: Wiss DA, Anglen JO, Bak SF, et al., editors. Master techniques in orthopaedic surgery: fractures. Philadelphia, PA: Lippincott Williams & Wilkins; 2006. p. 650–65.

41. Reilly MC. Fractures of the acetabulum. In: Bucholz RW, Heckman JD, Court-Brown CM, editors. Rockwood & Green's fractures in adults. Philadelphia, PA: Lippincott Williams and Wilkins; 2006. p. 1665–712.

42. Moed BR. Acetabular fractures: The Kocher-Langenbeck approach. In: Wiss DA, Anglen JO, Bak SF, et al., editors. Master techniques in orthopaedic surgery: fractures. Philadelphia, PA: Lippincott Williams & Wilkins; 2006. p. 686–706.

43. Matta JM, Reilly MC. Acetabular fractures: ilioinguinal approach. In: Wiss DA, Anglen JO, Bak SF, et al., editors. Master techniques in orthopaedic surgery: fractures. Philadelphia, PA: Lippincott Williams & Wilkins; 2006. p. 712–27.

44. Bartlett CS, Malkani AL, Sen MK, Helfet DL. Acetabular fractures: extended iliofemoral approach. In: Wiss DA, Anglen JO, Bak SF, et al., editors. Master techniques in orthopaedic surgery: fractures. Philadelphia, PA: Lippincott Williams & Wilkins; 2006. p. 730–45.

45. Egol KA, Koval KJ. Fractures of the proximal tibia. In: Bucholz RW, Heckman JD, Court-Brown CM, editors. Rockwood & Green's fractures in adults. Philadelphia, PA: Lippincott Williams and Wilkins; 2006. p. 2000–27.

46. Watson JT, Wiss DA. Tibial plateau fractures: open reduction internal fixation. In: Wiss DA, Anglen JO, Bak SF, et al., editors. Master techniques in orthopaedic surgery: fractures. Philadelphia, PA: Lippincott Williams & Wilkins; 2006. p. 408–35.

47. Stannard JP. Proximal tibia fractures: locked plating. In: Wiss DA, Anglen JO, Bak SF, et al., editors. Master techniques in orthopaedic surgery: fractures. Philadelphia, PA: Lippincott Williams & Wilkins; 2006. p. 440–51.

48. Court-Brown CM. Fractures of the tibia and fibula. In: Bucholz RW, Heckman JD, Court-Brown CM, editors. Rockwood & Green's fractures in adults. Philadelphia, PA: Lippincott Williams and Wilkins; 2006. p. 2079–143.

49. Winquist RA, Johnson K, Wiss DA. Tibial shaft fractures: intramedullary nailing. In: Wiss DA, Anglen JO, Bak SF, et al., editors. Master techniques in orthopaedic surgery: fractures. Philadelphia, PA: Lippincott Williams & Wilkins; 2006. p. 468–82.

50. Bolhofner BR. Tibial shaft fractures: open reduction internal fixation. In: Wiss DA, Anglen JO, Bak SF, et al., editors. Master techniques in orthopaedic surgery: fractures. Philadelphia, PA: Lippincott Williams & Wilkins; 2006. p. 454–66.

51. Borrelli J. Tibial pilon fractures: open reduction internal fixation. In: Wiss DA, Anglen JO, Bak SF, et al., editors. Master techniques in orthopaedic surgery: fractures. Philadelphia, PA: Lippincott Williams & Wilkins; 2006. p. 520–5.

52. Barei DP. Pilon Fractures. In: Bucholz RW, Heckman JD, Court-Brown CM, editors. Rockwood & Green's fractures in adults. Philadelphia, PA: Lippincott Williams and Wilkins; 2006. p. 1929–72.

53. Marsh JL, Saltzman CL. Ankle Fractures. In: Bucholz RW, Heckman JD, Court-Brown CM, editors. Rockwood & Green's fractures in adults. Philadelphia, PA: Lippincott Williams and Wilkins; 2006. p. 2147–242.

54. Hak DJ, Lee MA. Ankle fractures: open reduction internal fixation. In: Wiss DA, Anglen JO, Bak SF, et al., editors. Master techniques in orthopaedic surgery: fractures. Philadelphia, PA: Lippincott Williams & Wilkins; 2006. p. 552–65.

55. Sanders DW. Fractures of the talus. In: Bucholz RW, Heckman JD, Court-Brown CM, editors. Rockwood & Green's fractures in adults. Philadelphia, PA: Lippincott Williams and Wilkins; 2006. p. 2249–89.

56. Fortin PT, Wiater PJ. Talus fractures: open reduction internal fixation. In: Wiss DA, Anglen JO, Bak SF, et al., editors. Master techniques in orthopaedic surgery: fractures. Philadelphia, PA: Lippincott Williams & Wilkins; 2006. p. 570–82.

57. Early JS. Fractures and dislocations of the midfoot and forefoot. In: Bucholz RW, Heckman JD, Court-Brown CM, editors. Rockwood & Green's fractures in adults. Philadelphia, PA: Lippincott Williams and Wilkins; 2006. p. 2337–99.

58. Sangeorzan BJ, Benirschke SK, Gould MT. Tarsometatarsal lisfranc injuries: evaluation and management. In: Wiss DA, Anglen JO, Bak SF, et al., editors. Master techniques in orthopaedic surgery: fractures. Philadelphia, PA: Lippincott Williams & Wilkins; 2006. p. 606–17.

59. Warner JJ, Costouros JG, Gerber C. Fractures of the proximal humerus. In: Bucholz RW, Heckman JD, Court-Brown CM, editors. Rockwood & Green's fractures in adults. Philadelphia, PA: Lippincott Williams and Wilkins; 2006. p. 1162–204.

60. Koval KJ, Zuckerman JD. Proximal humerus fractures. In: Koval KJ, Zuckerman JD, editors. Handbook of fractures. Philadelphia, PA: Lippincott Williams & Wilkins; 2006. p. 165–71.

61. Cavanaugh JS, Cahil JB. Total shoulder arthroplasty. In: Cioppa-Mosca J, Cahill JB, Cavanaugh JT, et al., editors. Postsurgical rehabilitation guidelines for the orthopedic clinician. St. Louis, MO: Mosby Elsevier; 2006. p. 30–42.

62. Schmidt AH. Proximal humeral fractures: open reduction internal fixation. In: Wiss DA, Anglen JO, Bak SF, et al., editors. Master techniques in orthopaedic surgery: fractures. Philadelphia, PA: Lippincott Williams & Wilkins; 2006. p. 37–49.

63. Bigliani LU, Bak SF, Goldberg SS. Proximal humeral fractures: arthroplasty. In: Wiss DA, Anglen JO, Bak SF, et al., editors. Master techniques in orthopaedic surgery: fractures. Philadelphia, PA: Lippincott Williams & Wilkins; 2006. p. 51–64.

64. Robinson DE, O'Brien PJ. Humeral shaft fractures: open reduction internal fixation. In: Wiss DA, Anglen JO, Bak SF, et al., editors. Master techniques

in orthopaedic surgery: fractures. Philadelphia, PA: Lippincott Williams & Wilkins; 2006. p. 67–78.

65. Roberts CS, Walz BM, Yerasimides JG. Humeral shaft fractures: intramedullary nailing. In: Wiss DA, Anglen JO, Bak SF, et al., editors. Master techniques in orthopaedic surgery: fractures. Philadelphia, PA: Lippincott Williams & Wilkins; 2006. p. 81–94.

66. Gately CT. Distal radius fractures. In: Cioppa-Mosca J, Cahill JB, Cavanaugh JT, et al., editors. Postsurgical rehabilitation guidelines for the orthopedic clinician. St. Louis, MO: Mosby Elsevier; 2006. p. 110–4.

67. Koval KJ, Zuckerman JD. Pediatric wrist and hand. In: Koval KJ, Zuckerman JD, editors. Handbook of fractures. Philadelphia, PA: Lippincott Williams & Wilkins; 2006. p. 553–70.

68. Gately CT. Scaphoid fractures. In: Cioppa-Mosca J, Cahill JB, Cavanaugh JT, et al., editors. Postsurgical rehabilitation guidelines for the orthopedic clinician. St. Louis, MO: Mosby Elsevier; 2006. p. 118–22.

69. Koval KJ, Zuckerman JD. Hand. In: Koval KJ, Zuckerman JD, editors. Handbook of fractures. Philadelphia, PA: Lippincott Williams & Wilkins; 2006. p. 257–70.

70. Page C. Phalangeal and metacarpal fractures. In: Cioppa-Mosca J, Cahill JB, Cavanaugh JT, et al., editors. Postsurgical rehabilitation guidelines for the orthopedic clinician. St. Louis, MO: Mosby Elsevier; 2006. p. 126–32.

71. Freeman TL, Johnson E, Freeman ED, Brown DP. Electrodiagnostic medicine and clinical neuromuscular physiology. In: Cuccurullo S, editor. Physical medicine and rehabilitation board review. New York, NY: Demos Medical Publishing; 2004. p. 295–408.

72. Mackinnon SE, Novak CB. Compression neuropathies. In: Wolfe SW, Hotchkiss RN, Pederson WC, Kozin SH, editors. Wolfe: Green's operative hand surgery. Philadelphia, PA: Elsevier Churchill Livingstone; 2011. p. 990–1.

73. Barenholtz-Marshall A. Ulnar nerve transposition. In: Cioppa-Mosca J, Cahill JB, Cavanaugh JT, et al., editors. Postsurgical rehabilitation guidelines for the orthopedic clinician. St. Louis, MO: Mosby Elsevier; 2006. p. 194–9.

74. Glaser DL, Sher JS, Ricchetti ET, Williams GR, Soslowsky LJ. Anatomy, biomechanics, and pathophysiology of rotator cuff. In: Iannotti JP, Williams GR, editors. Disorders of the shoulder: diagnosis and management. Philadelphia, PA: Lippincott Williams & Wilkins; 2007. p. 3–33.

75. Craig EV. Mini-open and open techniques for full-thickness rotator cuff repairs. In: Craig EV, editor. Masters techniques in orthopedic surgery: shoulder. Philadelphia, PA: Lippincott Williams & Wilkins; 2004. p. 310–40.

76. Bowen JE, Malanga GA, Pappoe T, McFarland E. Physical examination of the shoulder. In: Malanga GA, Nadler SF, editors. Musculoskeletal physical examination: an evidence-based approach. Philadelphia, PA: Mosby Elsevier; 2006. p. 59–118.

77. Maschi R, Fives G. Rotator cuff repair: arthroscopic and open. In: Cioppa-Mosca J, Cahill JB, Cavanaugh JT, et al., editors. Postsurgical rehabilitation guidelines for the orthopedic clinician. St. Louis, MO: Mosby Elsevier; 2006. p. 501–9.

78. Reinold ML, et al. The effect of neuromuscular electrical stimulation of the infraspinatus on shoulder external rotation force production after rotator cuff repair surgery. Am J Sports Med. 2008;36(12):2317–21.

79. ICD9 Data.com. http://www.icd9data.com/2011/Volume1/default.htm. Accessed 24 Apr 2012.
80. Craig EV. Total shoulder replacement with intact bone and soft tissue. In: Craig EV, editor. Masters techniques in orthopedic surgery: shoulder. Philadelphia, PA: Lippincott Williams & Wilkins; 2004. p. 516–47.
81. Moholkar KD, Ziran BH. Local complications. In: Bucholz RW, Heckman JD, Court-Brown CM, Tornetta P, editors. Rockwood and Green's fractures in adults. Philadelphia, PA: Lippincott Williams & Wilkins; 2006. p. 569–84.
82. Hemmila MR. Pulmonary complications. In: Mulholland MW, Doherty GM, editors. Complications in surgery. Philadelphia, PA: Lippincott Williams & Wilkins; 2006. p. 157–72.
83. White T, Watts A. Systemic complications. In: Bucholz RW, Heckman JD, Court-Brown CM, Tornetta P, editors. Rockwood and Green's fractures in adults. Philadelphia, PA: Lippincott Williams & Wilkins; 2010. p. 590–9.
84. Wound Dehiscence. NYU Langone Medical Center. http://www.med.nyu.edu/content?ChunkIID=99918. Accessed 30 May 2012.
85. Doherty GM. Surgical site infections. In: Mulholland MW, Doherty GM, editors. Complications in surgery. Philadelphia, PA: Lippincott Williams & Wilkins; 2006. p. 114–24.
86. Ziran BH, Smith W, Rao N. Orthopedic infections and osteomyelitis. In: Bucholz RW, Heckman JD, Court-Brown CM, Tornetta P, editors. Rockwood and Green's fractures in adults. Philadelphia, PA: Lippincott Williams & Wilkins; 2010. p. 615–38.
87. Kilpadi DV, Cunningham MR. Evaluation of closed incision management with negative pressure wound therapy (CIM): hematoma/seroma and involvement of the lymphatic system. Wound Repair Regen. 2011;19(5):588–96.
88. Pachowksy M, et al. Negative pressure wound therapy to prevent seromas and treat surgical incisions after total hip arthroplasty. Int Orthop. 2012;36(4):719–22. Epub 15 Jul 2011.
89. Newman LA. Complications of breast surgery. In: Mulholland MW, Doherty GM, editors. Complications in surgery. Philadelphia, PA: Lippincott Williams & Wilkins; 2006. p. 606–30.
90. Patient Education Materials: Weight Bearing. UPMC. http://www.upmc.com/HealthAtoZ/patienteducation/R/Pages/weightbearing.aspx. Accessed 20 Jan 2012.

Chapter 5
Pediatric Rehabilitation

Sarah Khan and Colette Maduro

Initial Pediatric Evaluation

History

Prenatal/Perinatal history
- Prenatal complications
- Maternal health issues during pregnancy
- Delivery history: vaginal or C-section, and reason why C-section was performed
- Postnatal complications (e.g., sepsis, IVH, hyperbilirubinemia).

Developmental history: Age child achieved various developmental milestones
- Rolling, sitting alone, crawling, walking, first words, etc.

S. Khan, D.O. (✉)
Department of Physical Medicine and Rehabilitation,
Mount Sinai Medical Center, One Gustave L. Levy Place,
Box 1240, New York, NY 1029, USA
e-mail: dr.s.khan22@gmail.com

C. Maduro, D.O.
Department of Physical Medicine and Rehabilitation,
Elmhurst Hospital Center, 79-01 Broadway, Rm D2-81, Elmhurst,
NY 11373, USA
e-mail: maduroc@nychhc.org

K.A. Sackheim (ed.), *Rehab Clinical Pocket Guide:*
Rehabilitation Medicine, DOI 10.1007/978-1-4614-5419-9_5,
© Springer Science+Business Media, LLC 2013

Developmental Screening
- Denver screening: brief evaluation for accomplishment of appropriate developmental milestones.
- Bailey Infant Motor Scale
- PDMS-2 (Peabody Developmental Motor Scale)

Family history: medical diseases, genetic disorders, psychiatric diseases, neurological disorders.

Newborn/Infant Exam

HEENT:
- Anterior and posterior fontanelles should be open and flat
  - Sunken fontanelle–may signify dehydration
  - Bulging fontanelle–may signify hydrocephalus or meningitis
  - Widened anterior fontanelle–cretinism, hypothyroid
- Examine for plagiocephaly: flattening of posterior of side of head
- Note overriding sutures
- Note dysmorphic facial features: indicative of genetic syndromes (Fragile X, Down syndrome, Angelman syndrome, etc.) or fetal alcohol syndrome.
  - Widening of the eyes
  - Flattening of face
  - Jaw size
  - Size and position of ears
  - Brachiocelphalic
- Check for deformity of palate or tongue
  - Large tongue may be a sign of Pierre Robin syndrome or hypothyroidism
- Cry: Abnormal cries are characteristic of certain disorders
  - Genetic syndromes such as Cri de chat–high-pitched cat-like cry
  - Hypothyroidism–deep hoarse cry

Neck:
- Check for cervical masses or sternocleidomastoid tightness
  - May be due to fibromatosis coli or brachial cleft cyst
- Gently evaluate passive range of motion (PROM) of cervical spine
- Check that bilateral clavicles intact vs. depressed or discontinuity (suggestive of fracture)

Neuromuscular Exam:
- Evaluate posture: normal full-term baby should have midline flexor tone of trunk and extremities
  - Ex. of abnormal posturing: opisthotonus, asymmetric extremity posturing or motion, flaccidity
- Check infant moves all limbs equally and no palsy of one limb or one side
  - Check for asymmetric Moro
- Gently evaluate PROM of all limbs
- Evaluate tone: normal for newborn and premature babies to have some hypotonia at birth, limbs should not be flaccid or hypertonic.
  - On exam look for head lag when bringing infant from supine to sitting position, check degree of neck and elbow extension, and low tone or flaccidity in horizontal and vertical suspension.
  - Abnormal hypotonia is seen with disorders of the central nervous system (SMA, CP), neuromuscular junction disorder, neuropathy, myopathy.
  - Hypertonia is seen with central nervous system disorders.
- Check deep tendon reflexes: biceps, triceps, patella, crossed adductor and Achilles
  - Feel for tendon and tap with finger, do not necessarily need reflex hammer
- Check spine for any:
  - Spinal deformity: usually deep, with unidentifiable endpoint and above midline
  - Sacral dimple or dimple above gluteal crease
  - Fawn's patch
  - Any of the above findings may indicate spinal dysraphism
- Hip exam: r/o developmental dysplasia of hip
  - **Ortalani Test**: while abducting hip, index is over greater trochanter, pushing anteriorly
    - **Positive test:** indicated by a "clunk" as dislocated femoral head is lifted over the posterior acetabulum and relocated.
    - Relocating a dislocated hip
  - **Barlow Test**: hold hip in adduction and flexion, and apply lateral pressure to inner thigh with thumb
    - Dislocating a relocated hip
  - **Hip Abduction**: check with hips and knees flexed at 90° and look for symmetry of gluteal creases.
- Assess Primitive and Postural reflexes Table 5.1, 5.2, and 5.3

Table 5.1 Primitive reflexes [1, 5]

Primitive reflex	How to elicit	Normal response	Age of suppression
Palmar	Apply pressure to palm	Flexion of thumb and digits	5–6 months
Plantar	Apply pressure to sole of foot	Flexion of all toes	12–14 months or when child starts walking
Babinski	Lateral stroke from heel to base of toes	Extension and fanning of toes	When child starts walking
Moro	Lower head rapidly while cradling in arms	Shoulder abduction and upper extremity flexion, followed by upper extremity flexion and adduction	4–6 months
Rooting	Gentle stroking of lips or cheek near mouth	Lips and head turn to stimulus	4 months
Sucking	Place gloved finger or pacifier in mouth	Rhythmic stroking of tongue against palate	4 months
Galant	Stroking back just lateral to spine	Lateral trunk flexion toward stimulated side	4 months
Asymmetric tonic neck reflex	Turn head to side	Arm extends on face side and flexes on occiput side "fencer pose"	6–7 months
Symmetric tonic neck reflex	Neck flexion	Flexion of arms and legs	6–7 months
Placing	Tactile contact on dorsal foot	Leg flexion (to get over obstacle)	Before 12 months

Table 5.2 Postural reflexes [1, 5]

Postural reflex	How reflex is elicited	Normal response	Age of emergence
Head righting-prone	Place infant prone	Neck hyperextends to raise face	2 months
Head righting–supine	While supine, tilt infant to either side	Head to midline, opposite direction of body	4 months
Protective extensor tone: forward prop	Displacement of infant in anterior direction	Arms extend anteriorly to prevent loss of balance	5–7 months
Protective extensor tone: lateral prop	Displacement of infant in lateral direction	Arm extends laterally to prevent loss of balance	6–8 months
Protective extensor tone: posterior prop	Displacement of infant in posterior direction	Arms extend posteriorly to prevent loss of balance	7–8 months
Protective extensor tone: standing	Displacement of infant in any direction	Arms extend to prevent loss of balance	12–14 days
Parachute	Displace body downward quickly head first	Extension and abduction of arms for protection	9 months
Landau	When infant held in prone suspension, head and leg are in extension	If examiner flexes infant's neck, legs will flex. When released, head and legs go back into extension	4–5 months

Table 5.3 Developmental milestones [5, 12–14]

Age	Gross motor development	Speech development	Developmental play/fine motor	Signs of motor abnormality
By 3 months	While prone, pushes up on arms and lifts head	Cooing or vocalizing Smiles in response to voice Turns head to voice	Grasp rattle Following stimuli past midline	Difficulty lifting head Stiff legs with little or no movement Pushes back with head Persistent hand fisting Minimal arm movement
By 6 months	Sits using hand support Rolls from back to stomach Bears weight on legs when held in standing	Babbling Begins to eat cereals and pureed food	Transfers object from one hand to another Reaches hands to feet or nearby toys	Rounded back Poor head control Difficult to bring arms forward to reach out Arches back and stiffens legs
By 9 months	Sits unsupported Transitions from laying to sitting Crawling with alternate arm and leg movement Stands holding on	Increase variety of syllable combinations in babbling "dada"/"mama" nonspecific Looks at familiar objects and people when named Begins eating mashed table food	Holds bottle on own Examines objects using both hands Imitates simple acts during play Raking grasp	Favors use of one hand Poor use of arms in sitting Difficulty crawling Using only one side to move Rounded back Inability to bear weight on legs
By 12 months	Pull to stand Cruising along furniture Stand alone and take few steps independently	"mama"/"dada" specific Follows simple commands Jargoning/jabbering First words Begins using cup	Pincer grasp Finger feeds self Transfers objects to a large container	Trouble pulling to stand due to stiff legs and pointed toes Using only arms to pull to stand Sits with weight to one side Stiffness of arms in flexion or extension Use of hands to maintain sitting

By 15 months	Walks independently with good balance Able to stoop and recover	5–10 word vocabulary Tolerates eating chopped table food	Scribbles Stacks two cubes Imitates activities Independently hold and drinks from cup	Unable to take steps independently Poor standing balance or frequent falls Toe walking
By 2 years	Starts running Walks up steps using railing and step 2 gait Kick ball Throw ball overhand	Combine words Point to pictures Follows simple directions	Use spoon/fork Stack six cubes	Toe walking or difficulty with heel to toe gait Difficulty grasping objects Vocabulary of less 15 words Does not attempt to imitate sounds, words, or gestures Unable to follow one-step commands
By 3 years	Balance on 1 ft for 3 s Broad jump Catch ball	Name four pictures Three word phrases Knows three colors Knows full name	Build tower of ten cubes Copies a circle	Throwing or jumping with difficulty Unable to scribble Vocabulary of less than 50 words Unable to speak in sentences Does not interact with peers
By 4 months	Balance 5 s on 1 ft Throws ball underhand Walks up and down steps without railing	Uses adjectives, adverbs and past tense Knows opposites	Grasp marker w/thumb and index finger Can unbutton clothes Copies a cross Cut along line using scissors	Unable to jump or throws with difficulty Does not use multi-word sentences Unemotional and disengaged most of the time Difficulty with toileting

Toddler Exam

- Observation of a child's gait, play, and interaction with parents and peers (prior to exam) often provides a great deal of information.
- Important to establish a rapport with the child prior to exam by playing and talking to the child [1] and sitting or crouching to interact with the child at their height level.

HEENT:
- Examine for dysmorphic facies

MSK:
- Observation of posture, symmetry, muscle bulk
- Palpation of muscles and joints
- Range of motion (ROM) of all major joints
- Femoral Anteversion
- Genu varum is normal until age 2, then knee position changes to genu valgum [1]
- Genu valgum is normal until 5–7 years of age [1]
- Pes planus (aka flat foot) is normal up to 3–5 years

Neurological:
  Mental Status
  Cranial Nerves
  Deep Tendon Reflexes
  Motor: use a modified scale from the adult scale [1]
        0: No movement
        1: Trace movement
        2: Movement with gravity eliminated
        3: Movement against gravity
        4: Movement against resistance
- Also use functional activities like climbing stairs, climbing into a chair and throwing/kicking a ball to assess strength, as well as stoop and recover to assess antigravity strength.

  Coordination:
- Tandem walking: unstable at age 3, but should be able to do well by age 5 [1].
- Finger-to-nose test
- Handwriting and drawing to assess fine motor control

  Sensory:
- Assess behavioral responses in this age group: crying, withdrawing, stopping activity [1]

Speech:
- Receptive language: follows 1–2 step commands
- Expressive language: uses age-appropriate words and sentences
- Naming body parts, face, and color

Pre-teen/Teenager Exam

MSK:
- Observation of posture, symmetry, muscle bulk
- Palpation of muscles and joints
- ROM of all major joints

Neuro:
- Mental Status
- Cranial Nerves
- Deep Tendon Reflexes
- Motor Testing
- Coordination: tandem walking, finger to nose
- Sensory: light touch, pin prick, vibration; note sensory dermatomal levels of deficits

Back/Spine:
- Examine height of shoulders and pelvis, and scapular position both standing and seated
- Adam's forward bending test
- Paraspinal palpation for tenderness and/or hypertonicity

Developmental Delay

- No two children develop at the same rate, and a fair amount of variability is considered normal in acquiring developmental milestones.
- **Developmental Delay:** when a child does not achieve age-appropriate developmental milestones as expected
  - Developmental age differs from chronological age in premature infants.

- ○ To calculate:
  Developmental age = chronological age−(40 weeks−gestational age at birth)
  e.g., if child is born at 28 weeks gestational age and is currently 6 months (24 weeks) old, her developmental age is calculated as such:
  24 weeks−(40 weeks − 28 weeks)=24 −12=<u>12 weeks</u> or 3 months
- For at risk children, or if developmental delay is suspected, the child is often referred for a formal developmental evaluation. This evaluation assesses the child's strengths and weaknesses in five developmental areas [2]:
  1. **Physical development**: gross motor and fine motor skills
  2. **Cognitive development**
  3. **Communication development**: speech and language
  4. **Emotional and social development**
  5. **Adaptive skills development**
- Results from the developmental evaluation are used to determine if the child is a candidate for Early Intervention [2].
- **Early Intervention**:
  - ○ A state program for children ≤3 year old
  - ○ Provides them with an individualized treatment plan
  - ○ Services available include Physical Therapy, Occupational Therapy, Speech Therapy, Medical Services and Nursing Care, Family Counseling, Psychological Services, Nutritional Services, and a Teacher [2].
  - ○ Please check written results of the developmental evaluation for Early Intervention as those scoring greater than two standard deviations below normal will qualify for home services. Children scoring between normal and two standard deviations below normal should be referred for therapy (PT/OT/Speech) from other sources such as Homecare Agencies, Visiting Nurse Services, hospitals, or office-based treatment centers.
  - ○ Early intervention varies state to state: Please check for rules for your state.
- For children >3 year old, special education services are available through the public school system. An individualized educational program which may include therapy services at school is developed [2].

Rehabilitation Prescription:
DX: Developmental Delay ICD-9: 315.9

Co-morbidities:

Precautions: fall, sensory, cognitive

Impairment: Sensory processing delay, balance, gait, coordination, pain, visuospatial

Disability: Gait dysfunction, ADL dysfunction, cognitive disorder

Rehabilitation Program:

Sensory Integration:

- Theory based on three primary postulates [3]
  1. The proper intake and processing of sensory experience from the environment and movement is vital for learning to occur.
  2. Sensory processing delays or disorders may lead to motor planning and execution deficits
  3. Active participation in purposeful exercises can improve sensory integration processes and motor learning.
- Improve efficiency of neutral processing, and organization of adaptive responses [1]
- Guided by therapist, but child controls sensory input

Neurodevelopmental techniques:

- Emphasizes "gradual withdrawal of therapist's direct input"
- Use of facilitation techniques in which therapist directs toward and away to facilitate stability and mobility, respectively [3]

Developmental Play:

- Creative exercises to stimulate child's age-appropriate cognitive development
- Play design is developed to mimic or facilitate age-appropriate developmental milestones or positioning

Cerebral Palsy

- "Group of developmental disorders of movement and postures, causing activity limitations that are attributed to **non-progressive** disturbances that occurred in the developing fetal or infant brain" [4]
- Must adhere to the following criteria [4]:
  - Deficit in neuromuscular control resulting in an alteration of movement or posture

- ○ Static brain lesion
- ○ Acquired prenatally or within first few years of life
- **# 1 Risk Factor for CP is Prematurity** [4]

Types of Cerebral Palsy (CP)

1. **Spastic CP** (75%) [5]:
   - Monoplegia (rare)
   - Diplegia:
     - ○ Most common
     - ○ Spasticity affects lower extremities >> upper extremities
     - ○ Upper extremities may have coordination deficits
     - ○ History of prematurity
   - Triplegia: usually involves bilateral LE and one UE
   - Quadriplegia: affects all four extremities, often history of perinatal asphyxia
   - Hemiplegia: involves one side of body, usually arm more than leg
2. **Dyskinetic CP**: abnormal extrapyramidal movements and coordination deficits
   - Typically involve gray matter lesions of basal ganglia and thalamus [4]

Work-up:

- Complete prenatal and postnatal history focusing on risk factors for CP
- Family history of motor disorders
- Developmental history: motor and cognitive milestones
- High suspicion for CP if following [4]:
  - ○ Hand preference prior to 2 years or asymmetric extremity use
  - ○ Early head control, rolling, or standing may indicate increased tone
  - ○ Abnormal mobility preferences such as bunny hopping, commando crawl, scooting, toe walking or scissoring gait

Physical Exam:

- Evaluate deep tendon reflexes and central and peripheral tone:
  - ○ Severe hypotonia → tend to lay in frogleg position [4]
  - ○ Hypotonia or fluctuating tone may be a sign of dyskinetic CP [4]
  - ○ Persistent fisting, thumb in fist position (cortical thumb), or scissoring are signs of hypertonicity [4]
  - ○ Delay in suppression of primitive reflexes → often earliest sign [4]
  - ○ Primitive reflexes persist past 6 months, asymmetrical response, or obligatory response usually indicates motor impairment [4]
  - ○ Poor or absent postural reflexes

- Gait Abnormalities [1]:
  Spastic:
  ○ Scissoring or adducted hips
  ○ Hip internal rotation
  ○ Toe walking
    ▪ Associated with: CP, traumatic brain injury (TBI), or other upper motor neuron disorders
  Crouched:
  ○ Weakness of quadriceps and hip extensors or due to hamstring spasticity
  ○ Excessive dorsiflexion
    ▪ Associated with: CP, and Neuromuscular diseases
  Hemiparetic:
  ○ Circumduction or steppage pattern of affected lower extremity
  ○ Flexion posturing of upper extremity
  ○ Foot inversion or ankle equinovarus on affected side
    ▪ Associated with: CP and cerebrovascular accident (CVA)
  Ataxic:
  ○ Hip girdle weakness
  ○ Poor coordination
  ○ Wide-based gait
    ▪ Associated with: neuromuscular diseases, cerebellar ataxia, Fredreich's ataxia, ataxic type Cerebral Palsy, or post-TBI
  Vaulting:
  ○ Hyperextension and locking of affected side causing patient to vault over extremity [6]

Neuroimaging:
- Ultrasound of head in preterm infants <30 weeks at 7–14 days of age and at 36–40 weeks postmenstrual age [4]
- Grade 3 or 4 IVH, periventricular cyst lesions, or moderate to severe venticulomegaly signifies 10× increase in adverse outcome [4]
- For term newborns with suspected motor deficits: check CT of head, if inconclusive-check MRI at 2–8 days of age
- **MRI is the gold standard for pediatric CNS imaging**

Gross Motor Functional Classification System (GMFCS) [4]:
   I: Ambulation indoors and outdoors without limitations
   II: Ambulation indoors and outdoors, need railing for stair negotiation, limited ambulation on uneven surfaces
   III: Ambulation indoors and outdoors on level surfaces with assistive device

IV: Ambulation for short distances with assistive device, but require rolling walker or wheelchair for home and community ambulation

V: No independent mobility

Functional Prognosis:
- Independent sitting by age 2→high likelihood of independent ambulation
- Lack of independent sitting by age 4→poor likelihood of independent ambulation
- Children with the potential for independent ambulation will usually achieve this skill by age 8, rarely develop independent ambulation afterward [1].

Early Intervention:
- Individuals with Disabilities Act (IDEA): federally mandates early intervention for children with developmental delay given the importance of environmental influences in the early years [1]
- PT, OT, and Speech therapy team for not just treatment for the child, but provide support and education to the family as well as develop a team approach to care with the family [1].
- Direct Therapy Service Model: interdisciplinary, multidisciplinary, or transdisciplinary treatment in a center or home-based program [1]
- Consultation Therapy Model

Rehabilitation Prescription:
DX: Cerebral Palsy ICD-9: 343.9
Co-morbidities:
Precautions: sensory deficit, fall, cognitive, aspiration, seizure
Impairment: spasticity, hypertonia, decreased range of motion, motor weakness, gait impairment, cognitive impairment, speech impairment, dysphagia, visuospatial impairment
Disability: decreased ambulation, decreased ADLs, developmental delay
Rehabilitation Program:
- PROM/AROM
- Stretching to prevent contractures:
  - Shoulder adductors, elbow, wrist, finger flexors, hip flexors, hip adductors, knee flexors, and plantar flexors tend to be most susceptible to contractures [3]
- Sustained stretch preferred over manual stretching—use of orthotics, splints, and casting [3]
- Strengthening

- Daily Home Exercise Program
- Speech and Swallow evaluation
- **Constraint-Induced Movement Therapy (CIMT):** restraint of unaffected extremity for at least 3 h/day × at least two consecutive weeks [4]
- **Modified CIMT:** restraint of unaffected extremity for less than 3 h/day [4]
- **Forced use:** restraining unaffected limb without additional OT [4]
- CIMT may be labor intensive for families and uncomfortable and frustrating to child.
- **Neurodevelopmental techniques (Bobath):** involves inhibiting or modifying impairments of spasticity and abnormal reflex patterns [3], and facilitating automatic and normal movement patterns [1]
- **Sensorimotor Approach (Rood):**
  - Achieve stability through activation of postural responses
  - Once stability achieved, activate movement with the use of sensory stimuli such as tapping and brushing.
- **Sensory Integration Approach:** see section on Developmental Delay Rehabilitation Prescription above
- **Vojta:** European based
  - Proprioceptive information from the trunk and extremities is used to activate the CNS and guide the development of normal motor movements [3].
  - Encourages development of movement patterns by triggering reflex locomotive zones [1]
- **Patterning Therapy:**
  - Uses sensory and reflex stimulation and passive movement patterns to improve motor coordination, communication disorders, and intelligence
- **Conductive Education:**
  - Developed in Hungary and based on the idea that motor dysfunction is due to problems with learning.
  - Proactive and task-oriented learning in a highly structured program facilitated by a "conductor" [3, 4]
- **Partial Body Weight Supported Treadmill Training (PBWSTT):**
  - Treadmill ambulation with harness support
  - Theory based on activation of spinal and supraspinal pattern generators to promote development of locomotion

Infancy Prescription:
- Family education and Early Intervention
- Promote symmetry and movement that increase sensory variety and feedback in all activities (feeding, dressing, positioning, etc.) [3]
- ROM and stretching exercises
- Adaptive equipment to help promote functional development: e.g., seating system, adaptive toys, oromotor stimulation for babies who cannot do it themselves, feeding chair may need adaptive stroller for severe hypotonia or hypertonia [3].
- For infants with asymmetrical limb motion—position limbs so that infant can see hands, encourage midline play, reaching for feet, and oral stimulation with hands [3].
  - Helps promote self awareness
  - Promotion of trunk and neck muscle use: initially development of anterior and posterior control, and later lateral control
- Functional bracing as necessary

Preschool Prescription:
- Sensory feedback and biofeedback important in development of motor learning and control
- Formal standing programs started at 1 year if child cannot yet stand on own: 45 min 2–3 times/day to prevent the development of lower extremity contractures, or 60 min 4–5 times/day to promote bone development [3].
- Ambulation training important at this age
  - Initially start with prewalking skills involving weight bearing.
  - Posterior walkers are used to encourage a more upright posture and gait [3]
  - Power mobility: may be safely used starting at age 17 months [3].
  - Tricycle riding often helpful to strengthen lower extremity muscles
- Adaptive equipment: seating system, feeding chair, stander (supine vs. prone), adaptive stroller, gait trainer
- Functional orthotic bracing as necessary

School Age and Adolescent Prescription:
- Extremely prone to rapid development of contractures as bones growing faster than muscles
- Aggressive ROM, and force generation exercises
- Consider—E-stim to help improve ROM and improve tone, may be particularly useful after tendon lengthening surgery for muscular training and strength [3]

- Mobility [3]:
  - Usually children who ambulate independently also require an alternative form of mobility such as a manual wheelchair or power device to facilitate traveling greater distances to meet educational and social goals.
  - May have low endurance due to inefficient movement
  - Orthotics may significantly decrease energy demands
- Adaptive equipment and orthotic bracing as necessary

Spina Bifida

- Second most common childhood disability
- US incidence has decreased significantly since the fortification of grain with folic acid in 1996 [4].
- Guidelines for folic acid supplementation [4]
  - 400 mg/day for all women of childbearing age
  - 4 mg/day for women with history of prior pregnancy with a neural tube deficit or women with risk factors such as valproate acid use or diabetes

Types of Spina Bifida:

1. Spina Bifida Occulta
  - Failure of fusion of posterior elements of the spine
  - Most commonly L5-S1 [4]
  - No herniation of meninges or neural tube
  - Small percent may have clinical neurological deficits
  - Sacral dimpling or hairy tuft ("fawn's patch"); may also have sacral lipoma

2. Meningocele
  - Failure of fusion of posterior elements of spine
  - Cystic outpouching of thecal sac filled with CSF and herniation of meninges
  - No neural tube disruption
  - Usually normal neurological exam
  - Rare, <10% of cases [4]

3. Meningomyelocele:
  - Most common, involves herniation of both meninges and neural tube

- ○ Neurosurgical correction usually performed on day 1 after birth [4]

Associated Neurological findings/complications [4]:

1. Variable motor and sensory impairment
2. Arnold–Chiari malformation—caudal displacement of cerbellar vermis
3. Hydrocephalus: >90% of patients, 80% of patients will need ventriculoperitoneal shunt
4. Tethered cord: spinal cord becomes bound down at its distal end.
   - ○ Studies show extremely varied results of untethering surgery, 10–15% retether post-op
5. Syringomyelia: fluid filled cavity in the spinal cord, 5–40% of cases
6. Neurogenic bowel/bladder: timed bowel program recommended starting at 2–3 years, children may be able to perform intermittent catherization starting as age 5, medical management of bowel and bladder deficits
7. Skin care: daily skin inspection for breakdown and pressure reliefs to prevent decubitii
8. Paralytic Scoliosis: secondary to muscle imbalance and loss of trunk support, severity increases with higher lesions.
9. Latex Allergy: 18–40% of patients, due to early and frequent surgical exposure from a young age

- **Referral for Early Intervention**

Pediatric Rehabilitation Prescription:
DX: Spina Bifida, Myelomeningocele ICD-9: 741.0 (with hydrocephalus)
Co-morbidities: 741.9 (without hydrocephalus)
Precautions: sensory deficit/loss, fall, cognitive, latex allergy
Impairment: spasticity, decreased range of motion, motor weakness, gait impairment, cognitive impairment
Disability: decreased ambulation, decreased ADLs, developmental delay, incontinence

Infancy Rehabilitation Program:

- Family instruction in home exercise program
- Positioning, stretching, soft tissue mobilization
- Hypotonia: facilitation of head and trunk control, supported sitting by therapists and caregiver or seating system to encourage development of head and trunk control [3]

- Severe motor delay: Neurodevelopmental techniques and Proprioceptive Neuromuscular Facilitation techniques from 6 months to 1 year with emphasis on balance, trunk control, and development of upright posture [3].
- Teach caregivers daily skin inspection for pressure ulcers

Toddler/Preschool Prescription:
- Child's exploration of environment is limited due to impaired mobility which hinders learning and independence [3].
- Early teaching of ADLs to children to facilitate independence—often delays in ADL function persist due to low caregiver expectation and protective attitudes. Important that caregivers encourage development of independent ADL function as much as possible [3].
- Positioning, ROM/stretching, strengthening exercises
- Risk of contractures greatest around joints with muscle imbalances, or if child is in prolonged position for most of the day
- Functional electrical stimulation and biofeedback often helpful for learning optimal muscle function in new ROM achieved after stretching [3].
- Begin teaching children skin inspection and pressure reliefs.
- Instruct parents in urinary catheterization techniques.
- Mobility:
  - Prewalking skills should focus on balance, trunk control, and facilitation of upright posture using prone stander or gait trainer.
  - If not effectively mobile by 1 year, consider mobility device such as a walker or power wheelchair or rigid gait orthosis [3].
  - Important to counsel family that wheelchair use does not interfere with walking, but when necessary at an early age helps child explore environment and facilitates independence and social development and interest in other forms of mobility later in life [3].
  - *High-level lesions (thoracic to L2)*: PT prescription focus on preparation for wheelchair mobility →
    - Sitting balance, upper extremity strengthening, transfer training, manual or power wheelchair skills, safety training.
  - *L3 lesions and below*: much more likely to ambulate
    - Consider fitting for lower extremity orthotics for weight bearing alignment when children begin pulling to stand [3].
    - Lumbar lesions require upper extremity support for ambulation→Posterior walker is best for maintaining

upright posture once upright ambulation is achieved, may consider advancement to forearm or Loftstrand crutches.

○ *Sacral lesions*: may or may not require upper extremity support for ambulation.

School-Age Prescription:
• Stretching/ROM program focusing on low back extensors, hip flexors, hamstrings, and shoulder girdle muscles
• Positioning
• Strengthening
• Teach daily pressure reliefs
• Teach how to self-catheterize if cognitively capable
• Assessment for adaptive equipment in children with lack of independence in an ADL task in which 50% of normal peers perform independently [3]
• Promote efficiency in ADL performance as poor efficiency tends to cause caregiver to take over completion of ADL tasks, which should be avoided [3]
• When child starts school, may need to assess for alternative means of mobility to accommodate longer traveling distances for school and community ambulation.
   ○ Manual wheelchair with power-assist wheels vs. power wheelchair.
• May consider reciprocal gait orthosis or HKAFO
• Energy conservation strategies
• Encourage participation in recreational low-impact sports such as cycling, rowing, or swimming. Swimming is usually excellent option as children are able to perform competitively with normal peers and has minimal stress on joints [3].

Muscular Dystrophy

• Muscular dystrophies are a group of genetic disorders characterized by the abnormal development of muscle tissue and progressive muscular weakness.
• The two most common forms of this disease are Duchenne Muscular Dystrophy and Becker Muscular Dystrophy.

Duchenne Muscular Dystrophy

- X-linked recessive, Xp21 gene
- Disorder of plasma membrane protein dystrophin deficiency which causes membrane instability and susceptibility to injury from mechanical stresses and membrane leakage [4]
- Absent or <3% normal level of dystrophin
- Onset occurs between 3–5 years
- Relentlessly progressive replacement of muscle with fibrotic tissue and loss of motor function
- Loss of ambulation typically by 9–13 years of age [4].

History:

- Usually present with: delays in ambulation, frequent falls, trouble negotiating stairs, toe walking
- History of hypotonia and delayed motor milestones
- **Earliest sign of weakness is in neck flexors during preschool age [4]**
- Pelvic girdle weakness precedes shoulder girdle weakness by several years
- Loss of ambulation: 7–13 years (no corticosteroid treatment), 9–15 years (with corticosteroid treatment) [4].

Physical Exam:

- Pseudohypertrophy of muscles due to fatty and connective tissue infiltration
  - Myopathic Gait:
  - Hyperlordotic waddling gait
  - Anterior pelvic tilt due to weak back and hip extensors
  - Knee instability due to knee extensor weakness—compensate by limiting knee flexion during stance and plantar flexion
- Toe walking: initially compensation for hip and knee extensor weakness, but later persists due to progressive loss of anterior tibialis favoring plantar flexion [4]
- Unable to jump or run
- "Gower Sign": child rises from floor using a four-point stance on all extremities, and using arms to push off legs to reach standing in order to compensate for hip extensor weakness
- Scoliosis:
  - 50% of cases develop between 12 and 15 years of age or usually within 3–4 years after child becomes wheelchair dependent [4]

- ○ Referral to Orthopedics
- ○ Time as to when surgery appropriate dependent on pulmonary function rather than the progression of the scoliotic curve
- Contractures: mainly in plantar flexion, hip flexion, knee flexion, iliotibial band, elbow flexion, and wrist flexion
- Cardiac:
  - ○ EKG abnormalities developing around 13 years, dilated cardiomyopathy during first and second decades [4]
  - ○ Referral to Cardiology
- Respiratory:
  - ○ Linear decrease in FVC between 10 and 20 years, failure typically in second decade [4]
  - ○ Referral to Pulmonology
- Cognitive: mean IQ = 88
- Life expectancy: 15–25 years

Labs/Tests:
- ○ Very high CK (10–50 K)
- ○ Elevated ALT/AST
- ○ Myopathic EMG

Other referrals:
- Early Intervention
- Muscular Dystrophy Association (MDA) clinic

Becker Muscular Dystrophy
- X linked recessive
- Milder form of Duchenne Muscular Dystrophy: later onset and slower progression
- Variable course
- Variable levels of normal dystrophin
- Similar distribution of weakness as Duchenne

History and Physical Exam:
- Onset typically after 5 years of age, sometimes present during adolescence or adulthood.
- Usually present with difficulty running or climbing stairs, or muscle cramping with exercise [4, 5]
- Proximal muscle weakness
- Pseudohypertrophy
- Lordotic Gait
- Loss of ambulation: 16–18 years

- Contractures: mainly plantar flexion, but may have others
- Cardiac: Mild, variable EKG changes
  - Cardiomyopathy in third or fourth decade—may precede muscle weakness [4].
- Respiratory: small percentage may develop deficits
  - Usually no significant decrease in FVC until third or fourth decade [4]
  - Respiratory failure and ventilator dependence rare
- Cognitive: may have slight deficits

Labs/Tests:
- CK elevation (5–20 K)
- Myopathic EMG

Pediatric Rehabilitation Prescription:
DX: Duchenne Muscular Dystrophy ICD-9: 359.1
Co-morbidities:
Precautions: fall, cardiac, respiratory, cognitive
Impairment: decreased range of motion, motor weakness, gait impairment
Disability: decreased ambulation, decreased ADLs, developmental delay
Early School Age Rehabilitation Program:
- ROM/stretching primarily focusing on gastrocnemius, tensor fascia lata, and hip flexors [3]
- Night splints to limit progression of plantar flexion contractures
- Prone positioning at night to limit progression of hip and knee flexion contractures
- Submaximal exercise program focusing on abdominal, hip extensor and abductor, and knee extensor groups [3]
- Breathing exercises, such as blowing bubbles or inflating balloons, to limit progression of respiratory function compromise [3]
- Resistive exercise program controversial—potential risk of mechanical injury to muscular membranes, studies on resistive exercises have shown mixed results [4]
- Consider participation in MDA activities or summer camp
- Adaptive equipment:
  - Loftstrand crutch or walker
  - May need manual wheelchair (to be propelled by caregiver)
  - Power wheelchair may allow for more functional independence

Adolescence Prescription:
- Rapid progression of disability due to increasing muscle weakness and contractures
- Usually become wheelchair reliant by 10–12 years.
- ROM/Stretching exercises focusing on hip flexors, tensor fascia lata, and plantar flexors [3]
- Prone stretch of hip flexor, iliotibial band, and tensor fascia lata: hip is maximally extended and moved into hip adduction [3]
- Prone laying at night and as much as possible during the day
- Manual or power wheelchair mobility and skills
- Transfer training focusing on strengthening shoulder depressors and triceps
- ADL training at the wheelchair level
- Wheelchair prescription should include: lateral trunk and lumbar support, adductor pads, seat belt, chest harness, foot rests in a neutral position. May also consider reclining back to help slow progression of hip contractures, midline control stick to keep symmetric trunk alignment, tray, and head support [3].
- Upper extremity strengthening exercises focusing on shoulder flexors, abductors, and elbow flexors [3]
- Adaptive equipment:
  - Loftstrand crutch or walker
  - Most adolescents will need a power wheelchair
- Functional orthotic bracing as necessary

Congenital Muscular Torticollis

- AKA Infantile Torticollis
- Cervical ipsilateral side bending and contralateral rotation (e.g., Right Torticollis—right side bending with chin rotated to the left)
- 75% of cases involve right side [5]
- Most resolve within 4–6 weeks of age, but persistent torticollis remains in 10–20% [5]
- **Most common cause is Fibrosis of the Sternocleidomastoid (SCM) [3, 5]**
  - Believed to result from ischemia due to fetal malposition or compression in utero or birth trauma

- **Other Causes:**
  - **Cervical Hemivertebra**: will not respond to PT, requires surgical resection or fusion [4]
  - **Ocular Torticollis**: r/o ocular dysfunction (e.g., extraocular muscular paresis, ocular strabismus) when child has head tilt without limitation in range of motion (ROM) [3]
  - **Acquired Torticollis** may develop after brachial plexus injury secondary to prolonged positioning of infant on one side [3]
  - Multiple Gestation
  - Large for gestational age
  - Abnormal lie in utero
- MUST R/O HIP DYSPLASIA IN ALL INFANTS WITH MUSCULAR TORTICOLLIS, as there is a much higher than normal incidence of Developmental Dysplasia of the Hip in babies with muscular torticollis due to limited fetal motion in utero.

Physical Exam:
- Soft, non-tender thickening or lump, known as fibromatosis coli, may be palpable in the SCM [5]
  - Referred to as an "olive sign"
- Facial asymmetry and plagiocephaly (parieto-occipital flattening)
  - Frontal bossing on side of SCM tightness

Rehabilitation Prescription:
DX: Developmental Muscular Torticollis ICD-9: 723.5
Co-morbidities:
Precautions:
Impairment: decreased Range of Motion, contralateral sternocleido-mastoid weakness
Disability: decreased functional mobility
Rehabilitation Program:
- PROM and stretching to SCM: gently cradle occiput on the involved side and face on opposite side and slowly move into lateral flexion away from and rotation toward the tight SCM [3].
  - If child is strongly resistant to stretch, it may cause the tight SCM to become even stronger furthering muscular imbalance, in this case AROM will be better to use to stretch the tight SCM and strengthen the weak muscles.
- Strengthening of the weak SCM contralateral to the affected side is done by using visual tracking toward the affected SCM [3].

  - ○ Exercise should be performed in different positions such as supine, prone, reclined, and sitting
  - ○ May need to resist shoulder to prevent child from using trunk rotation to substitute for cervical rotation
- Functional activities that encourage simultaneous lateral cervical flexion and rotation to stretch the tight SCM [3]
  - ○ e.g., for a Left Torticollis, child encouraged to look and reach to the left. This promotes lateral cervical flexion against gravity to the right with simultaneous rotational stretch.
- Positioning:
  - ○ During sleep, position pillow under affected side to promote lateral SCM stretch [3].
  - ○ Can use towel or blanket folded like a wedge to increase rotation toward the tight SCM
  - ○ Position crib so infant must stretch SCM to gaze toward center of room, and place mobile on same side of tight SCM to encourage active cervical rotation [5].
  - ○ During play, position toys or child in a way to encourage rotation toward affected SCM [3].
  - ○ Persistent plagiocephaly often will require cranial helmet therapy or osteopathic manipulative therapy (OMT) to reshape skull.
    - ▪ Helmet is to be worn 23 h daily [4]
    - ▪ May refer to Cranial Academy Website Physician Finder to locate osteopathic physician for OMT (www.cranialacademy.com)
    - ▪ Family/caregiver daily Home exercise program instruction

Other Points:
- Facial asymmetry should resolve if normal ROM is obtained by 1 year of age
- If torticollis with significant deformity persists by 18–24 months, surgical intervention is considered—involves surgical resection of fibrotic SCM [5]
- May consider Botox treatment

Brachial Plexus Injury

- Usually due to birth trauma and obstetrical complications usually involving traction of the shoulder during delivery causing injury to the upper or lower trunks of the plexus

- Major Risk Factors: larger sized baby at birth, multiparous mothers, shoulder dystocia, maternal diabetes, prolonged labor, breech delivery, difficult cesarean extraction [4]

Upper Trunk Brachial Plexopathy: Erb-Duchenne Palsy
- Most common, ¾ of cases [4]
- Sudden neck traction during delivery of shoulder resulting in injury to the upper trunk of the brachial plexus affecting C5 and C6 innervated muscles in the upper extremity.
- Shoulder in extension, adduction and internal rotation, elbow extended, forearm pronated, and wrist and fingers flexed; "Waiter's tip" position
- Paralysis of rhomboids, levator scapula, serratus anterior, subscapularis, deltoid, supraspinatus, infraspinatus, teres minor, biceps, brachialis, brachioradialis, supinator, and wrist and finger extensors
- Grip strength is normal
- C5/C6 dermatomal sensory loss

Lower Trunk Brachial Plexopathy: Klumpke's Palsy
- Rarely due to birth trauma, but may be seen as a complication of vaginal delivery of breech position
- More commonly from fall onto hyperabducted shoulder [5]
- Sudden upward pull of shoulder resulting in injury to the lower trunk of the plexus affecting the C8-T1 innervated muscles
- Normal shoulder and elbow movements, forearm supinated at rest, and paralysis of wrist flexors and extensors and intrinsic muscles of the hand, weakened palmar grasp

Erb-Klumpke's Palsy:
- Combination injury to upper and lower trunks involving C5–T1 roots resulting in total arm paralysis and sensory loss [4]

History, Physical Exam, and Work-up for Brachial Plexus Injuries:
- Thorough prenatal and delivery history
- Exam: inspection of muscle bulk, asymmetry of motion, asymmetric reflexes in upper extremity, abnormal Moro—Erb's palsy, torticollis—face turned away from affected arm, ROM [3, 4]
- Consider NCS/EMG
- X-ray to r/o clavicular or humerus fracture [4]

Rehabilitation Prescription:

DX: Upper Trunk Brachial Plexopathy: Erb's Palsy ICD-9: 767.6

Co-morbidities:

Precautions: No overstretching of affected shoulder, Avoid I.V. puncture of affected extremity

Impairment: decreased range of motion of affected extremity, shoulder external rotation and flexion weakness, elbow flexion weakness, sensory deficit of affected arm

Disability: decreased functional mobility

Rehabilitation Program:

- Positioning: may begin immediately, during first 2 weeks, family instructed to gently position arm across abdomen, and avoid lying on involved arm [4].
  - Afterward, child's arm should be positioned in shoulder abduction and external rotation, elbow flexion, and forearm supination while sleeping and as much as possible during the day [3].
- ROM exercises: May begin after 2 weeks of age
  - Allows time for reduction of edema and hemorrhage around the injured plexus [3]
  - Avoid movement of affected extremity for first 2 weeks as much as possible to avoid pain [4]
  - After this may start gentle PROM—avoid overstretching as can cause harm to joints
  - Prevent scapulohumeral adhesions by allowing stretching of muscles between scapula and humerus by stabilizing the scapula up to 30° of rotation. Beyond this, scapula should rotate along with humeral motion to avoid impingement [3].
  - Avoid lifting child under axilla or pulling on arms as this can overstretch and damage shoulder joint [3]
- Sensory Awareness:
  - Position affected limb so it will be noticed by child [4]
  - Monitor affected limb closely for signs of injury due to sensory deficit
  - Promote sensory development by placing objects of different textures in hand [3]
  - Use affected limb to mimic movement of normal limb such as reaching, and bringing hand to mouth [4]
- Splinting:
  - Wrist splints to provide optimal tendon position in wrist drop [3]
  - Cock-up splint—keeps wrist neutral, while freeing fingers for play [3]

- ○ Resting night or day splints may be made to prevent wrist, finger, or elbow contracture
- Electrical Stimulation: 20 min. bid [3, 4]
  - ○ Used to increase muscle bulk and may improve motor strength after nerve regeneration
  - ○ May help increase sensory awareness of affected limb
  - ○ Controversial: may interfere with nerve regeneration
- Family/Caregiver Home Exercise Program Instruction

Surgical Intervention
- Infants with <3/5 elbow flexion strength at 6 months are surgical candidates [4].
- Neurosurgery [4]:
  - ○ Neurolysis—scar and fibrotic tissue removed from nerve
  - ○ Direct nerve transfer
  - ○ Neurorraphy—suturing of a divided nerve
- Orthopedic [3]:
  - ○ Latissimus dorsi and teres major tendon transfer to rotator cuff
  - ○ Derotational osteotomy for glenohumeral joint deformity with internal rotation contracture

Juvenile Idiopathic Arthritis

- Onset occurs <16 years of age
- Symptoms have >6 week course
- Formerly called Juvenile Rheumatoid Arthritis (JRA): which consisted of three subtypes - Systemic, Polyarticular, and Pauciarticular
- Reclassified by the International League of Associations for Rheumatology into seven subtypes [7]

Systemic Juvenile Idiopathic Arthritis (JIA)
- Diagnostic criteria [4, 7]:
  1. Arthritis
  2. Quotidian fever: alternating temperature spiking of >39°C and return to normal baseline temperature ×2 weeks
  3. At least one of the following: evanescent rash, general lymphadenopathy, hepatomegaly, splenomegaly, or serositis

- 4–17% of cases [7]
- Symmetrical and polyarticular
- About half of systemic JIA are relapsing-remitting course with good prognosis, with the other half affected by an unremitting course with severe joint destruction and poor prognosis [4].
- Imaging changes in joints within 2 years [4]
- Routine ophthalmology exams every 12 years to rule out iridocyclitis [7]
- Macrophage Activation syndrome:
  - Life-threatening condition affecting a minority of children with systemic JIA
  - Sudden onset of high fever, pancytopenia, hepatosplenomegaly, liver insufficiency, coagulopathy with hemorrhagic manifestations, and neurological symptoms [7]

Oligoarthritis JIA [4, 7]:
- 27–56% of cases
- Persistent type: four or fewer joints affected, mostly unilateral
- Extended type:
  - Greater than four joints affected after 6 months.
  - Involvement of an upper extremity joint and high ESR at onset predictor for extended oligoarthritis
- Onset <6 years of age
- Asymmetrical
- Preferentially affects females
- Lower extremities affected greater than upper extremities, preferentially affects knee and hip
- Check for leg length discrepancy: common due to increased blood circulation to the affected joints and growth plates
- Generally have the best prognosis of all JIA types
- Imaging changes in joints within 5 years
- ANA positive in 70–80% → high-risk factor for iridocyclitis
- NEED ROUTINE FOLLOW UP BY OPTHALMOLOGY AS SILENT UVEITIS IS COMMON
- Eye exams every 3–4 months for children with + ANA, and every 6 months for – ANA

Rheumatoid Factor Positive Polyarthritis JIA
- 2–7% of cases [7]
- Five or more joints affected in first 6 months [4]
- Positive IgM Rheumatoid factor on two occasions at least 3 months apart [7]

- Preferentially affects adolescent females [4]
- Symmetrical
- Mainly affects smaller joints of hands and feet, but also can affect large joints
- Severe joint deformity within 5 years of onset
- Rheumatoid nodules classically in forearm and elbow [7]

Rheumatoid Factor Negative Polyarthritis JIA
- 11–28% of cases [7]
- Five or more joints affected in first 6 months [4]
- Variable course
- Asymmetric
- 5–20% uveitis [4]

Psoariatic JIA [4, 7]
- 2–11% of cases
- DX: Arthritis and typical psoriatic rash
    - if no rash → need two of the following:
        1. Positive family history of Psoariasis in a first-degree relative.
        2. Dactylitis
        3. Nail Pitting
- Preferentially affects females
- Typically early onset, asymmetrical oligoarthritis
- Poorer prognosis in children diagnosed prior to 5 years of age

Enthesitis JIA
- 3–11% of cases [7]
- Tends to affect males >6 years of age
- Enthesitis: inflammation of tendon and ligament insertion
- Most common sites of enthesitis are the calcaneal insertion of the Achilles tendon, plantar fasciitis, and the tarsal region [7]
- Arthritis tends to mainly affect the joints of the lower extremities, especially the hip [4]

Undifferentiated Arthritis
- Any inflammatory joint arthropathy which does not fit into any of the above categories [7] or fit into more than one category.

Other points
- Be aware of risk for Atlantoaxial subluxation and check routine X-rays.
- If there is evidence of Atlantoaxial instability, hold exercise program and refer to orthopedics for evaluation. Patient should

wear cervical collar during vehicle transport to avoid potential cervical injury in event of rapid deceleration or motor vehicle accident [3].
- Routinely assess for leg length discrepancy, particularly in asymmetrical joint involvement: increased circulation to inflamed joints causes increased growth of limb [3].

Rehabilitation Prescription:
DX: Juvenile Idiopathic Arthritis ICD-9: 714.3
Co-morbidities:
Precautions: no aggressive ROM/stretching during acute flare
Impairment: decreased range of motion of affected extremity, pain
Disability: decreased functional mobility
Rehabilitation Program:
- Morning Stiffness:
  - Recommend warm bath in AM and water exercises
  - Resting night splints
  - Sleeping in sleeping bag to increase warmth during the night [3]
- Moist heat prior to PT/OT and daily exercise program
- Active ROM exercises essential
- PROM exercise (avoid during acute inflammatory periods)
- Prone positioning with feet left over edge of mat or bed to stretch hip and knee flexion contractures [3]
- Dynamic splinting for contractures for 2–3 times daily for 1 h each time and overnight, if tolerated [3]
- Serial casting used, usually for knee flexion contractures, if stretching, positioning, or dynamic splinting fails
- Concentric and eccentric strengthening program: elastic bands, 2–3 lb weights, cycling, swimming [3]
- Energy Conservation:
  - Teach patient to focus on using larger joints for activities when possible to avoid stressing smaller joints [3].
    - e.g., carry backpack correctly with straps on both shoulders rather than on one shoulder or briefcase
  - Built up utensils and grooming tools with larger handles to make for easier gripping [3]
  - Learning to pace one's ambulation and activities
  - Consider wheelchair ambulation for long distances in the community.

- Wheelchair Ambulation:
  - Manual vs. power wheelchair
  - Patient with moderate to severe involvement of the joints of the hands will likely require manual wheelchair with lowered seat to utilize foot propulsion, or a powered wheelchair [3].
- Assistive Devices for ADLs [3]:
  - Dressing stick to aid pulling up pants, hooks on zippers, velcro zippers, sock aid
  - Bathroom: tub bench, grab bars in shower or near toilet, shower hose, lever sink handles as opposed to knobs, raised toilet seat
- Heel lift to unaffected side if there is a leg length discrepancy [3]
- Recreation/Aerobic exercise:
  - Avoid gymnastics, running, contact sports, and other high-impact sports that may stress or damage joints.
  - Low-impact aerobics, cycling, and swimming are better exercise options for children with JIA

Common Orthopedic Disorders

Femoral Anteversion
- Measure hip ROM in prone position with the hip in neutral
- For a child who is upset and afraid, can examine with the parent holding child against their body while parent is standing [3]
- Version: angular difference between the transverse axis of the neck of the femur and the femoral shaft [3]
- Femoral anteversion: femoral head directed anteriorly, hip will have excessive internal rotation (IR)
- Excessive femoral anteversion causes intoeing gait
- There is 30–40° of femoral anteversion at birth and this gradually decreases to 15° by skeletal maturity [8].
- Torsional malignment syndrome: combination of excessive femoral anteversion and lateral tibial torsion; compensatory lateral tibial torsion develops in older child [9].

Exam:
- Place child prone, flex knees to 90° and palpate greater trochanter. In neutral position, greater trochanter will be posterior to normal lateral alignment. Rotate hip medially. The point at which the

greater trochanter becomes straight lateral is the degree of femoral ante torsion [9].
- Place child prone, flex knees to 90°, and examine foot angle—if medial deviation of forefoot (intoeing) corrects in this position, intoeing is due to femoral anteversion.
- Gait: increased medial rotation of foot and medially deviated patella [8]

Treatment:
- Avoid "W" sitting and encourage crossed leg sitting
- Most cases will resolve spontaneously
- Anteversion shorts
- Braces, twister cables, and special shoes are used by some, but have not shown proven benefit in clinical trials [3]
- If femoral anteversion is still problematic at age 10–14, femoral derotation surgery may be considered [3] if child has greater than 50° of femoral anteversion and greater than 80° of medial hip rotation.

Internal Tibial Torsion
- Medial rotation of the tibia resulting in an intoeing gait
- Unilateral tibial torsion is twice as common on the left than on the right side [9]

Exam:
- Thigh–Foot Angle:
  - Place child prone with knees flexed, then examine the angle of the foot relative to the thigh.
  - Internal tibial torsion is expressed as a negative value, and external tibial torsion is expressed as a positive value [8].
  - Infants normally have a negative thigh–foot angle, and in children the value ranges from +5 to +15° [9].
- Foot Progression Angle:
  - Angle between the longitudinal axis of the foot and a straight line of progression of the body when walking [3]
  - Observe the child when walking and note subjective deviation of the angle of the forefoot from the line of progression [9].
- Medial rotation of the foot with the patella in neutral [9]

Treatment:
- Debate exists regarding appropriate treatment of internal tibial torsion.
- Some clinicians recommend no treatment because the condition is usually self resolving [3].

- Others have recommended treatment starting at about 18 months with a Friedman counter splint (a flexible leather strap) or a Denis Brown bar (metal bar) for 6 months every night.
- Both these units are attached to the child's shoes and hold the foot in an externally rotated position [3].
- Wheaton Ankle Foot Orthosis (AFO): night AFO which gradually externally rotates lower leg and kept in 30–40° knee flexion.
- Surgery: supramalleolar osteotomy for extremely severe cases, rarely used [8]

Metatarsus Adductus
- Aka metatarsus varus
- Most common congenital foot deformity
- Due to either positional problems from restricted space in the uterine environment or true congenital abnormalities such as talipes equinovarus [3].
- Postural Metatarsus:
  - Usually due to positional problems from restricted space in the uterine environment [3]
  - Able to be corrected with passive manipulation [9]
  - Usually corrects spontaneously
- Congenital Metatarsus Adductus:
  - Rigid, unable to correct with passive manipulation and does not resolve spontaneously [9].
  - Crease present on medial plantar aspect of foot at tarsal metatarsal joint [9]

Exam:
- Medial rotation of the metatarsals on the cuneiform causing adduction of the forefoot [9]
- Normal slightly valgus positioning of the hindfoot
- Full ankle dorsiflexion ROM
- Examine child's feet statically and dynamically

Treatment [3]:
- Grade I (mild): usually resolves spontaneously by 4–6 months (85% of cases [8]), rarely requires treatment
- Grade II (moderate): stretching program, and corrective shoes–straight lace or reverse lace
- Grade III (severe): manipulation and serial casting followed by corrective shoes.
  - Casting most effective if implemented prior to 1 year of age [8]

- Casting is performed to above the knee with 20–25° of knee flexion to permit ambulation [8]
- Surgery: rarely indicated
  - Tarsometatarsal capsulotomy for patients 5 years and younger [8]
  - Proximal osteotomies of the lesser metatarsals for children older than 5 years [8]

Calcaneovalgus

- Abduction of the forefoot, hindfoot in valgus, and normal or excessive dorsiflexion
- Common foot disorder in infants most frequently due to positioning in a restricted intrauterine environment
- May also be due to muscle imbalance causing severe weakness of the plantar flexors
- Must be differentiated from congenital vertical talus, a condition in which the talus is vertical and the navicular is displaced onto the dorsal surface of the talus [3].
- Ability to dorsiflex the heel differentiates from congenital vertical talus where the forefoot is stiffer and the heel is in equines [8].
- Treatment [8]:
  - Most cases resolve spontaneously
  - Plantar flexion inversion casting may be used if no self correction in by a few months of age
  - Orthotics have not demonstrated any proven benefit
  - Surgery:
    - Difficult to surgically correct
    - May consider tibialis anterior transfer to os calcis or subtalar fusion to stabilize hindfoot [8]

Common Pediatric Orthopedic Gait Abnormalities [1]:
Intoeing:

- Internal tibial torsion-most common reason in toddlers [1]
- Femoral anteversion-most common reason in children up to age 10 [1]
- Metatarsus adductus-medial deviation of the metatarsal bones

Out toeing:

- External tibial torsion
  - Presents in children and pre-adolescents as pain in instep of foot or anterior knee pain [9]
  - Usually compensatory for excessive femoral anteversion or iliotibial band contracture [9]

- Exam: lateral thigh foot angle, Ober's test to rule out iliotibial band contracture; rule out triceps surae contracture by evaluating ankle dorsiflexion ROM [9]
- Femoral retroversion
  - Rare but often missed as a cause of hip pain
  - Cause is usually a primary developmental deformity (coxa valga) or due to slipped capital femoral epiphysis (femoral neck-shaft angle decreased) [9]
  - Exam: out-toeing gait, laterally deviated patella and foot progression angle, excessive lateral hip rotation [9]

Osgood Schlatter
- Partial avulsion of the tibial tuberosity secondary to repetitive stress on an immature skeleton [8]
- Activity related pain and swelling at patellar tendon insertion at the tibial tuberosity
- Most common in males during late childhood or early adolescence [8]
- Pain aggravated by palpation of tibial tubercle and jumping and running
- Treatment:
  - Rest and ice
  - Avoidance of exacerbating activities
  - Neoprene bracing or for severe cases, casting [3]
  - Most cases resolve spontaneously
  - Complete resolution usually occurs in 1–2 years

Painful Pes Planus
- Miserable malalignment syndrome: flexible flat foot causing pronation and ankle strain up to the knee
- Can present in any pediatric age group
- Often what is referred to "growing pains" in toddlers
- In school age children, more likely to present as knee problems
- Treatment: UCBL or semi-rigid orthosis

Idiopathic Scoliosis
History [9]:
- When was curve first noticed and by whom?
  - Parents, pediatrician, school screening, or incidental imaging
- What imaging or diagnostic studies have been performed?
- What treatment has patient had thus far?
  - Observation, physical therapy, exercises, bracing, surgery

- Has there been any change in the degree of scoliosis since it was first detected?
- Is there any pain in the spine?
  - Pain is usually not a feature of scoliosis. Patients with any painful spinal deformity need a thorough clinical exam and imaging studies including X-rays, bone scan, CT scan and/or MRI to rule out other spinal disorders such as bone lesions, inflammatory conditions, tumors, or spondylisthesis.

Exam [9]:
- Examine patient with back, iliac crests, and posterior superior iliac spines (PSIS) exposed
- Inspect for skin lesions: such as café au lait spots (suggestive of neurofibromatosis) and hair tufts (suggestive of spinal dysrhaphism)
- Examine spine while seated and standing, as well as from posterior, lateral, and anterior views
- Look for asymmetry of the shoulders, scapula, and iliac crests
- Check iliac crests and anterior superior iliac spine (ASIS) and PSIS in supine and prone positions to rule out pelvic obliquity.
- Gauge region (thoracic, thoracolumbar, etc.) and extent of curve visually
- Adam's forward bending test:
  - Examine patient while they are slowly bending forward at the hips
  - For thoracolumbar and lumbar curves, examine patient from posterior
  - For thoracic and cervical curves, examine patient from anterior
  - Note the degree and direction of vertebral rotation
  - Determine the degree of rotation measuring the height of the vertebral paraspinal prominence [9].
  - Direction of rotation [9]:
  - Structural scoliosis: spinous processes rotate toward concavity, prominence on convex side of the curve
  - Postural scoliosis: spinous processes rotate toward the convexity, prominence on concave side of curve
- Check lateral bending to assess the flexibility of the curve
- Assess degree of thoracic kyphosis, lumbar lordosis, and pelvic tilt
- Palpate for paraspinal tenderness and/or hyper tonicity

- Neuromuscular exam: deep tendon reflexes, motor strength, superficial abdominal reflex, cremasteric reflex—rule out paralytic scoliosis [9]

Imaging

- AP and lateral spinal standing X-rays for initial evaluation
- Flexed spinal X-rays should be ordered if orthotic or surgical intervention is under consideration [9]
- Check Cobb angle to measure curve degree [9]
  - Draw a perpendicular line from the superior border of the cephalad vertebrae of the scoliotic curve
  - Draw another perpendicular line from the inferior border of the caudal vertebrae of the scoliotic curve.
  - Angle formed by the intersection of these two perpendicular lines is the degree of the scoliotic curve
- Indications for MRI [9]:
  - Focal neurological deficit
  - No flattening or loss of lumbar lordosis when bringing knees to chest or forward flexion
  - Absent abdominal umbilical reflex or positive Beevor's sign
  - Skin lesions (spinal or sacral dimple, hair patch or pigmentation, hemangioma, etc.)
  - Paraspinal rigidity with Goldthwaite test (prone hip extension with 90° knee flexion).
  - Back pain
  - Aggressive curve progression
  - Left thoracic curve or other unusual curve pattern
  - Curve onset at younger age with progression.
  - Interpediculate space widening and/or pedicle erosion on X-ray (may indicate tumor, syringomyelia, diastematomyelia, or spinal dysrhaphism)
- Radiological assessment of skeletal maturity is determined by the Risser sign, which is a scale of the degree of ossification of the iliac crest on AP X-ray. Ossification starts from the ASIS and progresses posterior to the PSIS [9].
  - 0: No evidence of ossification
  - 1: Ossification of up to the anterior ¼ of the iliac crest
  - 2: Ossification of up to the anterior ½ of the iliac crest
  - 3: Ossification of up to the anterior ¾ of iliac crest
  - 4: Complete excursion of iliac crest
  - 5: Fusion of the ossification center apophysis to body of ilium

Treatment:
Observation
- For curves <20° and without progression do not require treatment but should be reevaluated every 3–4 months [9].
- Check new imaging if any change in physical exam from previous visit [9].

Rehabilitation Prescription:
DX: Juvenile or Adolescent Idiopathic Scoliosis ICD-9: 737.30
Co-morbidities:
Precautions:
Impairment: decreased spinal range of motion, weakness of paraspinals and trunk musculature
Disability: decreased functional mobility
Rehabilitation Program:
Schroth Method or Scoliosis Intensive Rehabilitation
- 3D treatment of scoliosis based on sensorimotor and kinesthetic principles with the goals of
  - Facilitating correction of asymmetric posture
  - Teach patient to maintain corrected posture in daily activities [10].
- Five Principles of Correction
  1. Active Axial Elongation: Stabilize pelvis to prevent trunk flexion or extension, and patient activates trunk muscles to achieve axial elongation [10].
  2. Deflexion: Uses concept of "system of blocks" in which shoulder girdle is the "upper block," thorax is the "middle block," and pelvis is the "lower block." Scoliotic curves corrected in frontal plane by translating deviated blocks against one another [10].
  3. Derotation: In the scoliotic spine, the convexities of the curve rotate dorsally, and the concavities rotate ventrally. For correction, the convexities are rotated ventrally and the concavities are rotated dorsally [10].
  4. Schroth's Rotational Breathing [10]:
  - Scoliotic curve affects proper breathing mechanics. Muscles along convexity are stretched and muscles along the concavity are contracted.

- ○ This muscle imbalance promotes abnormal respiratory mechanics which in turn leads to further muscle imbalance becoming a vicious cycle.
- ○ Stretched muscles in the convexity of the curve restrict full exhalation (so this region is "stuck" in inhalation), and the shortened muscles in the concavity of the curve retract to a greater degree of exhalation
- ○ Scoliotic deformity increases during exhalation and decreases during inhalation
- ○ This exercise focuses on tightening the convexity muscles and guiding breath into the concavity of curve
- ○ Utilizes proprioceptive sensation of detorsion on vertebrae.
  - 5. Stabilization: Maintenance of correction from Schroth's Rotational Breathing in exhalation with the goal of concentric contraction of stretched muscles along convexity and eccentric contraction of the shortened muscles along the concavity of the curve [10]

Lyonaise Method
- Focuses on 3D correction of posture using auto-elongation and sagittal correction by performing exercises within a spinal orthotic brace [10, 11]

Scientific Exercises Approach to Scoliosis (SEAS)
- Derived from Lyonaise school.
- 3D auto-correction focusing on postural spinal stability and balance reactions and improving sagittal spinal curvatures [11]

Side Shift Therapy
- Focuses on spinal correction in the frontal plane only and involves lateral trunk shift exercises [11]

Orthosis
- Indicated for skeletally immature patients with 30–45° scoliotic curve or 20–29° curve with evidence of progression
- Patient must have a minimum of 12 months of remaining skeletal growth for the orthosis to be effective. This is defined as [9]:
  - ○ Risser score less than or equal to 3
  - ○ Unfused vertebral apophyses
  - ○ For females: either premenarchal or recent menarche (within 6 months)

- Orthosis is contraindicated in skeletally mature patients, Risser score of 4 or 5, thoracic lordosis curves less than 45°, and psychiatric patients
- Types of Braces [9]:
  ○ Cervico-thoraco-lumbo-sacral orthosis (CTLSO) or Milwakee Brace
  ○ Thoraco-lumbo-sacral orthosis (TLSO): high brace for thoracic scoliosis and low brace for thoracolumbar or lumbar scoliosis
- Corrective Forces of Brace [9]
  ○ Transverse: directed at lateral or posterior apex of scoliotic curve using three point pressure system
  ○ Longitudinal traction
- Bracing Schedule [9]
  ○ Full-time: 22 h/day, removed only for bathing and exercise or physical therapy
  ○ Part-time: 16 h/day or only during night
  ○ Typical bracing period: 3–4 months
  ○ Wean from brace when Risser score is 4+, or vertebral growth completed, or 18 months post-menarche for females

Surgical Treatment
- Indications [9]:
  ○ Scoliotic curve greater than 45–50°
  ○ Scoliotic curve demonstrating progression despite orthosis
- Pre-surgical exam should include pulmonary function testing and complete neurological assessment
- Surgical Fusion
  ○ Should extend from the most inferior neutrally rotated vertebrae up to the most superior neutrally rotated vertebrae [9]
  ○ Proper fusion extends proximally enough to result in leveling of the shoulders [9]
  ○ May be performed from anterior or posterior approach or both
- Posterior Fusion: simplest and most common procedure for scoliosis [9]
- Anterior Fusion: indicated for single thoracolumbar or single lumbar curves [9]
- Anterior and Posterior Fusion: indicated for large rigid curves in skeletally immature to prevent loss of correction as child grows [9]
- Somatosensory evoked potentials (SSEP) and motor evoked potentials (MEP) is recommended during surgery to reduce risk of neurological complications, which still occurs at a rate of 0.5% in this procedure [9].

References

1. Braddom RL. Physical medicine and rehabilitation. 3rd ed. Philadelphia: Elsevier; 2007.
2. Developmental Delay. National Dissemination Center for Children with Disabilties. 2011. http://nichcy.trg/disability/specific/dd. Accessed 5 Oct 2011.
3. Campbell SK, Vander Linden DW, Palisano RJ. Physical therapy for children. 2nd ed. Philadelphia: W.B. Saunders; 2000.
4. Alexander MA, Matthews DJ. Pediatric rehabilitation. 4th ed. New York: Demos Medical; 2010.
5. Cuccurullo SJ. Physical medicine and rehabilitation board review. 2nd ed. New York: Demos Medical; 2010.
6. Leung AKC, Lemay JF. The limping child: pathophysiology. J Pediatr Health Care. 2004;18(5):219–23.
7. Ravelli A, Martini A. Juvenile idiopathic arthritis. Lancet. 2007;369:767–78.
8. Wheeless CR. Wheeless Textbook or Orthopedics. 2011. http://www.wheelessonline.com. Accessed 11 Oct 2011.
9. Tachdijian MO, Pediatric C. Orthopedics: the art of diagnosis and principals of management. Stamford: Appleton & Lange; 1997.
10. Grivas TB. The conservative scoliosis treatment. Amsterdam: Ios Press; 2008.
11. Negrini S, et al. Exercises reduce the progression rate of adolescent idiopathic scoliosis: results of a comprehensive systematic review of the literature. Disabil Rehabil. 2008;309(10):772–85.
12. Baby Growth and Development Chart. Pathways Awareness Foundation. np. http://pathways.org/awareness/parents/new-parents/monthly-milestones/. Accessed 31 Aug 2011.
13. Folio MR, Fewell RR. PDMS-2 Peabody developmental motor scales. 2nd ed. Austin: Pro-ed; 2000.
14. Ability Path. org. Milestone concerns. http://www.abilitypath.org/areas-of-development/milestone-concerns/. Accessed 6 Oct 2011.

Chapter 6
Cardiac Rehabilitation

Isaac Darko and Michelle Robalino-Sanghavi

Cardiac Rehab Prescription Writing:
- History and Physical with pertinent labs/tests/procedures/imaging
- Risk Stratify Patient (low, moderate, or high) while considering physical limitations according to the described parameters below
- Write Cardiac Rehab Protocol (Refer to Example of Cardiac Rehab Prescription) keeping in mind:
  - Acuity: Acute, Subacute, Transitional
  - Setting (Inpatient and/or outpatient)/or Phase of Cardiac Rehab
  - Special considerations in patients with specific heart disease including (CAD, Angioplasty and Stent, CABG/Heart Valve Surgery, CHF, Left Ventricular Assistive Device, Post-Heart Transplant, Arrhythmias)
  - Considerations/Precautions
  - General Goals
    - Short term
    - Long term
    - Length of stay and role of other members on the Rehab team including Exercise physiologist, PT, OT, Psychologist, Nutrition, and Rehab nurse.
- Patient Education on Cardiac Rehabilitation, which includes risk modification and management of complex medication regimen. Symptoms that may warrant calling the Rehab doctor such as worsening chest pain, severe sudden shortness of breath, sudden

I. Darko, M.D. (✉) • M. Robalino-Sanghavi, M.D.
Department of Rehabilitation Medicine, Mount Sinai Medical Center,
One Gustave Levy Place, Box 1240, New York, NY 10029, USA
e-mail: isaacdarko3@gmail.com; michellerobalino@gmail.com

K.A. Sackheim (ed.), *Rehab Clinical Pocket Guide:*
Rehabilitation Medicine, DOI 10.1007/978-1-4614-5419-9_6,
© Springer Science+Business Media, LLC 2013

chest pain, or an incision site draining unusual amounts or becomes increasingly erythematous
- Follow-up appointments with Rehab, Cardiology, and other needed services

Cardiac Rehabilitation (CR)
- Complex network aimed at aiding patients with limited function due to the sequelae of cardiac disease
- Cardiovascular disorders are the leading cause of mortality and morbidity in the industrialized world, accounting for almost 50% of all deaths annually
- According to US Public Health Services (USPHS), a CR program involves medical education, prescribed exercise, education, and counseling
- CR is useful for Patients (Pts) post-acute MI, chronic unstable angina, CHF, coronary revascularization, valve correction surgery, and cardiac transplantation
- Participation in CR has demonstrated an approximate 25% reduction in cardiac mortality during 3 years of follow-up versus those who do not attend [1]
- CR program typically begins with an intake evaluation that includes measurement of cardiac risk factors such as lipid measures, blood pressure, body weight, and smoking history
- A combination of different machines and muscle groups is recommended when designing an exercise program as training is muscle group specific
- An exercise stress test (EST) is done to help determine the exercise prescription
- An exercise physiologist, cardiac-trained nurse, or physical therapist closely monitors the patient (during exercise sessions)
  - Usual allowable maximal heart rate (HR max = 220-age), but for patients who have undergone cardiac event, this maximal HR is based on the type of cardiac event, premorbid conditions, comorbid conditions, and whether or not Pt is taking β(beta)-blocker
- CR is stratified into three phases
  - Phase I of CR is the inpatient phase which may begin on hospital day 2–4 and may last 7–14 days
  - Phase II is the outpatient phase which begins immediately post-discharge and may last 8–12 weeks
  - Phase III is the maintenance phase, and should be lifelong

Patients with Preexisting Cardiac Disease
- Symptomatic limitation of activity manifests as a steady decline in aerobic capacity
- Resting tachycardia is noted, and returns to normal after exercise completion is delayed
- Blood pressure responses are variable, and postural hypotension is common.

Physiologic Advantages of CR
- Substantial musculoskeletal, cardiovascular, and psychological adaptations are noted in 6–10 weeks of initiating training
- Pts must be educated that deconditioning and cardiac fatigue worsens with prolonged relative inactivity and improves with physical activity.
- Patients may also be hyper vigilant, anxious, and over report trivial symptoms, but physiologic and electrocardiographic data during CR can help allay fears and refocus on potential significant symptoms [2]
- The beneficial effects can be lost after lack of activity or bed rest extending over 2–3 weeks

Initial Evaluation Prior to Prescription Writing
- H&P (current hospital course; age, gender, admission date, pertinent events, lab/results/test, medications and heart rhythm, identification of cardiac risk factors)
- Patient interview and assessment (learning capabilities/deficits, psychosocial history, employment, recreation, physical limitations and limitations at work, musculoskeletal problems, and functional capacity using the Duke Activity Status index and/or Tinetti Balance/Gait Score. Also include risk modification needs, in addition to goals and plan of care. (*Adapted from Mount Sinai Cardiac Rehab document*)

Risk Stratification
- Patients are stratified into low, moderate, or high risk according to risk for complications.
- The risk stratification process serves as the basis for individualizing the prescription of exercise training. This is because exercise prescription [3] noncompliance and poor adherence to prescribed training HR [4] increase the risk of mortality. Even though, in patients with Heart Disease (HD), risk of cardiac events increases

during exercise, the overall mortality is significantly lower than in those who do not have cardiac disease [5].
- Risk Stratification is published by the American Association of Cardiovascular and Pulmonary Rehabilitation.

Guidelines for Risk Stratification *(Protocol and Guidelines adapted from Mount Sinai Cardiac Rehabilitation)*
- **Low**
  ○ No significant left ventricular dysfunction (i.e., EF > 50)
  ○ No resting or exercise-induced myocardial ischemia observed as angina or ST segment displacement
  ○ No resting or exercise-induced complex dysrhythmia
  ○ Uncomplicated myocardial infarction, coronary artery bypass, or angioplasty
- **Intermediate**
  ○ Mild to moderately depressed LVEF (i.e., EF 31–49%)
  ○ Functional capacity between 5 and 7 METS
  ○ Failure to comply with exercise intensity prescription
  ○ Exercise-induced myocardial ischemia (1–2 mm ST seg depression)
- **High**
  ○ Severely depressed left ventricular function (EF 30% or less)
  ○ Complex dysrhythmias at rest or increasing with exercise
  ○ Decrease in systolic blood pressure >20 mmHg or failure to rise with increasing work loads
  ○ Survivor of sudden cardiac death
  ○ Myocardial infarction complicated by CHF, cardiogenic shock, and/or complex ventricular dysrhythmias

Phases of Cardiac Rehabilitation [6]
- CR is useful for Pts post-acute MI, chronic unstable angina, CHF, coronary revascularization, valve correction surgery, and cardiac transplantation
- A physician-directed prescription is required for each Phase of CR program
- *Phase I:* Inpatient training (can begin on Hospital day 2–4 and lasts 1–2 wks)
  ○ Goals
    ▪ Prevention of sequelae of immobilization (DVT, PE)
    ▪ Promote self-care
    ▪ May also include Submaximal stress testing

- **_Phase II:_** Outpatient training phase (starts 2–4 wks after d/c, usually lasts 2–3 months)
  - Involves increasing CV capacity and gradual restoration to optimal baseline activity level
  - Modifications to exercise prescription and decisions on resuming work and sex are made after a functional exercise tolerance
  - Usual guidelines for safely resuming sexual activity after a cardiac event (MI or CABG) include asymptomatic pt, stable, and can tolerate 5–7 METs w/o abnormal ECG, BP or HR changes. The wait time period is usually 6 wks, but may vary. Some useful clinical test include the two-flight stair-climbing test: walking for 10 min at 2 paces/s (about 3 mi/h or 4.3 METS), then climbing two flight (~22 steps) of stairs in 10 s [7]
- **_Phase III:_** Maintenance Phase (typically lifelong program)
  - Usually done under minimal or no clinical supervision
  - Goal is to maintain and augment the benefits of phase I and phase II

Functional Exercise Stress Test
- The basis for the exercise prescription
- Used to assess the Pt's capacity to return to work
- May also be used as a guide for resumption of sexual activity
- Performed 6–8 weeks after an acute cardiac event
- Performed under the protection of the patient's cardiac medication
- Test begins at the lowest work level (2 METs) and is increased gradually at a 1 MET interval
- Modality used is similar to the activity to be performed

Absolute Contraindications to Functional Stress Testing
- Are comparable to contraindications to exercise sessions
- Recent change in ECG
- Serious cardiac arrhythmia
- LV dysfunction
- Uncontrolled HTN
- Systemic Illness
- Severe Aortic stenosis
- Severe physical disability precluding treadmill or arm ergometry use

Relative Contraindications
- Hypertrophic cardiomyopathy
- Electrolyte abnormalities
- Moderate valvular disease
- Significant arterial or pulmonary HTN

Contraindications for Inpatient Exercise Session (ACSM Guidelines)
- Unstable angina
- Resting SBP >200 mmHg or <80 mmHg (exception for end-stage heart failure/VAD patients)
- Resting DBP > 110
- Significant drop (≥20 mmHg in resting SBP from patient's average level which cannot be explained by mediations)
- Severe Aortic Stenosis
- Acute Systemic illness or fever (≥102)
- Uncontrolled atrial or ventricular dysrhythmia
- Resting HR > 120
- Symptomatic CHF at rest (Class IV NYSSHA)
- Second- or third-degree heart block without a pace maker
- Acute embolism which is not therapeutically anticoagulated
- Acute clinical thrombophlebitis
- Resting ischemic changes on telemetry
- Uncontrolled diabetes (blood glucose > 400 mg/dl)
- Orthopedic problems that would prohibit exercise
- SaO_2 < 86% (exception for the end-stage lung disease waiting for transplant; parameters to be established by pulmonologist)

Termination of an Exercise Session
- Anginal symptoms
- Significant increase in ventricular ectopy (>30% of complexes are ventricular)
- A significant drop in SBP >20 mmHg with an increased exercise workload
- Lightheadedness, shortness of breath, confusion, ataxia, pallor, cyanosis, and/or signs of severe peripheral circulatory insufficiency
- New ST segment changes
- Onset of second-/third-degree heart block
- Excessive rise in SBP >220 mmHg or >110 mmHg
- Chronotropic impairment
- New dysrhythmias

- New exercise-induced left bundle branch block
- Failure of monitoring system
- Borg rating >15

Borg's Rating of Perceived Exertion Scale (RPE) [6, 8, 9]
- Tool used to measure the degree of perceived physical exertion in a patient performing an exercise
- Fifteen point scale from 6 to 20 where the number 6 represents no perceived exertion or leg discomfort, 13 is "somewhat hard" and corresponds with a conversational level of exercise, and 20 represents the greatest amount of exertion that the patient has ever experienced [6, 9]
- Ratings of 15–16 suggest that the aerobic threshold has been exceeded, and greater than 18 indicates the patient has performed maximal exercise [9]
- Useful for Pts after cardiac transplant since denervation of the orthotopic heart makes HR parameters unreliable [2]

Borg RPE 15 Point Scale [8]
- 6–20% effort
- 7–30% effort—Very, very light (Rest)
- 8–40% effort
- 9–50% effort—Very light-gentle walking
- 10–55% effort
- 11–60% effort—Fairly light
- 12–65% effort
- 13–70% effort—Somewhat hard-steady pace; conversational level of exercise
- 14–75% effort
- 15–80% effort—Hard
- 16–85% effort
- 17–90% effort—Very hard
- 18–95% effort
- 19–100% effort—Very, very hard
- 20—Exhaustion

Six-Minute Walk Test [10]
- A functional capacity assessment that measures the distance a patient may quickly walk on a hard, flat surface in a period of 6 min
- Evaluates the global and integrated responses of all the systems involved during exercise (pulmonary and cardiovascular systems,

peripheral circulation, blood, neuromuscular units, and muscle metabolism)
- Self-paced (Patient chooses their own intensity), it assesses the submaximal level of functional capacity
- Pt is instructed to walk down a 100-foot hallway at their own pace and attempt to cover as much distance as possible in 6 min. The total distance walked is determined and the symptoms experienced are recorded [9]
- Consider this as complimentary to cardiopulmonary exercise testing

Five-Grade Dyspnea Scale [9]
- 0. No Dyspnea
- 1. Mild, noticeable
- 2. Mild, some difficulty
- 3. Moderate difficulty, but can continue
- 4. Severe difficulty, cannot continue

Five-Grade Angina Scale [9]
- 0. No Angina
- 1. Light, barely noticeable
- 2. Moderate, bothersome
- 3. Severe, very uncomfortable
- 4. Most pain ever experienced

Exercise Physiology [2, 6]
- Oxygen Consumption (VO_2): represents the oxygen consumption of the whole body; it characterizes the work of the peripheral skeletal muscles
- Aerobic Capacity (VO_2max): measure of the maximum amount of oxygen that a person can utilize; the higher the value of the VO_2max, the greater the aerobic fitness of the individual
  - Once aerobic capacity is reached, further increases in work are powered by anaerobic metabolism
  - Because cardiac patients do not feel well under anaerobic conditions, exercise intensities should be set below anaerobic threshold
  - The Fick equation can be used to calculate the aerobic capacity (VO_2max):
- Oxygen Consumption (VO_2) = Cardiac Output $(CO) \times$ Arteriovenous Oxygen Difference where Cardiac Output (CO) = Stroke Volume $(SV) \times$ Heart Rate (HR)

Metabolic Equivalents (MET) [11]

- One metabolic equivalent (MET) is defined as the resting metabolic rate; the amount of oxygen consumed while sitting at rest and is equal to 3.5 ml O_2/kg/min
- The MET concept expresses the energy cost of physical activities as a multiple of the resting metabolic rate
- MET is a consistent measure of function irrespective of exercise modality or program
- Metabolic equivalent energy use in different activities
  - Light (1–3 METS)–sleeping, shaving, sponge bathing, dressing/undressing, writing, typing, walking <3 MPH (strolling, level ground, very light effort), lifting <10 lbs.
  - Light to moderate (3–4 METS)–Showering, calisthenics, home exercise, light to moderate effort, walking 3 MPH, climbing stairs, driving, lifting <20 lbs
  - Moderate (4–5 METS)—walking 3.5 MPH, having sexual intercourse, bicycling <10 mph—light effort, lifting 20–50 lbs.
  - Heavy (5–7 METS)–walking 4–5 MPH, stationary bike-light effort, lifting 50–100 lbs.
  - Very Heavy (>7 METS)–jogging at 5 MPH, calisthenics (e.g., pushups, sit ups, pull-ups, jumping jacks) heavy, vigorous effort, running/jugging in place, rope jumping, playing soccer/basketball/horseback riding, lifting >100 lbs.

CR Education and Professionals' General Goals

- **Education**: Includes nutritional therapies, weight loss programs, management of lipid abnormalities, proper BP control, diabetes management, and stress management
- **Prevention:** physiologic deconditioning, achieve safe mobility, medical stability, functional independence, initiation of aerobic conditioning, and determine disposition (home versus acute rehabilitation)
- **Exercise Physiologist:** Exercise stress test, training heart rate prescription, supervision of aerobic training sessions, and progressive exercise tolerance (60 min of Telemetry monitored aerobic exercises)
- **PT:** functional independence measure (FIM) scoring, treatment of physical comorbidities; balance, gait, and stair training; supervision of aerobic training sessions; chest physical therapy; and home equipment (60 min/day)

- **OT:** functional independence measure (FIM) scoring, treatment of physical comorbidities, conservation and pacing education, relaxation and breathing exercises, use of assistive devices and home equipment (60 min/day)
- **Psychologist:** Cognitive and psychosocial evaluation and therapy, behavioral modification, and smoking cessation
- **Nutritionist:** dietary evaluation, education, and counseling
- **Rehabilitation Nurse:** Cardiovascular disease (CVD) and risk factor education
- **Physiatrist/Rehabilitation Doctor:** Prescription of CR program, team supervision and CR program modification, coordination of medical care, and patient education.

Inpatient CR (Lasts 10–14 days)
- Stretch before and after every exercise session
- Precautions
  - Avoid valsalva maneuvers, heavy resistance, inappropriate transfer techniques, and anaerobic exercise
  - Bleeding (from anticoagulation meds)
  - Beta blockers and heart transplant patients-blunted HR response to exercise intensity change
  - Sternal surgical wound-limit upper body exercise after CABG/heart valve surgery Heart Transplant (HT). After 6 wks can liberalize upper body exercise as post-op sternal wound knitting complete
  - Arrhythmias-especially in post-CABG patients with Diabetes, Hypertension, Hyperlipidemia, age > 70 [12], and discontinuation of amiodarone
- Physical therapist and exercise physiologist supervise the daily aerobic program (given according to risk stratification)
- 10 min callisthenic warm up (i.e., light workout, walking)
- 45–60 min low-impact aerobic training exercise (up to 15 min each of 3 or 4 modalities): Initially advance training duration, and then intensity.
- Exercise intensity and training HR as described by Karvonen [13]:
  - Training $HR = RHR + [(PHR - RHR) \times I]$
  - $RHR =$ Resting HR from EST, PHR is peak HR from the EST, and I a coefficient expressed as percentage if risk stratification class (low risk 70–85%; moderate risk, 55–70%, and high risk 40–55%). Remember that there are absolute and relative contraindications to exercise stress testing.
  - For patients on beta-blockers (or other blunted HR response to exercise), a training HR is set 10–20 beats above resting

- 10 min cool down (slow walk and stretching)
- Aerobic Modalities: Stationary bicycle, schwinn Airdyne, step machine, rowing machine, upper body ergometer, VersaClimber, and treadmill
- Perceived exertion: not to exceed 13–15 out of 20 on Borg scale

Outpatient Cardiac Rehabilitation
- Outpatient CR is ideally done in a setting in a hospital or close in proximity to a hospital to allow for rapid medical care in case of a cardiac emergency
- Goals include progressive aerobic conditioning, education on risk factor and lifestyle modification, and optimization for return to work and/or baseline functioning.
- Under the supervision of physical therapist or exercise physiologist, exercise sessions three to five times a week (a total of about 36 sessions, depending at times on insurance coverage) is needed to continue the training process.
- Self-directed exercise training three to five times a week is also recommended to maintain achieved gains.
- Pt education of behavioral and lifestyle modification, smoking cessation, psychosocial support, and nutrition continues during the outpatient program.

Protocol for Phase I Cardiac Rehabilitation in Low-Risk Patients
Plan: Phase I CR via physical therapy screening with nursing; progressing of activity level based on objective and subjective responses. Patient participation in medical and/or post-open heart surgery classes. All patients monitored by telemetry
Goals:
- Short term (1–3 days)
  - MET Level: 2–3
  - Activity: Self-care-dressing, washing, OOB to chair, ambulate 30–200 ft, UE/LE exercise, Incentive Spirometry, Patient/ Family education
  - Monitor: Symptoms, heart rate, BP, RR/SaO$_2$
  - Action: maintain muscle strength/tone, reduce orthostatic hypotension, maintain joint mobility
- Long Term (3–5 days)
  - MET Level: 3–5
  - Activity: Independent ADLs, independent transfers, CG to independent ambulation, Ambulation 2–5 min 3–5×, supervision 1

flight of stairs, continued patient/family education, independent in ambulation and exercise program, independent symptom monitoring
○ Monitor: Symptoms, HR, BP
○ Action: Improve muscle strength/tone, improved endurance, educate regarding cardiac risk factors, decrease patient/family anxiety, promote healthy lifestyle, and assess need for supervised phase II cardiac rehab program.

Protocol for Phase I cardiac Rehabilitation for Intermediate and High-Risk Patients
Plan: Phase I cardiac Rehabilitation via physical therapy (frequency 3–7× per week) with progression based on subjective and objective responses. Patient participation in medical and/or post-OHS education sessions. All patients will be on telemetry
Goals:
• Short Term (Variable)
  ○ MET Level: >2
  ○ Activity: self-care with assist, dangle sit with assist, OOB to chair BID, ambulate in place 1 min, UE/LE exercise, Incentive Spirometry, Patient/Family education
  ○ Monitor: Symptoms, HR, BP
  ○ Action: Maintain muscle strength/tone, reduce orthostatic hypertension, maintain joint mobility
• Long Term (Variable)
  ○ Activity
    ▪ MET Level 2–3: self-care with assist, OOB to chair TID, ambulation to bathroom with assistance, 5–10 min of UE/LE therapeutic exercise, ambulation 2–4 min with assist TID, Continued patient/family education
    ▪ MET Level 4–5: Independent with self-care, OOB to chair ad lib, Ambulate 4–5 min with min to no assist TID, Ascend/descend 1 flight of stairs with min assist to contact guard, Independent symptom monitoring
  ○ Monitor: Symptoms, HR, BP
  ○ Action: improved muscle strength/tone, improved endurance, educate regarding cardiac risk factors, decrease patient/family anxiety, promote healthy lifestyle, assess need for supervised phase II cardiac rehab program

Cardiac Rehab Prescription (Example)

Post-Myocardial Infarction Rehabilitation/Stable Angina

Note: Cardiac Rehabilitation is started as soon as Patient is medically stable following a cardiac event
Acute: 1st 3 days in CCU
- Precautions:
  - ○ HR→ between 50 and 120 bpm OR no >30 bpm from baseline
    - ▪ if on beta blocker no >20 BPM from baseline
  - ○ BP→ SBP not to decrease >10–20 mmHg
- Low-intensity activity (1–2 METS)
- PROM (1.5 METs)
  - ○ UE ROM→1.7 METs
  - ○ LE ROM→2 METs
- Can use bedside commode to avoid energy expenditure with bed pan
- Also avoid Valsalva maneuvers, heavy resistance, and anaerobic exercises.

Subacute: Ranges from 7 to 10 days, depending on medical stability, functional ability, insurance
- Calisthenics of known energy cost
- ROM, may add 1–2 lb resistance
- Early Ambulation (to prevent loss of cardiac reflexes associated with prolonged bed rest)
- Telemetry monitored seated activities, standing, and ambulation at 3–4 METs follows.
  - ○ 1 mph (1.5–2 METs)
  - ○ 2 mph (2–3 METs)
- Self-Care activities

Transitional: Community reintegration/activities
- Visiting nurse services for wound care, medical stabilization, and outpatient PT for continued functional gains and patient education.

Outpatient
- Ambulation increased to 30–60 min
  - ○ Slow walk 2 MPH 2 METs
  - ○ Regular walk 3 MPH 3 METs

- ○ Brisk walk 4.5 METs
- ○ Jogging 6+ METs
- Increase Calisthenics and mild resistance
- Stationary bike
- Progressive household activities
- Community ambulation (1.5 mph)
- Return to work for sedentary activities, must be able to do 3.5 mph × 30 min prior

Precautions/Special Considerations in Specific Heart Diseases
Cardiac Rehab Protocol for Patients with CAD/Stable Angina

- Exercise HR set 10 beats below the threshold HR from the Exercise Stress Test (EST)

Cardiac Rehab Protocol for Patients with MI

- Following a massive MI, delay initiation of exercise 4–6 weeks to allow for healing of heart tissues
- Implement low intensity level and frequent clinical and ECG monitoring
- Otherwise initiate exercise 2–4 weeks accordingly, as training soon after a small MI does not worsen remodeling [14]

Cardiac Rehab Protocol for Patients after Angioplasty and Stent

- Close monitoring for symptoms and signs of recurrent ischemia during CR

Cardiac Rehab Protocol for Patients after Coronary Artery Bypass Surgery (CABG)/Heart Valve Surgery

- Sternal wound precautions

Cardiac Rehab Protocol for Patients with Congestive Heart Failure CHF

- Continuous steady-state interval training [15] (short 60–120 s burst of intense exercise, with intervening 30–60 s recovery periods)
- CHF patients may need implantation of biventricular pacemaker with leads in order to significantly improve LV-EF

Cardiac Rehab Protocol for Patients with Left Ventricular Assist Device (LVAD)

- LVAD is usually a bridge to heart transplant for patients with end-stage CHF
- Initiate ambulation within 7–10 days of LVAD insertion

- Treadmill training by 3 weeks
- Resumption of ADL up to 5 METs within 6 weeks

Cardiac Rehab Protocol for Patients with Heart Transplant (HT)

- CR is recommended before and after HT
- CR is safe in patients on IV inotropic support awaiting HT
- Post-HT program is comparable to that of CABG. Patients have abnormal physiologic response to exercise, so HR in training intensities is unreliable
- Target training intensity 50–60% VO_{2max} (corresponds to a Borg rate of 11–13), then increasing to 13–15 [16].
- Include O_2 monitoring

Cardiac Rehab Protocol for Patients with Arrhythmias

- 1/3 patients develop atrial tachyarrhythmias immediately following cardiac surgery, most commonly atrial fibrillation
- If cannot cardiovert, then rate control is essential
- Can initiate exercise at HR < 100
- If asymptomatic, HR 100–120 is allowed
- HR >120 at rest, or >140 with light exercise is a contraindication
- Remember that after CABG or MI, risk of ventricular arrhythmias increase in the presence of HTN, DM, Hyperlipidemia, age >70 years old
- Prolonged warm-up and cool down before and after exercise training can reduce frequency of arrhythmia
- Decrease exercise intensity and increase duration and frequency if exercise capacity is limited by ventricular arrhythmias and poor EF [17]
- ICDs are used to manage malignant ventricular arrhythmias
- Upright exercise is preferred to supine in the setting of ventricular arrhythmias

Special Consideration for Patients Post-Thoracotomy

- Educate patient to expect slow return of strength and energy
- Instruct patient to avoid heavy lifting, yard work, and other activities that may stress the surgical incision.
- Can generally return to sexual activity after (6 weeks) unless otherwise specified
- Contact Physician if:
  - Incision draining unusual amount or becomes very red
  - Worsening pain

- ○ Sudden, severe shortness of breath
- ○ Sudden, sharp chest pain
- ○ Fever > 101
- ○ Experience rapid heartbeat or "fluttering" in chest

References

1. Suaya JA, Shepard DS, Normand SL, Ades PA, Prottas J, Stason WB. Use of cardiac rehabilitation by Medicare beneficiaries after myocardial infarction or coronary bypass surgery. Circulation. 2007;116:1653Y62.
2. Braddom LR. Physical medicine and rehabilitation. Third edition. 3rd ed. Physical medicine and rehabilitation, Braddom LR, editor. Saunders Elsevier; 2007. p. 42.
3. Roitman JL, LaFontaine T, Drimmer AM. A new model for risk stratification and delivery of cardiovascular rehabilitation services in the long-term clinical management of patients with coronary artery disease. J Cardiopulm Rehabil. 1998;18(2):113–23.
4. Hossack KF, Hartwig R. Cardiac arrest associated with supervised cardiac rehabilitation. J Cariac Rehabil. 1982;2:402–8.
5. Thompson PD. The benefits and risks of exercise training in patients with chronic coronary artery disease. JAMA. 1998;259(10):1537–40.
6. Choi HR, Fish S, Shatzer DE, Krabak M. Physical medicine and rehabilitation pocketpedia. Lippincott Williams and Wilkins; 2003.
7. Mallory GK, White PD, Sacedo SJ. The speed of healing of myocardial infarction: a study of the pathological anatomy in seventy-two cases. Am Heart J. 1939;18:14.
8. Borg GA. Psychophysical bases of perceived exertion. Med Sci Sports Exerc. 1982;14(5):377–81.
9. Delisa JA. Physical medicine and rehabilitation: principles and practice. 4th ed. Philadelphia, PA: Lippincott Williams & Wilkins; 2005.
10. American Thoracic Society. ATS statement: guidelines for the six-minute walk test. Am J Respir Crit Care Med. 2002;166:111–7.
11. Jette M, Sidney K, Blumchen G. Metabolic equivalents (METS) in exercise testing, exercise prescription, and evaluation of functional capacity. Clin Cardiol. 1990;13:555–65.
12. Galante A, et al. Incidence and risk factors associated with cardiac arrhythmias during rehabilitation after coronary artery bypass surgery. Arch Phys Med Rehabil. 2000;81(7):947–52.
13. Karvonen MJ, Kentala E, Mustala O. The effects of training on heart rate; a longitudinal study. Ann Med Exp Biol Fenn. 1957;35(3):307–15.
14. Cannistra LB, et al. Moderate-high intensity exercise training after myocardial infarction: effect on left ventricular remodeling. J Cardiopulm Rehabil. 1999;19(6):373–80.

15. Coats AJ, et al. Controlled trial of physical training in chronic heart failure. Exercise performance, hemodynamics, ventilation, and autonomic function. Circulation. 1992;85(6):2119–31.
16. Pina IL, et al. Exercise and heart failure: a statement from the American Heart Association Committee on exercise, rehabilitation, and prevention. Circulation. 2003;107(8):1210–25.
17. Kelly TM. Exercise testing and training of patients with malignant ventricular arrhythmias. Med Sci Sports Exerc. 1996;28(1):53–61.

Part II
Clinical Strategies

Chapter 7
Nutrition in Rehabilitation Medicine

Natalie Kretzer

Main Issues with Obtaining Proper Nutrition

1. Poor swallowing ability
2. Unintentional weight loss
3. PEG or NG tube dependence

Importance of Nutrition

While the outcomes of rehab medicine are typically focused on functional capability, nutrition is the fuel for helping patients accomplish therapy goals. Good nutrition leads to improved muscle strength and improved outcomes with therapy. Patients can receive adequate nutrition through oral intake, enteral nutrition, or a combination of both routes. Progressing a patient from dependence on enteral nutrition to eating by mouth can assist with an easier transition and less home care needs when the patient is ready for discharge. When a patient is assessed to have poor nutrition status, this means that there may be inadequate calorie and protein intake leading to low energy availability or ongoing muscle wasting. Long-term complications may include

N. Kretzer, R.D., C.D.N. (✉)
Department of Clinical Nutrition, Mount Sinai Medical Center,
One Gustave Levy Place, New York, NY 10029, USA
e-mail: nnkretzer@gmail.com

K.A. Sackheim (ed.), *Rehab Clinical Pocket Guide:*
Rehabilitation Medicine, DOI 10.1007/978-1-4614-5419-9_7,
© Springer Science+Business Media, LLC 2013

delayed wound healing or vitamin and mineral deficiencies such as iron or vitamin D. For patients with diabetes, poor nutrition, and variable intake can lead to difficulty managing blood glucose levels.

Poor nutrition status: there may be inadequate calorie and protein intake leading to low energy availability or ongoing muscle wasting
Long-term complications: delayed wound healing or vitamin and mineral deficiencies such as iron or vitamin D. For patients with diabetes, poor nutrition, and variable intake can lead to difficulty managing blood glucose levels.

Swallowing

- Decreased ability to swallow due to brain injury, stroke, or cognition with age
- Team collaboration between nutrition and speech language pathologist (SLP) to determine NPO status or appropriate liquid consistency and supplements
  - *Tests by SLP:* bedside exam with green dye to test for aspiration, trials with differing consistencies of food and liquids, Modified Barium Swallow, FEES
    - Indications that patient may need a SLP consult for diet consistency: coughing with swallowing, difficulty breathing and chewing, decreased intake, poor dentition, poor attention to meals

Diet Orders

Most options for each type of diet include additional diet restrictions such as diabetic, heart healthy, renal, and various restrictions for allergies, diet preferences, and religious beliefs. Diet modification may be necessary due to poor swallowing ability, poor dentition, or decreased ability to cut foods and feed self.

<u>Types of Diets:</u> (from least to most altered)

- **Regular**
- **Mechanical Soft/Altered**—chopped to smaller pieces with vegetables and meats cooked to a slightly softer consistency for ease of chewing. This is selected for patients as they progress from a puree diet to regular consistency. A patient may also receive this diet if they have limited functionality for cutting tougher pieces of food.

- **Soft**—depending on the hospital, this may be a GI soft diet or just a soft cooked diet. GI soft diets are low in fiber for ease of digestion. Soft diets are a step up from puree and would include regular types of food that can be cooked to a soft consistency but do not need to be altered by pureeing. (e.g., mashed potatoes, macaroni and cheese, pudding, and baked pasta dishes)
- **Pureed/Dysphagia**
- **NPO**—for patients you are really concerned about aspiration, they will require enteral or parenteral forms of nutrition

Liquid Orders

Methods to thicken: drinks can be thickened with powders such as "thicken up" or many hospitals have pre-thickened beverages (honey and nectar thick). If patients have an order for regular oral supplements, they must be thickened to the appropriate consistency before being given to the patient.

Types of Liquids: (from least to most modified)

- **Thins** (default order)
- **Nectar thick**—SLP determines when to place a patient on thins vs. thickened consistency based on aspiration risk. Nectar thick is slightly thicker than water but still runs off a spoon.
- **Honey thick**—the thickest liquid when the risk of aspiration is high. Most patients who start a PO diet after full PEG dependence start with honey thick liquids and advance to nectar thick and eventually thins. Fluid intake needs to be carefully monitored with honey thick liquids as most patients do not drink a sufficient amount and may need extra water flushes through the PEG even if they are eating enough solid foods to meet calorie and protein needs.
- **No liquids**—for patients you are really concerned about aspiration, they may need to have additional IVF depending on circumstances

Admissions at Night: what to do when Dietitians and Speech language pathologists are not present

Enteral Feeds

- Obtain a copy of the hospital formulary from the dietitian for enteral nutrition and supplements

- If the patient is admitted on a tube feed not available on the formulary, search the formula (that the pt was admitted with) online; the manufacturer should explain whether it is standard, semi-elemental, etc.
- Choose a similarly classified formula on the hospital's formulary
- If a patient was previously on 24 h feeds, run it at the same rate for 16 h overnight (to accommodate the rehab therapy schedule)
  - The RD can adjust the rate and plan to advance the next day to ensure that the patient is not overfed or experiences intolerance with volume

Oral diets
- If the patient is eating and you are concerned about the food and fluid consistency, check past SLP notes and choose the most conservative diet and liquid if there is any question regarding safety with swallowing
  - Place a consult for SLP to see patient the next day
- If you are unsure about the diet restrictions, choose what is logical (such as diabetic or renal) and the dietitian can liberalize the diet if appropriate
  - Place a consult for nutritionist to see patient the next day
- If you have any concerns about aspiration the safest thing to do is NPO or pureed diet overnight. You can always start IVF with glucose if needed and appropriate. caution with diabetics
- Occasionally dietitians are on call for immediate concerns

Caution with patients who have: stroke, traumatic brain injury, spinal cord injury, altered mental status, neuromuscular diseases, severe weakness, poor dentition, inattention to eating, advanced age, ongoing poor PO intake

Oral Supplements

- Used when a patient is able to eat but not meeting sufficient calorie needs
- Increase calorie and protein intake with less volume than typical food and fluids when a patient is malnourished or experiencing early satiety

Types of oral supplements: vary as tube feed formulas with standard, diabetic, renal

- Most are Kosher items and lactose free
- **Clear liquid or "juice based"** supplements used for patients with diarrhea or on a clear liquid (often post-op diet)
- **Thickened supplements**: puddings with increased calories and protein for patients with thickened liquid diet orders

Additives: used to alter standard oral supplements or formulas; can be mixed into the tube feed bag, added to water flushes with medications, or added to oral supplements

- **Fiber supplements:** used to treat empirically for diarrhea or constipation. If a patient has constipation, encourage increased fluid with fiber supplements.
- **Protein supplements:** increase protein without large increases in calories for enteral formulas; used when a patient has increased protein needs with multiple wounds or s/p surgeries. Protein modulars are often used in patients who are overweight/obese but need increased protein intake for medical issues such as dialysis but do not need additional calories.
- **Caloric additives:** powdered caloric additives; used when the tube feed volume cannot be increased due to pt tolerance but the formula is meeting the patient's protein needs. Can be used to increase caloric density of oral supplements when patients are severely malnourished or intake remains very minimal.

NPO: No nutrition by mouth

- Not safe to ingest any type of altered food or liquid by mouth because of high aspiration risk
- **Evaluate swallowing safety:** stroke, traumatic brain injury, spinal cord injury, altered mental status, neuromuscular diseases, severe weakness, poor dentition, inattention to eating, advanced age, ongoing poor PO intake

  If a patient requires NPO status because they are a high risk of aspiration, they will need nutrition by an alternative route:

    Enteral—nutrition provided via tube through the nose (NG), stomach (PEG) or small intestine (PEJ)

    Parenteral—nutrition provided intravenously, bypassing the GI tract

Enteral Routes:

- **Nasogastric tube (NGT):** used temporarily, typically ≤4 weeks), usually used to supplement a patient's oral intake if it appears that they will begin to meet their caloric needs soon

- **Percutaneous-endoscopic gastrostomy tube (PEG) or gastrostomy (G-tube)**: long-term management, used when a patient has very poor swallowing function and will take weeks to months to meet caloric needs PO. This can be used as a lifelong source of nutrition if the patient does not regain their ability to swallow or does not regain their appetite or attention to eat sufficient nutrients.
- **Percutaneous-endoscopic jejunostomy tube (PEG-J)**: inserted in the stomach and directed to the jejunum due to GI malabsorption or functional issues

Reasons for Combination of PO Diet and Tube Feeds (TFs)
- Patient unable to meet calorie and protein requirements PO but still able to eat, allowed for comfort measures
- Patient begins to eat but not yet meeting caloric requirements while weaning off the PEG
- Some Patients have a PEG for water and med administration but able to take puree PO without liquids

Tube Feed Orders

<u>Considerations when ordering TF</u>: Route of delivery, duration of tube feed, formula type
Route of delivery
- **Continuous:**
  - Requires a pump for ongoing administration of the tube feed for a set length of time
  - Usually run overnight and is the most common type of tube feed order due to good tolerance in patients and no disruption to the patient's therapy schedule.
  - Requires minimal attention from nursing staff besides intermittent checking of residuals
- **Bolus:**
  - Intermittent feeds given anywhere from 3–6 times per day.
  - Does not require a pump but a syringe or funnel to pour the formula into the PEG
  - Good option for a transitional feed from continuous to a PO diet. If a patient is to go home with a PEG, this is often easiest for the family and allows the pt to resume a more normal

"eating" schedule with intermittent periods of feeding to start signaling hunger and fullness.

- Young patients with high calorie needs may need additional bolus feeds with continuous feeds if unable to deliver enough nutrition overnight. This does not occur often but can happen when a patient is already receiving a concentrated formula or if a patient complains of hunger during the 8 h that no nutrition is being delivered on an overnight continuous schedule.
- Some issues with intolerance with large volumes of formula along with water flushes for adequate hydration flushed into the PEG at one time

Duration of tube feed
- Generally 16 h overnight for a rehab schedule to allow for maximum amount of uninterrupted time in therapy. Sixteen hour feeds overlap breakfast and dinner.
- As the patient weans off the PEG feed, shorter duration is needed to allow the patient to eat without receiving the tube feed at the same time

Formula type
- Each hospital has its own formulary card for the types available. Most hospitals have a contract with either Abbott and Nestle (see Web sites for their nutrition profiles for each tube feed).
  Formula Options:
  - **Intact, standard formula:** generally 1 kcal/mL formula, used in patients without any GI compromise with moderate protein needs
  - **Concentrated formulas:** any formula with greater than 1 kcal/mL (1.2–2 kcal/mL), often required in rehab due to the shortened duration of a tube feed for 16 h vs. 24 inpatient, can be with or without fiber
  - **Semi-elemental:** partially hydrolyzed amino acids for ease of absorption, usually higher in protein and better tolerated if issues with diarrhea persist with standard formulas
  - **Renal:** can be pre- or post-HD formulas. Pre-HD formulas will be lower in protein, whereas post-HD will be high in protein. Both types are fluid restricted and contain lower amounts of potassium and phosphorous.
  - **Diabetic:** lower percentage of carbohydrate in this formula.

Considerations for enteral formula selection

– Past medical history prior to rehab admission (diabetes, kidney disease, etc)
– Degree of stress: burns, fractures/breaks, wounds, recent surgeries that all increase protein needs
– fluid content of formula
– Amount of formula needed for amount of allotted time for tube feed administration
– Patient preferences for type (i.e. kosher) and what has been tolerated in the past

Starting tube feeds

– Start at 30–40 mL/h to monitor patient toleration
– Keep head of bed >45°
– Monitor for residuals >200 mL
– As patient tolerates TF, can increase by 15–30 mL every 6 h to reach goal
– Usually goal rates do not exceed 100–110 mL/h
– Consider patient size and toleration with goal rate

Fluids

– Depending on age and current condition, generally 25–35 mL/kg/day
– Calculate free water from TF (not all enteral formula volume counts as hydration), add water flushes to equal estimated fluid needs
– Generally do not exceed 250–300 mL/flush
– More concentrated formulas have less free water and require more water flushes
– Monitor labs and adjust off of "estimated needs," can use normal saline if patients have ongoing hyponatremia and they are already fluid restricted

Monitoring Labs

– Nutrition related labs
  • **Na, Creat, BUN:** monitor fluid status
  • **Phosphorus:** monitor for refeeding in malnourished patients with aggressive nutrition intervention, monitor in renal patients and consider phos binder if elevated on renal formula
  • **K:** monitor in refeeding in malnourished patients with aggressive nutrition intervention, monitor in renal patients and consider kayexalate if patient already on renal formula

- **Mg:** monitor in refeeding in malnourished patients with aggressive nutrition intervention
- **GFR:** monitor protein content of formula, if decreasing, monitor for increased K and phos
- **Albumin:** indicator of trends of protein status, half life of 21 days; not a good indicator for immediate delivery of protein and nutrition status
- **Prealbumin:** preferred nutrition lab for protein status, can check every 2–3 days to monitor adequacy of nutritional plan or delivery of tube feed

Tube Feed Trouble Shooting
- Diarrhea
  - check meds, even when bowel meds are held, the effect can be seen 2–3 days later
  - check formula: "carb steady" formulas can be malabsorbed
  - fiber: can cause or alleviate the problem, try adding it pt not receiving or vice versa
- Vomiting
  - position of patient during feeds: ensure pt is sitting upright
  - if ongoing, confirm that PEG has not been dislodged
- Clogged PEG
  - prevention: order water flushes of minimal volume (30 mL before and after) each feed to flush enteral residue out of tube; flush medications with water and choose liquid forms of medications when available over solid pill forms
  - attempt water flushes, historically ginger ale has worked but not medically accepted

References

1. Gottschlich MM, editor. The ASPEN nutrition support core curriculum: a case based approach—the adult patient. 2nd ed. Silver Spring, MD: American Society for Parenteral and Enteral Nutrition; 2007.
2. Merritt R. The ASPEN nutrition support practice manual. 2nd ed. Silver Spring, MD: American Society for Parenteral and Enteral Nutrition; 2005.
3. Abad-Jorge A, Banh L, Cumming C, et al. Adult enteral and nutrition handbook. 4th ed. Charlottesville, VA: University of Virginia Health System; 2008.

Chapter 8
Wheelchair Prescription Writing

Jenny Lieberman

A proper evaluation is essential for a wheelchair since improperly prescribed equipment can result in deformity, impairment in skin integrity, decreased function and pain. Simply ordering a wheelchair can have significant repercussions resulting in secondary disabling conditions such as ulcers which can incur significant expense to treat. For this reason, consideration need be made for accessories and seating. Additionally, when possible, patients with long-term conditions should be referred to a licensed medical professional, such as an occupational or physical therapist, who specializes in wheelchair seating and positioning.

Goals when providing a wheelchair:
- Facilitate function
- Ensure proper respiration
- Facilitate proper alignment
- Halt the progression of deformity
- Encourage independent mobility
- Promote good skin integrity

Wheelchair Considerations:
- **Length of need**
  - *Short term*—(<1 year) can use rental, e.g., fracture and recent surgery etc.

J. Lieberman, M.S.O.T. (✉)
Mount Sinai Hospital, Department of Rehabilitation,
Wheelchair Seating and Positioning Clinic, 17 East 102nd Street, 2E
New York, NY 10029, USA
e-mail: jenny.lieberman@mountsinai.org

K.A. Sackheim (ed.), *Rehab Clinical Pocket Guide:*
Rehabilitation Medicine, DOI 10.1007/978-1-4614-5419-9_8,
© Springer Science+Business Media, LLC 2013

- ○ *Long term*—may need to purchase through insurance; refer to a wheelchair clinic for specialized assessment for mobility and seating needs
- **Reimbursement**
  - ○ **Cost:** can vary depending on needs
    - ▪ Standard manual wheelchair with basic seating to custom manual wheelchair with rehab seating = $350–$6,000
    - ▪ Manual reclining wheelchair to manual tilt in space wheelchair with rehab seating = $1,000–$8,000
    - ▪ Scooters = $1,500–$4,000
    - ▪ Basic power wheelchair with Captains Seat to high-end power wheelchair with power seating and rehab seating = $5,500–$27,000
  - ○ *Reimbursement requires use of the device for 5 years*, unless there is a dramatic change in diagnosis/condition.
  - ○ **Medicare:** focus is on ability to complete MRADL (mobility-related activities of daily living) in the home safely and in a timely fashion [1]
    - ▪ If device is needed in the home, refer to the mobility paradigm: walking (if can't walk, address use of cane and/or walker), use of manual wheelchair, scooter, or power wheelchair.
    - ▪ For powered mobility devices (scooter and power wheelchair), additional paperwork must be generated to support the need for the mobility device. The physician is responsible for the face to face evaluation:
      - • The face to face evaluation consists of an office visit note (or medical chart if patient is inpatient) addressing why the user cannot walk even with a device (cane or walker) or propel a manual wheelchair. If a scooter is appropriate, indicate need of scooter for function, if for power wheelchair, indicate that they cannot use a scooter in the home and will only be able to complete MRADL in the home with a power wheelchair. Note must indicate that the visit is a face to face evaluation for a powered mobility device.
      - • Date of completion of face to face: if referred to a licensed/certified medical profession (OT or PT), the date of completion is the date the letter of medical necessity is signed (this is different with many managed Medicare programs; refer to the vendor for specifics).
- **Documentation:** For persons with disabilities, requiring the use of a mobility device now or in the future, chart documentation

should indicate functional mobility (i.e., patient can take steps with walker, but cannot walk while completing function, in place of: patient can walk with walker).

- All wheelchairs should be prescribed as far in advance of discharge as possible so patient receives the equipment for use at home.

Patient Considerations:
- Do they live in a house or apartment?
- Are there steps to enter? Ramp? Elevator? If steps, where will the wheelchair/Scooter be stored?
- Access in the home: doorway widths, location of doors off of hallways (can determine the type of wheelchair based upon turn required; front versus mid wheel drive)
- Transportation:
  - Do they drive or are they transported?
  - Van or car?
  - Bus or subway? (can determine type of wheelchair based upon clearance required: rear wheel for subway, front and mid for bus)
- Employment
  - Are there issues of access in the workplace: work station, bathroom, elevators?
- Family
  - Are there children? Are they a caretaker?

Classification of Wheelchairs

- **Amputee axle wheelchair:** rear axles are placed posterior the frame to shift center of gravity to compensate for the loss of one or both lower extremities. This increases balance and stability.
- **Basic wheelchair:** manual wheelchair with minimal modifications, used when patient has a temporary disability or when patient still has ability to stand and transfer
- **Custom wheelchair:** requires structural changes with possible change in depth, width and height, as well as change in axle position to move rear wheel for easier access and change center of gravity for improved balance
- **Lightweight or ultra-lightweight:** constructed of aluminum or titanium; some are rigid while others fold. These are recommended for full time wheelchair users, especially those with postural

asymmetry and upper limb dysfunction. Rigid is lighter in weight and often clinically more appropriate but folding is easier for some clients to disassemble [2, 3].

- **Manual:** propelled by hand
- **Motorized:** propelled by electric motor, compensates for patients inability to use manual propulsion, patients who have decrease or inability to use both lower extremities, combined with a decrease or inability to use at least one upper extremity, also used in patients with severe COPD, MS, SCI, Stroke, amputation, DJD, RA, and severe cardiovascular disease, must be able to use without endangering self or others. Allows for the addition of power seating (power tilt, recline, seat elevator, or elevating leg rests). Can also allow for power standing feature. These are considerations for patients with limited range of motion, ulcers, dependence with weight shift, pain, and deformity [4–6].
- **Power Assist:** power attachments to manual wheelchair provide assistance with propulsion. Motor is both placed in the wheels and accessed by activating the Rims, or there is a Joystick attachment. Good for patients who require a manual wheelchair for access, but lack strength or range of motion to propel.
- **Scooters:** electrically motorized device, enable impaired patients increased mobility, must be able to use without endangering self or others.
  - ○ Scooter requires good upper limb range of motion and strength as well as good balance and postural alignment; there are no modifications that can be made to a scooter. For patients with postural asymmetry, upper limb weakness, and decreased range of motion, a power wheelchair is recommended since there are adjustments that can be made (seating, location of joystick, electronics to decrease sensitivity).
- **Sports model:** built to be used during sports activities

Equipment Considerations

- **Cushions:**
  - ○ General use—Only recommended for short-term use due to lack of support or pressure relief.
  - ○ Pressure relieving—Consideration is presence of wound and ability to maintain.

- Air is the best support surface, but requires maintenance [7]. Otherwise, consider fluid/gel supports
  - Supportive—Level of contour dependent on need for lateral thigh support (adductors) or ease of transfers (flat top).
    - Another consideration is viscosity of foam: forgiving versus solid
- **Seat height, seat dump, and seat to back angle**
  - Front seat to floor height must be high enough to accommodate to lower leg length: front seat to floor height = lower limb length—cushion height + 2 in. for ground clearance (this 2 in. is customary but dependent on skill of wheelchair user to tip back over obstacles during propulsion).
  - Seat dump is the difference between rear and front seat to floor heights, with front being higher. Often recommended for patient with imbalance or spinal deformity.
  - Seat to back angle can be squeezed or open
    - Squeeze is an angle less than 90° where the seat meets the back, resulting in the hips being flexed. This is often recommended for patients with high extensor tone but they MUST have hip range to accommodate.
    - Open seat to back angle is recommended for patients who cannot flex to 90° and for patients with imbalance. Also, research has indicated −10° with lumbar support is ideal for pelvic and lower back position.
- **Back Supports:**
  - Upholstery and general use—Only recommended for short-term use.
    - They provide no support and are generally not recommended for persons using wheelchairs full time.
  - Level of contour—Consideration: Lateral transfers can be impacted with increased contour.
- **Foot/Legrests:**
  - Elevating Legrests versus Swingaway Footrests
    - Elevating Legrests only recommended for limitations in knee flexion and contracture.
      - Consideration: They are heavy and increase turning radius. Also consider hamstring length: contraindicated for tight hamstrings.
- **Armrests**
  - Consideration: Request removable armrests
    - Non-removable interferes in transfers and function

- **Headrests**
  - Recommended with tilt and recline and for use on transportation
  - Consideration: Single Contour versus Bi-Pad dependent on cervical spine lateral versus anterior/posterior curve
- **Caster**
  - Size is dependent on two factors: Lower leg length and terrain
  - The smaller the Caster, the lower to the floor and the tighter the turn but the more difficult it is to maneuver rough terrain.
  - The larger the Caster an increase in seat to floor height, turn and length but easier to maneuver rough terrain.
  - Must also consider Caster clearance of the feet during mobility so the Caster does not hit the patient's heels.
- **Tires**
  - *Solid* tires are solid urethane tires with or without tread. They are a not shock absorbing so the ride is not as smooth.
  - *Pneumatic tires*
    - Pneumatic with foam-filled inserts do not go flat but are not as soft a ride as pneumatics alone.
    - High pressure tires are tires that hold higher pressures and are more durable than standard pneumatics resulting in a smoother ride. Often used with ultra-lightweight and sports wheelchairs.
- **Wheels**
  - Mag Wheels are heavier in weight, requiring no maintenance. Not recommended for full time wheelchair user.
  - Metal Spokes are the standard option on lightweight and ultra-lightweight wheelchairs. Spokes can require maintenance.
  - Fiber Spokes are much lighter in weight, more shock absorbing and more durable, but can cost up to $900.
- **Wheel locks**
  - Push to lock versus pull to lock is standard. Throw dependent on what is easier for patient. Push allows for Lock to be below the cushion for transfers. However, when unlocked they are close to the wheel and can interfere in propulsion (hand hits lock).
  - Scissor locks are below the seat frame so they do not interfere with transfers and are out of the way during propulsion but require balance to reach under the seat.

- ○ Electronic locks are new to the market. They are ideal for persons with upper limb dysfunction or impaired prehension, but can add a bit more weight to the frame since they lock to the wheelchair at the hub.
- **Hand rims**
  - ○ Aluminum is the standard option
  - ○ Plastic Coated recommended for impaired prehension
  - ○ Projections can be requested with Plastic Rims for persons who require something to push off of
  - ○ Oblong are new to the market (Natural Fit Rims) allowing for a more natural wrist position. These are recommended for persons with CTS and other upper limb dysfunctions.
- **Frame**
  - ○ Folding—more easily can fit into car trunk, heavier
  - ○ Rigid—easier to propel, lighter, more maneuverability
- **Pelvic Support (Lapbelt)**
  - ○ Padded for high tone to stabilize pelvis without increased anterior pelvic pressure; 4-Point Lapbelt for greater tone to provide support at thighs and pelvis.
  - ○ Push Button versus Airline dependent on ability to pinch versus lift off

Diagnostic Considerations

- **Spinal cord injury (SCI)**
  - ○ Level of injury:
    - *Paraplegia*—Manual wheelchair unless presence of upper-limb dysfunction, severe postural deformity, pressure ulcer, or cardiac/respiratory issues affecting endurance and/or health
    - *Tetraplegia*—Power wheelchair unless there is:
      - Functional hand use
      - Issues of access
      - Special mobility and environmental needs
  - ○ Skin integrity:
    - Sensation—Greater risk with loss of or decrease in sensation
    - Incontinence—Decreased wound healing with incontinence.
      - Consider referral for colostomy or super-pubic catheter if wound is non-healing.

- History of impairment—increased risk for impairment with presence of scar tissue; scar tissue more prone to breaking up resulting in recurrence of ulcer
  ○ Postural alignment and range of motion:
    - Spine—Consideration: flexible versus fixed
      • Goal is to correct spine as best as possible for respiratory function, digestion, and elimination
    - Pelvis—Obliquity designated by the lower side
      • Goal is equal pressure distribution to decrease peak pressures and promote good skin integrity
    - Heterotopic ossification (H.O.)—H.O. in hips can limit flexion, requiring significant extension (very rarely limits extension)
      • Risk of severe impairment in skin integrity from shearing as the body repositions itself. Also, high risk for plantar ulcers from force into footplates.
      • H.O. in knees requires specific foot support dependent on block in flexion or extension (elevating leg rest versus tucking foot platform).
      • Consideration: If non-healing wounds or severe complaints of pain refer to orthopedics for surgical evaluation.
- Back pain
  - Consideration: lumbar space
    • Lumbar kyphosis: Correlated with increased complaints of back pain. Relief with lumbar support.
  - Consideration: Trapezium and levator scapulae pain.
    • Scapular protraction and elevation, thoracic kyphosis, and cervical lordosis associated with pain. Possible relief with spinal extension, scapular retraction and neutral cervical spine.
- Upper limb injury
  - Posture
    • Poor alignment: scapular protraction and elevation, thoracic kyphosis, and cervical lordosis results in shortening of pectoral muscles. This is correlated with shoulder impingement.
  - Wheel location in Manual Wheelchair
    • The rear wheel should be forward of the rear frame with the middle finger in close proximity to the hub of the wheel.
  - Propulsion technique
    • Want long fluid strides

◦ Consider referral to OT or PT for mobility skills training

- **Stroke**
  - ◦ Tone and asymmetry—Asymmetry can be due to tone
    - ▪ Consider anti-spasmodic medications or muscle injections to decrease spasticity
  - ◦ Cognitive and perceptual function—Power wheelchair not indicated if impairment in cognition and perception unless supervised full time.
  - ◦ Functional limb use—Considerations for manual wheelchair: foot propulsion or one-armed drive
    - ▪ May allow for some mobility but not necessarily functional for completion of activities of daily living.
- **Neuromuscular disease** (e.g., MD, ALS, PLS, SMA)
  - ◦ Progression—Results in muscle atrophy or spasticity. Can be rapid, necessitating urgent equipment needs.
    - ▪ Consider loaner equipment from local loan closets (ALSA and MDA)
  - ◦ Postural presentations—Certain postures are common requiring custom support (i.e., lordosis in MD, scoliosis in SMA)
- **Multiple sclerosis (MS)**
  - ◦ Type—Rate of progression impacts equipment recommendation.
    - ▪ If Progressive, recommend power wheelchair in place of manual wheelchair or Scooter based upon needs now and within 5 years.
    - ▪ Consider seating needs over time: ability to shift weight and risk for impairment in skin integrity (if need power wheelchair, consider a model that allows for the addition of power seating within the next few years).
  - ◦ Cognition—Power wheelchair not indicated if impairment in cognition and perception unless supervised full time.
  - ◦ Postural alignment and range of motion—Consider spinal, pelvic alignment, contracture and tone
- **Rheumatoid arthritis (RA)**
  - ◦ Joint involvement—Joint subluxation results in inability to self propel, requiring power wheelchair for functional mobility
  - ◦ Organ involvement—Bladder and bowel involvement can result in the need for incontinence-proof seating supports
- **General medical diagnoses** (e.g., cardiac disease, pulmonary hypertension, osteoarthritis)

○ Oxygen—Insurance often requires that the oxygen company provide the oxygen tank holder, which does not integrate with a manual or power wheelchair.
○ Fatigue and pain—Can indicate need of power wheelchair for mobility for completion of activities in a timely fashion.

Scooters

Considerations
- Recommended for patient with decreased endurance and strength who is unable to operate a manual wheelchair but does not require a power wheelchair.
- Covered by insurance based upon needs
  ○ Medicare if needed in the home
  ○ Medicaid for outdoor mobility (if secondary to Medicare)
- **Diagnostic considerations:** Arthritis, respiratory disease (emphysema, COPD), cardiovascular disease (CAD, CHF), amputation, early MS (not recommended for later stage MS with postural deformity, impaired skin integrity, and imbalance)
- **Contraindications:**
  ○ Not for patient with impaired skin integrity or potential for impairment (SCI)
  ○ Not recommended for single limb use (stroke)
  ○ Cardiac or respiratory disease with worsening symptoms with bilateral limb use; consider where oxygen tank will be placed (check saturation levels with pulse oxymeter if possible).
  ○ Joint instability in hands
  ○ Must be able to use without endangering self or others
  ○ Must have balance and postural stability to remain upright
  ○ Must have upper extremity range of motion and strength to control tiller
  ○ Must be able to safely transfer onto and off of the device

Types of scooters
- 3-Wheel:
  ○ More maneuverable (32" to 42" turning radius)
  ○ Reimbursed by Medicare and insurances following Medicare guidelines (non-covered under Medicaid)

- 4-Wheel:
    - Larger turning radius (44" to 54" turning radius)
    - Reimbursed by Medicaid (non-covered by Medicare)

Wheelchair Replacement

Reasons to replace: Insurance can be strict with the 5 year rule, but there are circumstances they will consider:
- Current wheelchair no longer meets the needs of the patient due to change in condition or new diagnosis
- Repair costs >1/2 the replacement costs
- Loss or destruction due to circumstances beyond patient's control
    - Stolen: Require a police report
    - Airline damage: Airline will pay to replace if damage is identified prior to leaving the airport

Helpful pearls:
- List of specialty wheelchair clinics and Assistive Technology Practitioners (ATP) available from RESNA (Rehabilitation Engineering and Assistive Technology Society of North America) at http://www.RESNA.org.
- The equipment user should be an active participant in the entire evaluation and order process to ensure goals are met and to decrease incidence of abandonment of equipment [8].

Wheelchair Prescription

Date:

Name:
Date of birth:

Diagnosis: □Stroke □TBI □SCI □Multiple Sclerosis □LE Amputation □s/p TKR/THR □s/p spine surgery □Arthritis □Other _____

Prescription/Referral: □Rental (13 month or less) □Purchase □Refer to Wheelchair Clinic for evaluation if for long-term use

Type of Wheelchair: □Amputee Wheelchair □Basic Manual Wheelchair □Reclining Manual Wheelchair □Manual Tilt In Space Wheelchair □Lightweight Manual Wheelchair □Custom Ultra-Lightweight Wheelchair (**Frame:** □Folding □Rigid) □Scooter □Motorized Wheelchair □Custom Motorized Wheelchair (□Power Tilt □Power Recline □Elevating Legrests □Elevating Platform □Power Elevating Seat)

Modifications:
Seat Width: □16" □18" □20" □22"
Seat Depth: □16" □18" □20" □22"
Foot/Legrests: □Swingaway Footrests □Elevating Legrests (only if cannot flex knee or requires mild elevation) □Angle Adjustable Plates □Composite Plates
Armrest: □Height Adjustable Armrests □Removable Armrests
Pelvic support: □Push Button Lapbelt □Airline Lapbelt □Padded □Non-Padded

Seating:
Back: □General Use □Positioning (□Mild Contour □Max Contour)
Cushion types: □General Use □Pressure Relieving □Pressure Relieving and Positioning
Model: □Roho High Profile □Roho High Profile Quadtro Select □Jay 2 □Jay2 Deep Contour □Other _____

Accessories
Headrest: □10"size Pad □14" size Pad □Removable
Feet: □Foot Straps □Ankle Straps □Heel Loops
Upper Extremity Support: □Hemi □Full

Estimated length of need: □weeks □months □<5 years □>5 years □lifetime

Justification:

_____
_____
_____

Wheelchair Justification Examples

Pressure reliefs

Patient is dependent for weight shift with presence of stage II skin
ulcer at the sacrum, requiring a *pressure relieving seat cushion*.
There is no less costly option to support the asymmetrical
deformity and promote wound healing and good skin
integrity.

Patient is dependent for weight shift with presence of stage II skin
ulcer at the sacrum, requiring a *tilt in space wheelchair*. The
patient is unable to sustain a lift up weight shift for more than
2 min due to weakness/decreased range of motion/etc. In addition, due to spasticity/imbalance the patient can't perform a
forward flexion weight shift. Furthermore, a manual reclining
wheelchair is not recommended due to the incidence of shearing with positional change which will result in greater damage
to impact skin integrity.

Ultra-lightweight chair

Patient presents with paraplegia and shoulder impingement,
resulting in dependence for propulsion in a standard wheelchair. Patient requires a wheelchair with rear wheel able to be
moved forward 2 in. for improved hand to wheel ratio, ruling
out a standard (K0001), lightweight (K0003), and active duty
lightweight wheelchair (K0004). Only with a properly
configured *ultra-lightweight wheelchair* (K0005) will the
patient be able to independently access the kitchen for food or
bathroom for hygiene.

Lateral trunk support

Patient presents with a spinal scoliosis with apex on the right,
necessitating *aggressive lateral trunk support*. There is no less
costly option to support the asymmetrical deformity.

Height adjustable arm rests

Due to long seat to elbow length, the patient requires *height
adjustable armrests*. They cannot be properly supported by
non-adjustable armrests, resulting in lateral spine flexion and
worsening the existing deformity.

Brake extensions

Due to limitations in elbow extension, the patient requires *brake
extensions*. They cannot independently access the brakes without extensions. These are therefore required for safe transfers.

Seat cushions:
Positional:
Due to asymmetrical pelvic deformity (e.g., obliquity, pelvic tilt, pelvic rotation) the patient requires a positional seat cushion. They cannot be supported by a General Use Seat Cushion. There is no less costly option to halt the progression of the asymmetrical deformity.

Pressure relieving:
Due to impairment in skin integrity with a stage (e.g., 2) ulcer, this patient requires a pressure relieving seat cushion. The (e.g., air, fluid, viscous foam) cushion results in immersion into the seat cushion with peak pressures decreased, circulation encouraged and wound healing and good skin integrity promoted. There is no less costly option to promote wound healing and good skin integrity.

Pressure relieving and positional:
Due to the existing asymmetrical deformity with pressure ulcer present, this client requires both a pressure relieving seat cushion as well as a positioning seat cushion. There is no less costly option to halt the progression of the asymmetrical deformity while simultaneously promoting wound healing and good skin integrity.

References

1. Local Coverage Decision (LCD) for Power Mobility Devices (L21271). CMS pub. 100–3, *Medicare National Coverage Determination Manual.* Chapter 1, Section 280.3.
2. Paralyzed Veterans of America Consortium for Spinal Cord Medicine. Preservation of upper limb function following spinal cord injury: a clinical practice guideline for health care professionals. J Spinal Cord Med. 2005;28(5):434–70.
3. Rehabilitation Engineering and Assistive Technology Society of North America. RESNA position on the application of ultralight manual wheelchairs. Arlington: RESNA; 2012.
4. Arva J, Paleg G, Lange M, Lieberman J, Schmeler M, Dicianno B, Babinec M, Rosen L. RESNA position on the application of standing wheelchair devices. Assist Technol. 2009;21(3):161–8.
5. Arva J, Schmeler MR, Lange ML, Lipka DD, Rosen LE. RESNA position on the application of seat-elevating devices for wheelchair users. Assist Technol. 2009;21(2):69–72.

6. Dicianno BE, Arva J, Lieberman JM, Schmeler MR, Souza A, Phillips K, Lange M, Cooper R, Davis K, Betz KL. RESNA position on the application of tilt, recline and elevating legrests for wheelchair users. Assist Technol. 2009;21(1):13–22.
7. The ROHO Group High Profile Quadtro Select Cushion. Cushion maintenance. http://www.youtube.com/watch?v=Dd37symdvYo.
8. Cook A, Hussey S. Assistive technologies: principles and practice. 2nd ed. St. Louis: Mosby; 2002.

Chapter 9
Modalities

Paul Lee

Additional Abbreviations for this Chapter:

A   Alpha
AC   Alternating current
CV   Conduction velocity

Thermotherapy

- Thermotherapy uses physical agents to transfer thermal energy, raising soft tissue temperature to treat injuries and pathological conditions
- Therapeutic range when heating soft tissue:
  ○ Between 40°C and 45°C (104°F to 113°F) [1]
- Typically heats superficial tissues but also has the ability to penetrate deeper muscles and joints
- Modalities used in rehabilitation transfer thermal energy by way of:
  ○ **Conduction:** transmission of energy from direct contact of thermal source.
    ▪ Moist heat packs
    ▪ Paraffin-wax baths

P. Lee, P.T. (✉)
Department of Physical Medicine and Rehabilitation
Phillips Ambulatory Care Center, Beth Israel Medical Center,
10 Union Square East Suite 5N, New York, NY 10002, USA
e-mail: paullee@chpnet.org

K.A. Sackheim (ed.), *Rehab Clinical Pocket Guide:*
Rehabilitation Medicine, DOI 10.1007/978-1-4614-5419-9_9,
© Springer Science+Business Media, LLC 2013

- ◦ **Convection:** transmission of energy through movement of fluid or gases resulting in a variation of temperature
  - ▪ Hot whirlpool
  - ▪ Fluidotherapy
- ◦ **Radiation:** energy transfer where energetic particles travel through medium or space in the form of electric and magnetic fields that make up electromagnetic waves [2]
  - ▪ Most commonly used modality is infrared lamp

Ultrasound and shortwave diathermy are also modalities with thermal abilities but are not indicated as their sole function. These modalities will be discussed in a separate section.

Physiological Effects of Thermotherapy: Vasodilates increases metabolic rate, increases collagen extensibility, increases nerve conduction, decreases conduction latency of sensory and motor nerves, increases pain threshold, and decreases muscle tone and spasms [1, 3–10].

Thermal Conduction Agents: Hot packs and paraffin wax baths
Type of heat: Wet/moist
Indications: Management of chronic pain/joint stiffness, and muscle guarding [1, 3–6]
Primary effects: promotes soft tissue healing, promotes relaxation, and reduces joint stiffness [1, 3–6]
Temperature range:
- Hot packs: 71–77°C (160–170°F)
- Paraffin wax baths: 51–53°C (124–127°F), raise temperature to >93°C (>200°F) to kill bacteria in the equipment

Duration: Hot packs: 20 min, paraffin wax baths: 30 min
Application Methods:
- **Hot packs:** Towels are used as a coupling media, approximately 1-in. thickness between the heat pack and the skin (typically about 6 towels), more towels can be added depending on surface area being covered.
- **Paraffin wax bath:** [7–10]
  1. *Raise cutaneous temperature:* Seven consecutive dips in the wax, providing a few seconds to harden in between each dip, then immerse in the paraffin wax for 30 min without wrapping after removal from the bath.
     - Indication: superficial/cutaneous heating
  2. *Dip immersion with wrapping*: Ten consecutive dips in the wax, providing a few seconds to harden in between each dip then

wrap with a plastic bag, towel, or wax paper for 20–30 min (traditional method)
- Indication: Heating cutaneous and subcutaneous tissue structures
3. *Raise subcutaneous and musculature temperature*: Seven consecutive dips in the wax, providing a few seconds to harden in between each dip, then immerse in the paraffin wax for 30 min. Follow by wrapping in a plastic bag, towel, or wax paper and maintain for 30 min.
   - Indications: Heating deeper structures at muscular level or superficial joints

Contraindications: [11]
- Over malignant areas
- Open wounds
- Skin with impaired sensation to heat
- Severe or acute inflammatory conditions
- Swollen areas
- Thrombophlebitic areas
- Confused and unpredictable patients

Thermal Convection Agents: Hot whirlpools and fluidotherapy
Modality: Fluidotherapy
Type of heat: Dry
Indications: pain in distal extremities, wounds, acute injuries, swelling, joint stiffness, and blood flow insufficiency [1, 8]
Primary effects: relieves pain, increases in tissue temperature, increases in blood flow, increases in metabolic rate, facilitates tissue healing, increases temperature in joint capsules and muscles, and desensitizes skin [1, 8]
Temperature range: Maximum temperature 47.8°C/118°F
Duration: 20 min
Application Methods:
Patient is placed comfortably close to the machine. Place the limb to be treated in the sleeve of the unit. Fasten the sleeve or place a protective towel between the patient and the machine. Set the air speed and pulse time to an appropriate agitation. Patient may perform ROM or use splints or stretching devices during the treatment. Assess the patient after the initial few minutes of treatment.
Contraindications: [11]
- Over malignant areas
- Skin with impaired sensation to heat

- Thrombophlebitic areas
- Confused and unpredictable patients

Precautions/Recommendations: place protective dressing over open wounds/lesions and frequently reassess if treating a severe or acute inflammatory conditions

Modality: Hot whirlpool

Type of heat: Wet

Indications:

1. Neutral temperature: exercise for weakness
2. Neutral-warm: open wounds (necrotic, ischemic, moderate/heavy exudative lesions) circulatory and sensory disorders, and hypertonicity
3. Warm: mobility and ROM limitations with burn patients, and muscle and joint stiffness
4. Hot: pain, and muscle and joint stiffness
5. Very hot: chronic conditions, increase soft tissue extensibility, recommended uses for only distal extremities

Primary effects: increases core temperature, vasodilation, increases blood flow, loosens necrotic tissue, increase leukocytes and antibodies, aids phagocytosis, stimulates granulation tissue formation, decreases muscle tone, increases pulse rate, decreases blood pressure, and provides a relaxing/sedative effect. [1, 8, 10]

Temperature range:

1. Neutral: 32–34°C/90–93°F
2. Neutral-warm: 33–35.5°C/92–96°F
3. Warm: 35.5–37°C/96–98°F
4. Hot: 37–40°C/99–100°F
5. Very hot: 40–43°C/104–110°F

Duration: 15–20 min

Application Methods: Depending on the purpose of the treatment, adjust the temperature of the whirlpool to the appropriate range. Place the involved body segment into the whirlpool approximately 7 in. away from the direct flow of current. The patient may perform ROM or exercises with the body segment being treated.

Contraindications:

- Clean granulating wounds
- New skin grafts or tissue flaps
- Venous ulcers
- During the first trimester of pregnancy
- Multiple sclerosis

- Severely mental impairment
- Full body immersions with urinary or fecal incontinence

Thermal Radiation Agents: Infrared lamps
Indications: Pain
Primary effects: increases temperature of superficial tissue and mild pain relief
Radiation wavelength: 780–1,500 nm
Duration: 15–20 min
Application method: Place a moist towel over the area to be treated. Lamp beam is perpendicular to the specific area being treated for optimal intensity. The lamp is distanced approximately 20 in. from the target treatment area to prevent any skin burns.
Disadvantage: does not penetrate deeper than 3 mm of the skin [10]
Contraindications:
- Severe mental impairment
- Insensate skin

Cryotherapy

- Form of thermal energy modality that decreases tissue temperature
- Typically used for acute and subacute conditions to help reduce inflammation and pain
- The modalities in rehabilitation transfer heat away from tissue by way of:
  - Conduction
    - Ice pack
    - Ice massage
    - Cold pack
    - Cold whirlpool
    - Cold compression units
  - Evaporation
    - Vapo-coolant spray (i.e. Flouri-Methane)
  - Convection
    - Cold whirlpool

Physiologic effects: vasoconstriction, decreases cell metabolism, decreases blood flow, decreases gamma motorneuron activity, decreases muscle spasm and spasticity, decreases nerve conduction velocity, decreases pain, decreases leukocytes and phagocytes, and decreases formation of edema. [1, 6, 10, 12–15]

Stages with continuous application between 0–18°C/32–65°F:
1. Cold and stinging within ~3 min
2. Burning within ~4–7 min
3. Analgesia within ~8–15 min
4. Numbness within ~15–30 min

Conductive Cryotherapy: Ice massage, ice/cold pack, and cold whirlpool

Modality: Ice massage
Indications: contusions, acute and chronic pain, muscle strain, sub-acute tendonitis, tenosynovitis, and bursitis
Primary effects: analgesic, decreases muscle spasm and spasticity, and decreases blood flow
Temperature range: 0–10°C/32–50°F
Duration: 5–15 min
Application method: Position the patient in a comfortable resting posture and place a towel under the area being treated. Rub the ice pack in a continuous circular motion without using excessive pressure until analgesia is reached. Skin temperature must be reduced to 14°C/58°F to reach analgesia.

Modality: Ice pack/gel pack
Indications: acute musculoskeletal injury, acute to chronic pain, and postsurgical edema
Primary effects: all four stages of continuous application of cryotherapy and decreases formation/accumulation of edema
Temperature range: <0°C/32°F
Duration: 20 min
Application method: may place towel between skin and cold pack

Modality: Cold compression unit
Indications: Post-surgical pain and edema
Primary effects: all four stages of continuous application of cryotherapy and decreases formation/accumulation of edema
Temperature range: 10–15°C/50–59°F
Duration: 20 min, but may be applied continuously for 24–48 h with acute injuries or postsurgical conditions.
Application method: Cover treated segment with stockinet if possible. Wrap the sleeve of the unit to the body segment. Set the machine for either continuous or intermittent (20 min every 2 h).

Modality: Cold whirlpool
Mechanism: Conduction with non-circulating, convection with circulating whirlpool
Indications: Acute and subacute injuries
Primary effects: all four stages of continuous application, decreases core temperature, decreases pulse rate, increases blood pressure, decreases respiratory, and increases muscle tone
Temperature range: [10, 12, 13]

1. *Limb immersion:* 10–15°C/50–60°F
2. *Total body immersion:* 13–26°C/65–60°F

Duration: 5–15 min
Application method: Set the whirlpool to the appropriate temperature. Use ice to assist in bringing the whirlpool to the target temperature. The patient may perform exercises with the immersed limb during treatment.

Evaporation Cold Agent: Vapo-coolant spray
Indication: Trigger point, trauma, pain, muscle spasm, and muscle guarding
Primary effects: reduces muscle spasm, inhibits muscle spindle, stimulates the Aβ fiber
Temperature range: 15°C/60°F
Duration: NA
Application method: Spray Flouri-Methane 14–17 in. from the specific treatment area. Spray 3–5 in. lines, 2–5 times in one direction only. Apply a stretch to muscle fibers that are being targeted. Stretch should be held for 30–60 s. Perform the "spray—and—stretch" technique until desired muscle length is gained or pain is reduced.

Electrotherapy

- Multiple clinical applications due to the electrical currents direct and indirect physiological effects on the tissues of the human body.
- The desired effect and outcome of electrotherapy can be influenced specifically by the current type, intensity, voltage, duration, and density of the electrical current. The characteristics and type of tissue involved or being targeted will also influence the outcome of electrotherapy.
- The placement and size of the electrodes are important factors to consider when determining the type of treatment with electrotherapy.

Electrode placement: The clinician needs to consider the target tissue, nerve, and the desired response to determine the best size and placement of the electrodes.

- For deeper structures (i.e. Joints, deep muscles, nerves, or bone), electrodes should be placed further apart.
- When attempting to stimulate a nerve, motor point, trigger point, or compact area, a smaller electrode is recommended over a larger dispersing electrode.
- When using interferential currents, one must consider centralizing the target area with the quadripolar electrode placement.

Current type: The commonly used electrical currents are direct (DC), alternating (AC), and pulsatile (PC). There are different uses of these currents depending on:
- *Waveform:* sinusoidal, rectangular, twin spike
- *Amplitude:* intensity
- *Pulse duration:* width or one pulse length time, a shorter duration is more comfortable
- *Charge:* duration and amplitude of a phase, pulse, or cycle are the determining factors
- *Frequency:* rate or number of pulses or cycles delivered in per unit time; pulse per second (pps) for PC, or cycles per seconds (cps) for AC.

DC electrotherapies, also referred to as monophasic, are typically used with iontophoresis and monophasic direct current.
- **Indications for monophasic DC**: wound healing [16–18], bacterial inhibition [16, 18–21], bone healing [22], and to increase blood flow [17]
- **Indication for iontophoresis**: refer to section on iontophoresis

PC electrotherapies are commonly used with asymmetric biphasic, high volt current, and pulsed galvanic current. These currents, depending on the parameters settings, are commonly used in rehabilitation for (TENS), and neuromuscular electrical stimulation (NMES).
- **Indications for TENS:** analgesic effects and pain management [23–31], increases blood flow [31], and healing bone fractures
- **Indications for High Volt Pulsed Current (HVPC):** wound healing [21, 32, 33], acute edema (negative polarity) [34–37], pain management [35], muscle spasm, and to increases blood flow (negative polarity) [34, 36]
- **Indications for NMES**: muscle reeducation [38–41], strengthening [40–44], spasticity management (limited evidence) [38],

functional electrical stimulation [45], and atrophy prevention [40, 41, 43, 44]

AC currents that are commonly used in electrotherapies are IFC and Russian, but are also known as medium frequency currents with beats (IFC) or bursts (Russian) in cycles.

- **Indications for IFC**: pain [46–48], urinary incontinence disorders [49, 50], and edema management [48].
- **Indication for Russian**: functional electrical stimulation [10], strengthening [51–54], and muscle reeducation [39]

Contraindications for Electrotherapy

Pacemakers, malignancies, pregnancy, deep brain stimulators (DBS), active epiphysis, active bleeding tissue, active DVT, transcranially, near reproductive organ, anterior neck, carotid sinus, implantable cardioverter defribillator (ICD), and patients suffering from mental confusion [11].

1. ELECTROTHERAPY FOR PAIN
Waveform/Current Type: Asymmetric Biphasic Currents for transcutaneous electrical nerve stimulation (TENS)

Acute Pain Settings:
Mechanism: Gate control
Stimulation: Sensory level
Pulse duration: 75–200 µs
Frequency: 80–150 pps
On time: continuous mode
Time: approx 30 min
Amplitude: Produce maximum tolerated tingling
Location: Near or over painful area, may include trigger points and acupuncture points
Treatment time: variable depending on level of pain, minutes to hours
Analgesic affects: Pain relief in the initial 30 min, last < few hours
Optional waveform: Symmetric biphasic

Chronic Pain Settings:
Mechanism: Release of enkephalin
Stimulation: Low frequency/Motor level

Pulse duration: 100–300 ms
Frequency: <20 pps, (1–5 pps for acupuncture-like TENS)
On time: 30 s to 1 min
Amplitude: Elicit tingling and muscle contraction
Location: Electrode over motor points, acupuncture, and trigger points
Treatment time: 15–60 min
Analgesic affects: Pain relief in the initial hour, last greater than an hour

Waveform/Current Type: High Volt Pulsed Current
Chronic Pain Settings:

Mechanism: Release of B-endorphins
Type: Low frequency/Noxious level
Duration: Continuous
Frequency: 1–5 pps
Current: pulsed high volt
On time: 30–45 s
Amplitude: High intensity/muscle contraction
Location: Trigger or acupuncture points
Treatment time: Few minutes to 60 min, typically a brief treatment
Analgesic affects: 6–7 h

Waveform/Current Type: Interferential (IFC)
Acute Pain Settings:

Mechanism: Nonopiate senory level
Type: IFC Conventional TENS treatment
Current: Medium Frequency Beat Alternating Current Waveform
Cycle duration: Constant or sweep mode
Frequency: 50–120 bps
Current Amplitude: 1–140 mA, produce tingling to maximum tolerated tingling
Location: Quadripolar placement, centralizing painful region
Treatment time: ≤2 h

Acute Pain Settings:

Stimulation: Sensory level
Type: Premodulated IFC
Current: Medium Frequency Beat Alternating Current Waveform
Frequency: 4,000 Hz sinusoidal waves
Modulated Frequency: 100–250 Hz
Current Amplitude: 4–29 mA, "strong but comfortable" maintained

Location: Quadripolar placement, centralizing painful region
Treatment time: ~20 min

2. ELECTROTHERAPY FOR FUNCTIONAL ELECTRICAL STIMULATION (FES)

Waveform/Current Type: Frequency Burst Alternating Current Waveform/Russian

FES Settings:

Mechanism: Forceful muscle contraction to perform a functional movement

Cycle duration: 50% duty cycle

Frequency: 2,500 Hz or 5,000 Hz

Current Amplitude: >25% of maximum voluntary isometric contraction (MVIC), to patient's tolerance or until desired movement is achieved

On:Off time: 1:5–1:1 ratio (6–15 s on)

Ramp time: Variable (<1–6 s), to patient's tolerance and specific to movement

Electrode placement: motor point, parallel to muscle fibers

Waveform/Current Type: Symmetric Biphasic Pulse Current

FES Settings:

Mechanism: Forceful muscle contraction to perform a functional movement

Pulse Duration: 100–600 μs

Frequency: 12–50 pps

Current Amplitude: activity specific (patient's maximum tolerance)

On:Off time: Activity specific/1:1 (6–15 s)

Treatment time: Activity specific

3. ELECTROTHERAPY FOR MUSCLE REEDUCATION

Waveform/Current Type: High Volt Pulsed Current (HVPC)

Muscle Reeducation Settings:

Mechanism: comfortable tetanic muscle contraction (without fatigue)

Pulse duration: 100–600 μs

Frequency: 35–55 pps

Current Amplitude: typically up to patient's tolerance

On:Off time: 1:1–4 s or 5:10 s depending on patients fatigue level and goals

Ramp time: 1 s ramp up, 0.5 s ramp down, but variable to patient's tolerance

Electrode placement: Motor points, parallel to muscle fibers

Treatment time: 15–30 min, multiple times per day

Waveform/Current Type: Symmetric Biphasic Pulse Current
Sports Specific and Strength Training Setting: [55, 56]
Mechanism: Forceful contraction
Pulse duration: 100–400 μs
Frequency: 50–100 pps
Current Amplitude: Patient's tolerance
Evoked force: 40–70% of MVIC (maximum voluntary isometric contraction)
On:Off time: 1:4 (5:20 s)
Treatment time: 20 min, 2–3 days/week for 4 weeks, followed by sports specific training with each session.

4. ELECTROTHERAPY FOR MUSCLE STRENGTHENING
Waveform/Current Type: Medium frequency Burst AC (Russian)
Muscle Strengthening Settings:
Mechanism: Forceful contraction
Cycle duration: 50% Duty cycle
Current Amplitude/Evoked Force: ≥50% MVIC (maximum voluntary isometric contraction) for healthy muscles, ≥10% MVIC (of uninjured muscle on opposite limb) for injured muscles
Frequency: 2,500–10,000 Hz carrier frequency delivered in 75 bursts per second
Pulse duration: 400 μs
Burst duration: 6.7 s
On/Off time: 6–10/50–120 s
Treatment time: 10–20 reps, 3 days/week for 6 weeks

Waveform/Current Type: Asymmetric Biphasic Pulse Current
Muscle Strengthening Settings:
Incompete Class D Spinal Cord Injury: [44]
Mechanism: Forceful contraction
Pulse duration: 200 μs
Frequency: 50 pps
Current Amplitude: 78% of MVIC (maximum voluntary isometric contraction)
On:Off time: 3:5 s
Treatment time: 60 min, 6 days/week for 6 months

Electrotherapy for Edema (Acute):
Waveform/Current Type: High Volt Pulsed Current (HVPC) Acute Edema Settings:

Mechanism: Sensory level stimulation
Polarity: Negative
Pulse duration: 20–100 μs
Frequency: 120 pps
Current Amplitude: Lower the intensity by 10% after the first visible muscle contraction is observed to maintain below motor threshold
Treatment time: 30 min, every 4 h immediately after the injury (up to 4/day)

5. ELECTROTHERAPY FOR WOUND HEALING
Waveform/Current Type: High-voltage pulsed current (HVPC)
Wound Healing Settings:
Current Amplitude: 75–260 V
Frequency: 80–100 pps
Treatment time: 45–60 min
Application: Positive polarity is used in the initial three days of treatment on the wound to augment migration and proliferation of epithelial cells to accelerate wound healing and closure. Negative electrode is placed on wound for antibacterial effects or infections until the signs of infection are absent.

Waveform/Current Type: Monophasic DC
Wound Healing Settings:
Current Amplitude: 200–800 μA (>400 μA for denervated skin)
Frequency: Continuous
Duration: 1:2 ratio on:off time (i.e. 2 h on: 4 h off, as to patients tolerance)
Application: Positive polarity is used in the initial three days of treatment on the wound to augment migration and proliferation of epithelial cells to accelerate wound healing and closure. Negative electrode is placed on wound for antibacterial effects or infections until the signs of infection are absent.

6. ELECTROTHERAPY FOR FRACTURE HEALING
Waveform/Current Type: Biphasic symmetric current
Fracture Healing Settings:
Indication: Post 6-month nonunion fractures
Pulse duration: highest pulse duration (>200 μs if possible)
Frequency: 5–10 pps
Treatment time: 30–60 min, four times/day
Location: Negative electrode distal to fracture site or immobilizer, positive electrode placed proximal to fracture or immobilizer.

Iontophoresis:

Iontophoresis uses continuous direct current to provide transcutaneous delivery of ionized medication using ion repulsion in the created electrical field. Depending on the polarity of the medication, the electrode will have a positive (anode) or negative (cathode) charge to deliver the medication. The charged electrode will then repel the ionized medication into the skin. The dosage of medication being delivered is measured in milliampere-minutes (mA-min). Total dose delivered (mA-min) equals the current (mA) times the treatment time (min). Most iontophoresis machines have current intensity between 1 and 5 mA. Typically, 40 mA-min total drug dosage is used and the current intensity is set to the patient's tolerance.

Indications: Inflammation of superficial muscles or tendons, calcium deposits, scar tissue, localized pain, burns, analgesia, and fungi [42].

Intensity: <1–5 mA, depending on patient tolerance

Duration: dependent on the intensity

Frequency: Recommended frequency is typically 3–4 times per week and most medications are used for 5–6 weeks. Beneficial results should be seen within approximately 4 treatments, and should be stopped if no or adverse reactions are observed within that time frame.

Medications and indications used in rehabilitation: [57, 58]
Negative polarity medications:

Acetic acid 2% solution for acute or chronic calcific deposits

Dexamethasone Sodium Phosphate 0.4% for acute and chronic inflammatory conditions

Potassium Citrate 2% solution for rheumatoid arthritis

Ketoprofen 10% for inflammatory musculoskeletal conditions (alternative to corticosteroids)

Iodine 4.7% for adhesive capsulitis

Diclofenac Sodium 1% pain and inflammation (alternative to corticosteroids)

Naproxen Sodium 2% pain and inflammation (alternative to corticosteroids)

Sodium Chloride 2% for keloids, burns, and scar tissue

Sodium Salicylate 2–3% pain and inflammation (alternative to corticosteroids)

Positive polarity medications:
Zinc oxide ointment, 20% for open lesions
Magnesium Sulfate 2% for vasodilation and muscle relaxant (as needed)
Lidocaine 4–5% for soft tissue pain, inflammation, and anesthesia (as needed)
Calium Chloride 2% solution for spasmodic conditions
Tolazoline Chloride 2% aqueous solution for indolent cutaneous ulcers

Ultrasound

Ultrasound is high frequency acoustic vibrations that produce greater than 20,000 cycles per second (Hz).

- Therapeutic ultrasound is known to be frequency between 0.7 and 3.3 MHz.
- The depth of the penetration range from 2 to 5 cm, which depends on the frequency of sounds waves, most machines are set to 1 or 3 MHz.
- Lower frequency (1 MHz) can penetrate to the deeper soft tissue structures
- Higher frequency (3 MHz) is used for superficial tissue to absorb the sound waves
- The ability to regulate the thermal or nonthermal effects of ultrasound is also another important clinical asset when treating various biological tissue structures.
- Absorption coefficient is different for each tissue type. The rate of temperature rise in the tissues with higher collagen content has the highest coefficient and increases in proportion to the ultrasound frequency.
- The intensity, duration, and duty cycle are also important factors to consider when increasing the amount of heat being delivered to the tissue.
- Higher the intensity and continuous treatments results in greater molecular vibrations, causing more micro friction and heat, which in turn lead to increases in tissue temperature.
- Thermal effects of ultrasound are achieved with continuous mode (100% duty cycle)
- Non-thermal effects with pulsed (typically 20–50% duty cycle).

Thermal effects of ultrasound: refer to thermal/heat therapy section for physiological effects of thermal therapy.
Indications: increases extensibility of collagen, decreases pain and muscle spasms

Non-thermal ultrasound is associated with modulating membrane permeability to accelerate the healing process.

- Non-thermal ultrasound has been understood to be clinically effective with treating tissue injuries, which is accredited to its influence in stimulating fibroblast activity resulting in an increase of protein synthesis.
- increases in intracellular calcium, chemotactic factor and histamine release, mast cell degranulation and macrophage responses are also other effects of pulsed ultrasound that stimulate the cellular processes that are critical to tissue healing.

Indications: Clinically, pulsed ultrasound is indicated with soft tissue healing and repair, acute and post acute injuries, dermal ulcers, tendon injuries, bone fractures (within initial 2 wks), nonunion fractures, surgical skin incisions, and chronic inflammation [59–63].

Effective radiating area (ERA): approximately the size of transducer but slightly smaller

Treatment area: twice the size of the ERA

Ultrasound settings:

Bone Growth (initial 2 wks of injury) Settings: [60–63]
Intensity:0.5 W/cm^2
Duty cycle: 20%
Duration: 5 min, four times per week

Intensity:0.03 W/cm^2 (low intensity pulsed ultrasound device required)
Frequency: 1.5 MHz, ultrasound wave pulsed at 1 kHz
Duty cycle: 20%
Duration: 20 min daily

Acute Injury (3–4 h after injury) Settings:
Pulsed:
Intensity: 0.5 W/cm^2
Duty cycle: 20%
Duration: 5 min

Continuous:
Intensity: US 0.1 W/cm^2
Duty cycle: Continuous
Duration: 5 min

Muscle Spasms Settings:
Intensity: 1.0–1.5 W/cm^2
Frequency: 3 MHz for superficial muscles, 1 MHz for deeper muscles

Duty cycle: continuous
Duration: 5 min

Wound Healing Settings: [64]
Periulcer skin:
Intensity: .5–1 W/cm^2
Frequency: 3 MHz
Duty cycle: 20%
Duration: 5 min, area of 5 cm^2

Phonophoresis

Ultrasound is used as a medium for transcutaneous drug delivery of a topically prepared drug. It provides a painless, effective, and conservative method of delivering medication to a specific area. Hydrocortisone is often used for musculoskeletal inflammatory conditions, however due to the consistency of the typical cream base, it acts as a poor conductor and becomes less effective [64, 65].

Medications:
Dexamethasone (0.4% ointment dexamethasone sodium phosphate): anti-inflammatory agent [65, 66]
Lidocaine (5% ointment): soft tissue pain and inflammation, i.e. bursitis and tenosynovitis [66]
Salicylates (10% trolamine salicylates ointment or 3% sodium salicylate ointment): for analgesia, muscle, and joint pain in acute and chronic conditions [66, 67].
Contraindicated: applying ultrasound over cancerous lesions, hemorrhagic legions, epiphyseal plates, orbital cavities [11].
Settings for *superficial* tissue:
Intensity: 0.5–1.3 W/cm^2
Duty cycle: depending on desired effects
 1. Non-thermal, Pulsed (20–50% duty cycle) for anti-inflammatory effects
 2. Thermal effects, Continuous (100% duty cycle)

Duration: typically 5–7 min per 16 square inches

Settings for *deep* tissue:

Intensity: 1.0–2.0 W/cm^2

Duty cycle: depending on desired effects
1. Non-thermal, Pulsed (20–50% duty cycle) for anti-inflammatory effects
2. Thermal effects, Continuous (100% duty cycle)

Duration: typically 5–7 min per 16 square inches

Shortwave Diathermy

SWD is a form of thermal modality that is typically used to increase temperature in the tissue by way of high frequency oscillating alternating current with electromagnetic energy [68, 69].
Thermal effects are achieved with use of continuous setting.

1. **Capacitance technique:**
   - Greater electrical field versus magnetic field, known to be more effective on regions with less adipose tissue and high in electrolytes
   - Electromagnetic power produced: >38 W
   - Treatment depth: Superficial
   - Uses capacitor electrodes:
     - ○ Air space plates: recommended for hands, feet, wrist, ankles, ribs, and spine where there are typically low subcutaneous fat content
     - ○ Pads: target treatment area should be centered between the pads and sufficient layer of towels is needed to protect the skin

2. **Induction technique:**
   - Greater magnetic field versus electrical field, using the limb or area being treated as part of the circuit
   - Electromagnetic power produced: >38 W
   - Treatment depth: deep and superficial
   - Uses inductor electrodes:
     - ○ Drums: towel covering the skin should be in contact with the structure covering the drum electrode for the best results
     - ○ Cables: two arrangements, pancake coil or wraparound coil

Non-thermal effects are achieved with use of pulsed setting.
1. **Pulsed shortwave diathermy (PSWD):** periodically interrupted delivery of electromagnetic energy [70, 71].

- Typically inductive technique with drum electrodes
- Pulse duration: 20–400 μs
- Pulse Frequency: 1–7,000 Hz
- Electromagnetic power produced: <24 W
- PSWD can also have thermal effects, such as increasing the temperature of the knee joint capsule when producing >38 W of electromagnetic power.
- Treatment depth: deep to superficial

2. **Pulsed Electromagnetic Fields (PEMFs):** Primarily used for healing for nonunion bone fractures [72, 73]
    - Only uses magnetic fields
    - Pulse Frequency: 1–1,000 Hz
    - Physiological effects: bone growth

Thermal
- Indications: Joint stiffness, decreased ROM, muscle spasms, scarring, fibrosis, osteoarthritis, synovitis, chronic pain, and decreased blood circulation [69].
- Primary effects: Increases oxygenation to tissue, increases deep tissue temperature and muscular circulation, increases metabolic response, removes metabolic waste, increases soft tissue healing, and increases.

Non-thermal:
- Indications: Edema, acute injury, acute pain, wound healing, nerve healing, and bone healing [70].
- Primary effects: Increases local tissue oxygenation, phagocytosis, increases microvascular perfusion, alters cellular activity, and stimulates ATP and protein synthesis.

Frequencies:
- Three frequencies bands used with SWD devices are 13.56, 27.12, and 40.68 Hz.
- 27.12 Hz is the most commonly used bandwidth.

Treatment time: 15–30 min
Application:
Inductive Cable:
1. Place a towel to cover the region being treated
2. Space the cable turns ≥ 3 cm from each other (use a stiff spacer to prevent tangling of coil and to ensure even spacing)

3. Place approximately 2–3 cm of toweling from the coil, when placing the coil over the treatment area

Caution: Operator of the machine should stay at minimum of 1 m from the unit [74].

Drum Applicator:

1. Place a towel over the treatment area
2. Have the applicator on the towel of the target treatment area
3. Applicator should be angled parallel to the tissues being treated

Caution: Operator of the machine should stay at minimum of 1 m from the unit [74].

Air space plates (Capacitors):

1. Place the two plates evenly over the target treatment area, approximately 2–10 cm apart. (i.e. each plate must be 5 cm away from the surface of the area being treated and the treated limb should equally interpose the plates)

Caution:

- If the plates are not evenly spaced from the skin, the plate closer to the skin will become hotter and may cause a burn.
- Operator of the machine should stay at minimum of 2 m from the unit [74].

Pads (Capacitors):

1. Place 2–3 cm of toweling between the pads and the skin
2. The distance separating the pads from each other should equal the diameter of the pad (i.e. if the pad is 10 cm in diameter across, the pads should placed 10 cm away from each other)

Caution: Operator of the machine should stay at minimum of 2 m from the unit [73].

Contraindications:

Non-thermal: Pacemakers, active DVT, thrombophlebitis, hemorrhagic conditions, anterior neck or carotid sinus, chest, heart, and tuberculosis-affected area [11].

Thermal: Pacemakers, over metal implants, plastic or cement implants, anterior neck or carotid sinus, chest, heart, active DVT, thrombophlebitis, acute injury, over pelvic regions of women during menstruation, malignancy, eyes, pregnancy, hemorrhagic conditions, impaired cognition, area with impaired sensation, infected region, eczema, recently radiated tissues, tuberculosis-affected area, testes, regenerating nerves, regenerating organs, and over growing epiphyses [11].

LASER: Light Amplification for the Stimulated Emission of Radiation

- Low-level laser therapy (LLLT) uses electromagnetic light energy with photons to transfer energy and influence change in tissue structures.
- Two most common types of laser devices are:
  - **Helium-neon (HeNe) laser**: uses two gases (Helium and Neon) as a medium
    - Wavelength: 632.8 nm
    - Direct penetration (direct absorption): 0.5 cm of tissue
    - Indirect penetration (lesser response that occurs deeper in the tissue, effects of the reaction from the energy absorbed in the superficial tissue): 1 cm of tissue
    - Pulse rate: Continuous wave
    - Pulse width: Continuous wave
    - Energy density/treatment time recommendations vary per condition. Refer to suggested treatment protocols provided by companies of FDA approved low-level laser products.
  - **Gallium-Arsenide (GaAs) lasers**: uses a semiconductor diode as its medium
    - Wavelength: 904 nm
    - Direct penetration (direct absorption): 2 cm
    - Indirect penetration (lesser response that occurs deeper in the tissue, effects of the reaction from the energy absorbed in the superficial tissue): 5 cm
    - Pulse rate: 1–1,000 Hz
    - Pulse width: 200 ns
    - Energy density/treatment time recommendations vary per condition. Refer to suggested treatment protocols provided by companies of FDA approved low-level laser products.

Indications: Wound healing; post-operative and diabetic ulcers, inflammation, scar tissue healing, pain, osteoarthritis, and trigger point [75–82]

Primary effects: Increases in fibroblast proliferation, increases tensile strength of wounds, influences prostraglandins levels, increases epithelialization, decreases exudates, and increases the distal latency of distal peripheral nerves [75–82]

Contraindications: Malignancy, active DVT, hemorrhagic conditions, reproductive organs, tuberculosis-affected area, directly over eye, cancerous tumors, and over pelvic/abdominal areas when pregnant [11]

Diagnoses to Treat with Modalities

I. Pain:
1. Electrical Stimulation- TENS Asymmetric biphasic
2. Electrical Stimulation–Interferential
3. Electrical Stimulation–High Volt Pulsed Current
4. Ultrasound
5. Shortwave and microwave diathermy (analgesia)
6. Cryotherapy—cold packs, ice massage (analgesia)
7. Thermatherapy—moist heat, hot whirlpool, paraffin, infrared lamps (analgesia)
8. Low-power laser

II. Wound healing:
1. Electrical Stimulation—HVPC
2. Electrical Stimulation—Monophasic DC
3. Ultrasound
4. Shortwave and microwave diathermy
5. Thermotherapy—moist heat, hot whirlpool, paraffin, infrared lamps
6. Low-power laser

III. Muscle spasms/guarding
1. Ultrasound
2. Electrical Stimulation—Russian
3. Shortwave and microwave diathermy
4. Cryotherapy
5. Thermotherapy
6. Biofeedback

IV. Fracture healing
1. ES—High Volt
2. ES—Low volt

    3. ES—Weak Biphasic
    4. Ultrasound-Pulsed
    5. Electrical bone growth stimulator (EBS)
    6. Ultrasonic bone growth stimulator

V. Trigger Point
    1. Low-power laser
    2. Phonophoresis
    3. Manual myofascial release

VI. Muscle re-education
    1. ES—high volt
    2. ES—interferential
    3. ES—Russian
    4. Biofeedback

VII. Acute Inflammation
    1. Ultrasound
    2. Phonophoresis—Pulsed
    3. ES—monophasic DC
    4. Low—power laser
    5. Cryotherapy
    6. Compression

References

1. Lehmann JF, DeLateur BJ. Therapeutic heat. In: Lehmann JF, editor. *Therapeutic heat and cold*. 4th ed. Baltimore: Williams & Wilkins; 1990. p. 448.
2. Electromagnetic Radiation. Britannica Web site. http://www.britannica.com/EBchecked/topic/183228/electromagnetic-radiation. Accessed 18 June 2012.
3. Robertson VJ, Ward AR, Jung P. The effect of heat on tissue extensibility: a comparison of deep and superficial heating. Arch Phys Med Rehabil. 2005;86(4):819–25.
4. Draper et al. Hot packs and 1-MHz ultrasound treatments have an additive effect on muscle temperature increase. J Athl Train. 1998; 33(1):21–4.
5. Cetin et al. Comparing hot pack, short-wave diathermy, ultrasound, and TENS on isokinetic strength, pain, and functional status of women with osteoarthritic knees: a single-blind, randomized, controlled trial. Am J Phys Med Rehab. 2008;87(6):443–51.
6. Garra et al. Heat or cold packs for neck and back strain: a randomized controlled trial of efficacy. Acad Emerg Med. 2010; 17(5): 484–9.
7. Abramson et al. Effects of paraffin bath and hot fomentation on local tissue temperatures. Arch Phys Med Rehab. 1964;45:87–94.
8. Borell et al. Comparison of in vivo temperatures produced by hydrotherapy, paraffin wax treatment, and fluidotherapy. Phys Ther. 1980;60(10):1273–6.

9. Ayling J, Marks R. Efficacy of paraffin wax baths for rheumatoid arthritic hands. Physiotherapy. 2000;86(4):190–201.
10. Cameron MH. *Physical agents in rehabilitation*: From research to practice. Philadelphia: W.B. Saunders; 1999.
11. Houghton et al. Electrophysical agents—contraindications and precautions: an evidence-based approach to clinical decision making in physical therapy. Physiother Can. 2010 Fall;62(5):1–80. Epub 2011 Jan 5.
12. Rupp et al. Intramuscular temperature changes during and after 2 different cryotherapy interventions in healthy individuals. J Orthop Sports Phys Ther. 2012 Mar 23. [Epub ahead of print]
13. Merrick MA, Jutte LS, Smith ME. Cold modalitites with different thermodynamic properties produce different surface and intramuscular temperature. J Athl Train. 2003;38(1):28–33.
14. Knight KL. *Cryotherapy in sports injury and management*, Champaign, IL: Human Kinetics; 1995.
15. Brosseau et al. Thermotherapy for treatment of osteoarthritis. Cochrane Database Syst Rev. 2003;(4):CD004522.
16. Kloth LC. Electrical stimulation for wound healing: a review of evidence from in vitro studies, animal experiments, and clinical trials. Int J Lower Extremity Wounds. 2005;4(1):23–44.
17. Rowley et al. The influence of electrical current on an infecting microorganism in wounds. Ann NY Acad Sci. 1974;238:543–551.
18. Asadi M, Torkaman G, Hedayati M. Effect of sensory and motor electrical stimulation in vascular endothelial growth factor expression of muscle and skin in full-thickness wound. J Rehabil Res Dev. 2011;48(3):195–201.
19. Ong et al. Antibacterial effects of a silver electrode carrying microamperage direct current in vitro. J Clin Electrophysiol. 1994;6(1):14–18.
20. Thibodeau et al. Inhibition and killing of oral bacteria by silver ion generated with low intensity direct current. J Dent Res. 1978;57:922–926.
21. Kinaid C, Lavoie K. Inhibition of bacterial growth in vitro following stimulation with high voltage, monophasic, pulsed current. Phys Ther. 1989;69(8): 651–5.
22. Nelson et al. Use of physical forces in bone healing. Am Acad Orthop Surg. 2003;11(5):344–54.
23. Pietrosimone et al. Immediate effects of TENS and focal knee joint cooling on quadriceps activation. Med Sci Sports Exerc. 2009;41(6):1175–81.
24. DeSantana J et al. Effectiveness of transcutaneous electrical nerve stimulation for treatment of hyperalgesia and pain. Curr Rheumatol Rep. 2008;10(6): 492–9.
25. Sluka KA, Chandran P. Enhanced reduction in hyperalgesia by combined administration of clonidine and TENS. Pain. 2002;100:183–90.
26. King EW, Audette K, Athman GA, et al. Transcutaneous electrical nerve stimulation activates peripherally located alpha-2A adrenergic receptors. Pain. 2005;115:364–73.
27. Johnson M, Tabasam G. An investigation into the analgesic effects of interferential currents and transcutaneous electrical nerve stimulation on experimentally induced ischemic pain in otherwise pain-free volunteers. Phys Ther. 2003;83(3):208–23.

28. Facci et al. Effects of transcutaneous electrical nerve stimulation (TENS) and interferential currents (IFC) inpatients with nonspecific chronic low back pain: randomized clinical trial. Sao Paulo Med J. 2011;129(4):206–16.

29. Johnson MI. Tabasam G An investigation into the analgesic effects of interferential currents and transcutaneous electrical nerve stimulation on experimentally induced ischemic pain in otherwise pain-free volunteers. Phys Ther. 2003;83(3):208–23.

30. Milne et al. Transcutaneous electrical nerve stimulation (TENS) for chronic low back pain. Cochrane Database Syst Rev. 2001;(2):CD003008.

31. Denegar C. Influence of transcutaneous electrical nerve stimulation on pain, range of motion, and serum cortisol concentration in females experiencing delayed onset muscle soreness. J Orthop Sports Phys Ther. 1989;11: 100–103.

32. Faghri et al. Venous hemodynamics of the lower extremities in response to electrical stimulation. Arch Phys Med Rehabil. 1998;79:842–8.

33. Goldman et al. Electrotherapy promotes healing and microcirculation of infrapopliteal ischemic wounds: a prospective pilot study. Adv Skin Wound Care. 2004;17(6):284–94.

34. Unger PG. Update on high-voltage pulsed current research and application. Topics Geriatric Rehab. 2000;16(2):35–46.

35. Snyder et al. The influence of high-voltage electrical stimulation on edema formation after acute injury: a systematic review. J Sport Rehabil. 2010;19(4): 436–51.

36. Mendel F. Influence of high voltage pulsed current on edema formation following impact injury in rats. Phys Ther. 1992;72(9):668–73.

37. Sandoval et al. Effect of high-voltage pulsed current plus conventional treatment on acute ankle sprain. Rev Bras Fisioter. 2010;14(3):193–9.

38. Lin Z, Yan T. Long-term effectiveness of neuromuscular electrical stimulation for promoting motor recovery of the upper extremity after stroke. J Rehabil Med. 2011;43(6):506–10.

39. Lake DA. Neuromuscular electrical stimulation. An overview and its application in the treatment of sports injuries. Sports Med. 1992;13(5):320–36.

40. Maffiulett N. Physiological and methodological considerations for the use of neuromuscular electrical stimulation. Eur J Appl Physiol. 2010;110(2): 223–34.

41. Sheffler L, Chae J. Neuromuscular electrical stimulation in neurorehabilitation. Muscle Nerve. 2007;35(5):562–90.

42. Wallis et al. Effects of preoperative neuromuscular electrical stimulation on quadriceps strength and functional recovery in total knee arthroplasty. A pilot study. BMC Musculoskeletal Disord. 2010;11:119.

43. Lyons et al. Differences in quadriceps femoris muscle torque when using a clinical electrical stimulator versus a portable electrical stimulator. Phys Ther. 2005;85(1):44–51.

44. Johnston T, Smith B, Betz R. Strengthening of partially denervated knee extensor using percutaneous electrical stimulation in a young man with spinal cord injury. Arch Phys Med Rehabil. 2005;86(5):1037–42.

45. Peckham PH. Functional electrical stimulation for neuromuscular applications. Ann Rev Biomed Eng. 2005;7:327–60.

46. Fuentes et al. Effectiveness of interferential current therapy in the management of musculoskeletal pain: a systematic review and meta-analysis. Phys Ther 2010;90(9)1219–38.
47. Johnson MI, Tabasam G. An investigation into the analgesic effects of interferential currents and transcutaneous electrical nerve stimulation on experimentally induced ischemic pain in otherwise pain-free volunteers. Phys Ther. 2003;83(3):208–23.
48. Jarit et al. The effects of home interferential therapy on post-operative pain, edema, and range of motion of the knee. Clin J Sport Med. 2003;13(1): 16–20.
49. Laycock J, Jerwood D. Does premodulated interferential therapy cure genuine stress incontinence? Physiotherapy. 1993;79(8):553–60.
50. Vahtera et al. Pelvic floor rehabilitation is effective in patients with multiple sclerosis.1997;11(3):211–9.
51. Rooney JG, Currier DP, Nitz AJ. Effects of variation in the burst and carrier frequency modes of neuromuscular electrical stimulation on pain perception of healthy subjects. Phys Ther. 1992; 72(11):800–6; discussion 807–9.
52. Stevens JE, Mizner RL, Snyder-Mackler L. Neuromuscular electrical stimulation for quadriceps muscle strengthening after bilateral total knee arthroplasty: a case series. J Orthop Sports Phys Ther. 2004;34:21–9.
53. Ward AR. Alternating current electrical stimulation using Kilohertz-frequency. Phys Ther. 2009;89:181–90.
54. Snyder-Mackler et al. Use of electrical stimulation to enhance recovery of quadriceps femoris muscle force production in patients following anterior cruciate ligament reconstruction. Phys Ther. 1994;74(10):901–7.
55. Maffiuletti NA. The use of electrostimulation exercise in competitive sport. Int J Sports Physiol Perform. 2006;1:406–7.
56. Seyri KM, Maffiuletti NA. Effects of electromyostimulation training on muscle strength and sports performance. Strength Conditioning J. 2011;33(1):70–5.
57. Ciccone CD. Pharmacology in rehabilitation. 4th ed. Philadelphia, PA: F.A. Davis Company; 2007.
58. Alternative Iontophoresis Medications. Physical Therapy Products page. Available at: http://www.ptproductsonline.com/issues/articles/2005-09_04. asp. Accessed November 10, 2011.
59. Speed CA. Review: therapeutic ultrasound in soft tissue lesions. Rheumatology. 2001;40:1331–6.
60. Pounder NM, Harrison AJ. Low intensity pulsed ultrasound for fracture healing: a review of the clinical evidence and associated biological mechanism of action. Ultrasonics. 2008;48(4):330–8.
61. Adalberto L, et al. Effect of low-intensity pulsed ultrasound on the cartilage repair in people with mild to moderate knee osteoarthritis: a double-blinded, randomized, placebo-controlled pilot study. Arch Phys Med Rehabil. 2012;93(1):35–42.
62. Dyson M, Brookes M. Stimulation of bone repair by ultrasound (abstract). Ultrasound Med Biol. 1983;Suppl 2:61–6.
63. Hantes M, et al. Low-intensity transosseous ultrasound accelerates osteotomy healing in a sheep fracture model. J Bone Joint Surg Am. 2004;86-A(10):2275–82.

64. Franek et al. Application of various power densities of ultrasound in the treatment of leg ulcers. J Dermatolog Treat. 2004;15(6):379–86.

65. Kuntz A, Griffiths C, Rankin J. Cortisol concentrations in human skeletal muscle tissue after phonophoresis with 10% hydrocortisone gel. J Athl Train. 2006;41(3):321–4.

66. Ciccone CD. Pharmacology in rehabilitation. 4th ed. Philadelphia, PA: F.A. Davis Company; 2007.

67. Ciccone C, Leggin B, Callamaro J. Effects of ultrasound and trolamine salicye phonophoresis on delayed-onset muscel soreness. Phys Ther. 1991;71(9): 666–75.

68. Cetin et al. Comparing hot pack, short-wave diathermy, ultrasound, and TENS on isokinetic strength, pain, and functional status of women with osteoarthritic knees: a single-blind, randomized, controlled trial. Am J Phys Med Rehab. 2008;87(6):443–51.

69. Goats GC. Continuous short-wave (radio-frequency) diathermy. Br J Sports Med. 1989;23(2):123–7.

70. Al-Mandeel M, Watson T. The thermal and nonthermal effects of high and low doses of pulsed short waved therapy (PSWT). Physiother Res Int. 2010;15(4):199–211.

71. Low J. Dosage of some pulsed shortwave clinical trials. Physiotherapy. 1995;81(10):611–6.

72. Midura et al. Pulsed electromagnetic field treatments enhance the healing of fibular osteotomies. J Orthop Res. 2005;23(5):1035–46.

73. Okada et al. Upregulation of intervertebral disc-cell matrix synthesis by pulsed electromagnetic field is mediated by bone morphogenetic proteins. J Spinal Disord Thech. 2011;18.

74. Shields N, O'Hare N, Gomley J. An evaluation of safety guidelines to restrict exposure to stray radiofrquency radiation from short-wave diathermy units. Phys Med Biol. 2004;49(13):2999–3015.

75. Sanati et al. Effects of Ga_As (904 nm) and He-Ne (632.8) laser on injury potential of skin full-thickness wound. J Photochem Photobiol B. 2011; 103(2):180–5.

76. Mester E, Mester A, Mester E. Biomedical effects of laser application. Laser Surg Med. 1985;5:31–9.

77. Houreid N, Abrahamse H. Low intensity laser irradiation stimulates wound healing in diabetic wounded fibroblasts cells (WS1). Diabetes Technol Ther. 2010;12(12):971–8.

78. Surinchak J, Alago M, Bellamy R. Effects of low-level energy lasers on the healing of full thickness skin defects. Lasers Surg Med. 1983;2:276–4.

79. Alfredo et al. Efficacy of low level laser therapy associated with exercises in knee osteoarthritis: a randomized double-blind study. Clin Rehabil. 2011; 14.

80. Vasilenko et al. The effect of equal daily dose achieved by different power densities of low-level therapy at 635 and 670 nm on wound tensile strength in rats: a short report. Photomed Laser Surg. 2010;28(2):281.

81. Snyder-Mackier L, et al. Effects of helium—neon laser irradiation on skin resistance and pain in patients with trigger points in the neck or back. Phys Ther. 1989;69(5):336–41.

82. Snyder-Mackier L, Bork CE. Effect of helium-neon laser irradiation on peripheral sensory nerve latency. Phys Ther. 1988;68(2):223–5.

Chapter 10
Medical Complications and Emergencies in Rehabilitation

Lauren Stern

ANEMIA
- Hb < 13.5 in men, Hb < 12.0 in women

Differential Dx:
- Bleeding
- Hemolysis
- Decreased production of RBCs

Workup:
- Check vital signs—is the patient hemodynamically stable?
- Check stool for occult bleeding
- Labs:
  - ° Repeat CBC
  - ° Check MCV
    - MCV > 100: *Macrocytic*–B12 or folate deficiency
    - MCV < 70: *Microcytic*–iron deficiency (low iron, high TIBC, low ferritin)
    - MCV 70–100: *Normocytic*–anemia of chronic disease, anemia of CKD
  - ° Iron, TIBC, ferritin, transferrin saturation
  - ° B12, folate levels

L. Stern, M.D. (✉)
Department of Medicine and Nephrology,
Boston University School of Medicine,
650 Albany Street, #540,
Boston, MA 02118, USA
e-mail: lstern@bu.edu

K.A. Sackheim (ed.), *Rehab Clinical Pocket Guide:*
Rehabilitation Medicine, DOI 10.1007/978-1-4614-5419-9_10,
© Springer Science+Business Media, LLC 2013

- ° Reticulocyte count
- ° *If you suspect hemolysis*: LDH, haptoglobin, d-dimer
- ° Just in case transfusion may be needed:
  - ▪ PT/PTT
  - ▪ Type and cross

Special situations:
- Does the patient have liver disease?
  - ° May need FFP to correct elevated INR
- Does the patient have advanced renal disease?
  - ° May need DDAVP to correct uremic platelet dysfunction

Treatment:
- When to transfuse?
  - ° This is dependent on each patient and their symptoms, but the following can be utilized as a guide
    - ▪ Cardiac patients: Hb < 10
    - ▪ Noncardiac patients: Hb < 7
    - ▪ Sickle cell disease patients: discuss with heme
- How to transfuse?
  - ° *# units*? 1 unit will raise Hb ~ 1 g
  - ° *Rate*? Over 2–4 h (4 h for patients at risk of volume overload; i.e., cirrhotics, CHF, CKD)
  - ° *What to transfuse*? Packed RBCs
- Iron Deficiency Anemia
  - ° Ferrous Sulfate 325 mg po tid
  - ° This medication can turn stool black
  - ° Don't forget to prescribe a stool softener to prevent constipation from this medication
- Folate Deficiency
  - ° Folic acid 1 mcg po qday
- Vitamin B12 deficiency
  - ° Vitamin B12 1,000 mcg SC/IM qday × 1 week, then qweek × 1 month, then q month
- Hemolysis
  - ° Discuss with hematology consultant

ALTERED MENTAL STATUS

- Altered state of sensorium from baseline

Differential Dx:
- Delirium
- Dementia
- CNS—stroke, seizure, tumor, infection
- Infection
- Toxic/metabolic—hepatic encephalopathy, uremia, electrolyte abnormality
- Medication induced—(anticholinergics, benzodiazepenes, narcotics, etc.)
- Endocrine—hypoglycemia, hyperthyroidism, hypothyroidism, adrenal crisis
- Respiratory—hypercapnea, respiratory failure, pulmonary embolism
- Urinary retention

Workup:
- Call neurology consult if needed
- Check ABCs + blood glucose level
   ° Airway—can the patient protect their airway?
   ° Breathing—any respiratory distress?
   ° Circulation—are they maintaining pulse and blood pressure
   ° Blood glucose—hypoglycemia? Hyperglycemia?
- If CNS etiology is a concern—stat noncontrast head CT
- Seizure—diazepam 0.1–0.3 mg/kg IV push stat, lay patient on side
- Check vitals—Febrile? Hypoxic? Hypotensive?
- Review medications
   ° Are they taking anticholinergic meds, benzodiazepenes, narcotics?
- Check for urinary retention
- Check comprehensive metabolic panel (renal function, liver function, electrolytes)
- Check CBC
- Check blood and urine cultures if infection is suspected
- Consider full infection workup if needed

FEVER

- Temperature > 38 °C, > 100.4 °F

Differential Dx:
- Infection
- Medication
- Malignancy
- Endocrine—hyperthyroidism
- Malignant hyperthermia
- Neuroleptic malignant syndrome
- Postoperative
- DVT/PE

Workup:
- CBC with diff
- Urinalysis
- Blood culture×2 (from 2 different sites), Urine Culture, stool culture/c diff (if diarrhea and leukocytosis)
- Always culture before starting empiric antibiotics!!
- Chest X-ray—PA and Lateral, unless not stable can get portable
- Assess for old indwelling lines/catheters

Treatment:
*** These are suggestions of possible regimens, please consult antibiotic therapy guides for updated recommendations, alternative agents for allergies, and dosing for renal and hepatic dysfunction***

UTI
- Urinalysis will be positive for white blood cells, leucocyte estevase, and nitrite
- Typically caused by (E. coli, S. Saprophyticus, Enterococcus sp.)
- Uncomplicated treat for 3 days
- Complicated treat for 5–7 days
  - Examples of regimens (consult antibiotic therapy guides for updated recommendations and alternative agents for allergies)
    - Bactrim DS 1 tab po bid×3 days (for complicated UTI increase to 7–14 days)
    - Ciprofloxacin po 250 mg po bid×3 days (for complicated UTIs increase to 500 mg po bid×7–14 day)
    - Levofloxacin 250 mg po qday×3 day (for complicated UTI increase to 750 mg po qday×5 day)

PNEUMONIA (PNA)
- Community Acquired Pneumonia (CAP)
  - Typical organisms
    Strep pneumoniae

- ▪ Atypical organism
    Legionella
    Chlamydia psittaci
    Mycoplasma
- ▪ Third-generation cephalosporin + macrolide
    - • Ceftriaxone 1 g IV qday × 7 days + azithromycin 500 mg po qday × 5 days
- ▪ Flouroquinolones
    - • Levofloxacin 750 mg po qday × 5 days
- ○ Health care-associated pneumonia (pseudomonas, staph aureus, klebseilla; can be multi drug resistant)
    - ▪ Include coverage for pseudomonas
        - • i.e., Cefepime 1 g IV q12 h or Zosyn 2.375 g IV q 6 h × 7 days

BACTEREMIA
- – If signs of sepsis (hypotension, tachycardia) and indwelling lines
    - ○ Consider vancomycin 1 g IV q12 h for MRSA
    - ○ Consider third- or fourth-generation cephalosporin for gram negative coverage (E. coli, Klebsiella, pseudomonas)
        - ▪ i.e., cefepime 1 g IV q12 or Ceftriaxone 1 g IV q12
    - ○ Consult internists or infectious disease specialist once cultures are resulted or if patient is unstable. You may also need a medicine consult.

CHEST PAIN

Differential Dx:
- – Always rule out life-threatening causes first!!!
    - ○ MI
    - ○ PE
    - ○ Aortic Dissection
- – Pericarditis
- – Costochondritis / Muscular
- – Trauma
- – PNA
- – Referred pain
- – CHF

Workup:
- – Vital signs (including pulse ox)

- ° Values to be cautious about? Extremes of BP (very hypertensive or very hypotensive), tachycardia (P > 100), bradycardia (P < 50), hypoxia (PaO$_2$ < 60)
- Is it reproducible with palpation?
  - ° May be indicative of costochondritis but does not exclude MI
- Is it pleuritic?
  - ° May be indicative of pericarditis, PE
- EKG—ST elevations/depressions? Q waves? T inversions?
- Chest X-ray

Treatment:
- *If you suspect an MI:*
  - ° Call cardiology immediately
  - ° Morphine 1–2 mg IV push, Oxygen (titrate to SaO$_2$ > 96 %), Nitroglycerin (0.3–0.6 mg SL q 5 min × 3 doses or 2 % oint 0.5–2 in topical q4–6 h prn) monitor for hypotension, Aspirin 325 mg po stat, Beta-Blocker (metoprolol 5 mg IV q 2 min × 3)
- *If you suspect a PE:*
  - ° Hypoxic? Tachycardic? Immobile? Malignancy? Hypercoagulable?
  - ° Start heparin gtt (ensure no allergies or contraindications) 80 u/kg bolus, then 18 u/kg gtt, check PT-PTT q 6 h and adjust based on hospital nomogram (see below for dosing table) (Table 10.1)
  - ° Can check a d-dimer, but elevation can be nonspecific in chronic inflammatory states (normal 250 ng/mL or 0.50 mcg/mL FEU)
  - ° Imaging:
    - V/Q scan—useful if no underlying pulmonary disease, infiltrates, effusions

Table 10.1 Heparin protocol

Adjust rate based on aPTT:		
Lab result	Infusion rate change	Next aPTT
aPTT < 30 s	Increase rate by 1 mcg/kg/min	aPTT in 2 h
aPTT 30–40 s	Increase rate by 0.5 mcg/kg/min	aPTT in 2 h
aPTT 40–70 s	Same rate	aPTT repeat in 2–4 h, if in range aPTT in am
aPTT 71–90 s	Decrease rate by 0.5 mcg/kg/min	aPTT in 2 h
aPTT > 90 s	Decrease rate by 1 mcg/kg/min	aPTT in 2 h

Max dose is 10 mcg/kg/min. No initial dose adjustment needed with renal impairment and in absence of hepatic dysfunction
Hepatic elimination. Not renally cleared
Heparin references: [1–3]

- CT angiogram—discuss with consultant if pt has CKD or iodine allergy. May not detect peripheral small subsegmental emboli
- If you suspect aortic dissection:
  ○ Symptoms—Tearing chest pain that radiates to the back
  ○ Alert medical consultant
  ○ Stat CT angiogram
  ○ If CT angiogram is contraindicated (IV contrast allergy, kidney injury), consider Transesophageal echocardiogram (TEE)

SHORTNESS OF BREATH (SOB)

Differential Dx:
- MI
- CHF
- PNA
- Pleural effusion
- PE
- Asthma
- COPD
- Anemia

Workup:
- Check ABCs
  ○ Can patient protect their airway?
- Check oxygen saturation
  ○ If < 95 % concerning (but take into consideration if the patient is hypoxic at baseline, i.e., are they on home O_2?)
- Check ABG
  ○ Normal values are:
    ▪ pH 7.40; pCO_2 40; $PaO_2 > 60$
- *Does the patient retain CO_2 chronically?*
  ○ High oxygen supplementation may worsen hypercarbia and cause patient to lose respiratory drive (Keep SaO_2 92–94 %)
  ○ These patients need bipap or cpap along with oxygen
- *Do you suspect flash pulmonary edema? (Wet rales throughout lung fields)*
  ○ Call medical consultant
  ○ Stat loop diuretics (consider lasix 40 mgIV×1), nitroglycerin (apply nitropaste as above or SL NG), and morphine (consider 2 mg IV push×1)

- Check EKG
- Check CXR

Treatment:
- Supplemental oxygen
- Bipap for CO_2 retainers
- Asthma:
  - Bronchodilators (albuterol)—caution if arrhythmia
  - Steroids? (Consider starting at 40 mg po qday with quick taper over 5 days; if severe discuss dosing of IV solumedrol with consultant)

DIABETES MELLITUS

- Order diabetic diet
- Check finger stick qac and qhs
- Consult internal medicine/endocrinology if blood glucose is poorly controlled (hypo/hyperglycemia)
- Insulin sliding scale (see below for scale) (Table 10.2)
- Inpatient blood glucose goals:
  - < 140 pre-meal, < 180 at other times

Type I:
  - Always give *basal insulin* (glargine, levemir, lantus)
    - 0.25 U/kg/day or use home dose!!
  - *Mealtime insulin* (aspart, humalog, lispro, regular)
    - 0.05–0.1 U/kg/meal, or 1/3 of basal dose per meal
    - **if poor po intake or NPO, decrease insulin and give after part of meal is eaten

Type 2:
  - Order Hemoglobin A_1C (if none in the past 3 months)
  - Oral Meds
    - Hold the following when:
      - Metformin—Cr > 1.4, prior to and post-IV contrast or surgery
      - Thiazolidinediones (pioglitazone)—CHF, volume overload
      - Sulfonylureas—NPO, poor po intake, renal failure
  - Insulin
    - *Basal* dose (glargine, levemir, lantus)
      - Home dose if glucose is controlled and no hypoglycemia
      - Decrease dose if NPO, poor po intake
    - *Mealtime* dose (aspart, humalog, lispro, regular)
      - Give if eating

Table 10.2 Insulin sliding scale: use for regular/lispro/aspart/humalog. http://diabetesinstitute.pitt.edu/files/RegHumulinISS.pdf

Regular insulin (e.g., Humulin-R®) sliding scale-standard orders

Recommended indications:

- As a *supplement* to a patient's usual diabetes medications (long-acting insulin or oral agents) to treat uncontrolled high blood sugars
- For short-term use (24–48 h) in a patient admitted with an unknown insulin requirement

Regimens:

- Low-dose scale: Suggested starting point for thin and elderly, or those being initiated on TPN
- Moderate-dose scale: Suggested starting point for average patient
- High-dose scale: Suggested for patients with infections or those receiving therapy with high-dose corticosteroids

Blood sugar (mg/dL)	Low-dose scale	Moderate-dose scale	High-dose scale	Patient-specific scale
<70	Initiate hypoglycemia protocol	Initiate hypoglycemia protocol	Initiate hypoglycemia protocol	Initiate hypoglycemia protocol
70–130	0 units	0 units	0 units	___ units
131–180	2 units	4 units	8 units	___ units
181–240	4 units	8 units	12 units	___ units
241–300	6 units	10 units	16 units	___ units
301–350	8 units	12 units	20 units	___ units
351–400	10 units	16 units	24 units	___ units
>400	12 units and call MD	20 units and call MD	28 units and call MD	___ units and call MD

- • If not eating a lot, decrease dose and give after some of meal is eaten
  ◦ **Initiating insulin**
    ▪ *Basal* dose
      • 0.2 U/kg/day
      • If frail, ESRD, elderly—0.1 U/kg
    ▪ *Mealtime* insulin
      • Only give if the patient is eating and blood sugar is still elevated with basal insulin
      • 1/3 basal dose with each meal

CONSTIPATION

Workup:
– Is patient on narcotics?
– Is the patient paraplegic?
– Does the patient have hypothyroidism that is not adequately replaced?
– Does the patient have abdominal pain?
– Abdominal sounds present?
– Is the patient vomiting feculent material?
– Is the patient on peritoneal dialysis (PD catheters do not work properly if the pt is constipated)

Treatment:
  ◦ If SBO is suspected (abdominal distension, decreased bowel sounds, constipation, obstipation):
    ▪ Stat KUB
    ▪ Surgical consult
  ◦ Bowel regimen for all patients who are on narcotics, peritoneal dialysis, paraplegia
  ◦ Medications:
    ▪ Senna—1–2 tabs po qhs prn (max 4 tabs); increases peristalsis
    ▪ Colace—100–300 mg po qday-tid; stool softener
    ▪ Docusate—5–10 mg po or pr prn; stool softener, also comes in suppository form
    ▪ Miralax-1 capful po qday prn; osmotic laxative
    ▪ Lactulose—15 mL po qday prn; osmotic laxative, ideal for ESLD as it promotes excretion of ammonia
    ▪ Magnesium hydroxide—30–60 mL po qday prn; osmotic laxative, caution in renal failure (can cause hypermagnesemia)

- Go-lytely—osmotic laxative
- Enema
  - Tap water
  - Mineral oil
  - Fleet phosphasoda—caution in CKD/AKI, can cause irreversible kidney failure (phosphate nephropathy)!
  ○ Increase fiber intake
  ○ Increase fluid intake

DIARRHEA

Differential Dx:
- Stool softener
- Infectious (C diff, etc.)
- IBD (Inflammatory Bowel Disease)
- Lactose intolerance
- Bacterial overgrowth
- Antibiotic-associated diarrhea
- Post-ileostomy (takes ~ 1 month for ileum to hypertrophy and reabsorb fluid that the colon normally would)

Workup:
- Is the patient hemodynamically stable?
- Does the patient have abdominal pain?
- Bloody diarrhea?
- Is the patient immunocompromised (AIDS, etc.)?
- Is the patient being given stool softeners?
- Has the patient traveled recently?
- Has the patient been on antibiotics recently?
- Send stool for clostridium dificile toxin, immunocompromised Ova and Parasites (if indicated), stool culture (if hospitalized < 3 days)

Treatment:
- IVF if evidence of volume depletion
- Check chemistry (assess for electrolyte abnormalities and Acute Kidney Injury)
- d/c stool softerners
  ○ Clostridium difficile:
    - Place patient in contact isolation bed
    - PO flagyl (500 mg po q8h) ± po vancomycin if severe (125 mg po q6 h)

- If other etiology determined, treat appropriately
- Severe? (Hemodynamically unstable, severe abdominal pain, abdominal distension)
  - Call surgical and internal medicine consult
  ○ Imodium/Lomitil is only okay to administer if infectious etiology has been ruled out
  - If stool is positive for ova and parasites, may need to consult medicine and/or infectious disease service.

HYPOTENSION

Differential Dx:
- Infection/sepsis
- Cardiogenic shock
- Cardiac tamponade
- Volume depletion (vomiting, diarrhea, diuretics)
- Adrenal insufficiency
- Autonomic dysfunction
- End-stage liver disease
- Medication induced

Workup:
- Check ABCs
- Repeat BP on both arms with a manual cuff
- Is the patient mentating at baseline? This will help to determine if there is adequate cerebral perfusion.
- Check medications
  ○ Hold antihypertensive medications
  ○ Was the patient previously on steroids and at risk for adrenal insufficiency?
    - Yes →check a cortisol level at 8 am
- Any evidence of infection? (Don't forget to check decubitus ulcers and indwelling catheters)
  ○ Check blood cultures, urine cultures, urinalysis, CXR
  ○ Consider empiric antibiotics
- Does the patient have decompensated cirrhosis?
  ○ These patients are typically hypotensive (SBP< 100)
  ○ Ensure that they are mentating
- Does this patient have decompensated heart failure?
  ○ Are they cool and wet?

– Does the patient have distant heart sounds, elevated JVP, and tachycardia?
  ○ Transthoracic echo to rule out impending tamponade
Treatment:
  ○ Hold antihypertensives and diuretics
  ○ IVF bolus-start with 250–1,000 mL of normal saline depending on volume status
    ▪ Use caution when administering IVF to patients with edematous states (CHF, nephrotic syndrome, cirrhosis). Consider medicine consult for assistance with treatment to avoid complications.

HYPERTENSION

  ○ BP > 140/90 on 3 separate occasions
  ○ *Hypertensive urgency*
    ▪ BP > 180/120, no end-organ damage
  ○ *Hypertensive emergency*
    ▪ Call medical consultant
    ▪ BP > 180/120, evidence of end-organ damage
      • Hypertensive encephalopathy (AMS, seizure)
      • Papilledema
      • CHF/pulmonary edema
      • MI
      • Kidney injury
    ▪ Do not lower blood pressure too aggressively in the first 24 h, need to maintain cerebral perfusion
  ○ **Antihypertensive Medication Classes**
    ▪ *Diuretics:*
      • Thiazides—very effective in African Americans, do not use if eGFR <30 (does not work), h/o hyponatremia
        ○ i.e., HCTZ 12.5 mg po qday (25 mg po qday max)
      • Loop Diuretics—effective in hypertensive and volume-overloaded patients
        ○ i.e., furosemide 20 mg po qday as a starting dose if normal kidney function and loop diuretic naïve. Discuss with medicine consult about increasing dose.
    ▪ *Beta-Blockers*
      • Caution in bradycardia, cocaine abusers, and patients with history of bronchospasm

- Labetalol is most effective anti-hypertensive in the class
- Metoprolol (i.e., metoprolol 25 mg po twice daily, or metoprolol XL 25 mg po qday and titrate up) and Carvedilol (3.125 mg po bid and titrate up to 25 mg po bid max)are beneficial in CHF

▪ *Calcium channel blockers*
  - Dihydropyridines can cause LE edema; no effect on heart rate
    ○ i.e., amlodipine 5 mg po qday (10 mg po qday mx); nifedipine XL 30 mg po qday (120 mg po qday max)
  - Non-dihydropyridines—caution in bradycardia (i.e. verapamil, diltiazem)

▪ *Ace-inhibitors (ACE-I)*
  - Beneficial in CHF and proteinuric renal disease
  - Can cause hyperkalemia
  - Discuss with nephrologist before starting in patients with CKD, caution in acute kidney injury
  - Can cause cough, angioedema
    ○ i.e., lisinopril 10 mg po qday (40 mg po qday max)

▪ *Angiotensin Receptor Blockers (ARB)* (losartan, valsartan, olmasartan, telmisartan)
  - See above, similar to ACE-I
  - Does not cause cough, can cause angioedema
    ○ i.e., losartan 25 mg qday (100 mg po qday max)

▪ *Centrally acting agents*
  - Clonidine—very effective antihypertensive, but causes rebound hypertension if doses are missed (do not use as a one-time agent)
    ○ Clonidine 0.1 mg po bid (can titrate up to 0.3 mg po tid)

▪ *Vasodilators*
  - Hydralazine—short half-life, can cause reflex tachycardia
    ○ Start with 10 mg po q6 h (titrate up to maximum dose 100 mg po q6 h)
    ○ Can cause drug-induced lupus syndrome at high doses
  - Minoxidil—very effective agent, caution in volume-overloaded patients, can cause reflex tachycardia
    ○ Start 2.5 mg po qday (titrate up to 100 mg po qday)

Management of Hypertension Over Night

Consider short-acting agents (i.e., Labetalol, Hydralazine, Captopril)
Must think about the possible side effects listed above before dosing.
If frequent prn dosing is needed, daily BP medications should be ti-
trated up to avoid additional prn dosing

LOWER EXTREMITY (LE) EDEMA

Differential Dx:
– CHF
– Nephrotic syndrome/proteinuria
– End-stage liver disease
– DVT
– Lymphatic/venous obstruction
– Cellulitis
– Internal bleed in lower extremity
– Malnutrition (hypoalbuminemia)

Workup:
– Is it bilateral or unilateral?
– Is it chronic or acute?
– Consider LE dopplers
   ○ If dopplers are negative
      ▪ Check urinalysis to asses proteinuria
      ▪ Consider echocardiogram to rule out heart failure
      ▪ Check liver function tests to rule out heart texture including albumin
   ○ If all of the above are negative and edema is persistent and se-
     vere consider imaging of the pelvis to assess for lymphatic/ve-
     nous obstruction

Treatment:
– Treat underlying cause as outlined in this chapter

HYPONATREMIA

– Serum Na < 135

Workup:
- Is Na < 120? Call renal consult immediately
- Check serum osmolality
  - ° Differentiate between hypotonic, isotonic, hypertonic hypo-natremia (normal serum osm ~ 280–310)
- Check urine osmolality
  - ° Differentiates SIADH from low solute intake states
    - ▪ U osm > 300 more c/w SIADH
    - ▪ U osm < 200 more c/w beer potomania, psychogenic poly-dipsia, tea and toast diet
- If hypotonic: check volume status
  - ° **Hypovolemic Etiologies**
    - ▪ Renal vs GI loss
      - • *Treatment:* IVF (discuss rate of repletion with consultant)
  - ° **Euvolemic Etiologies**
    - ▪ SIADH (pulmonary, intracranial pathology)
    - ▪ Hypothyroidism
    - ▪ Glucorticoid deficiency
    - ▪ Beer potomania (low solute intake)
    - ▪ Psychogenic polydipsia
    - ▪ Tea and toast diet (low solute intake)
    - ▪ Drugs (antipsychotics, SSRIs)
      - • *Treatment:* Free water restriction, liberalize Na in diet
  - ° **Hypervolemic Etiologies**
    - ▪ CHF
    - ▪ Nephrotic syndrome
    - ▪ Cirrhosis
      - • *Treatment:* loop diuretics, Na restricted diet, free water restriction

HYPERNATREMIA

- Serum Na > 145

Workup/Differential:
- Hypertonic sodium infusion?
- Decreased water intake?

– Water loss?
  ○ GI losses—osmotic diarrhea
  ○ Renal losses
    ▪ Osmotic diuresis (glucose, mannitol)
    ▪ Diabetes insipidus (suspect if polyuria and very dilute urine)
      • Central—No ADH production
        ○ *Treatment:* DDAVP
      • Nephrogenic—kidney does not respond to ADH
        ○ *Treatment:* HCTZ, DDAVP

Treatment: Discuss repletion rate of IV Fluids with consultant
  ○ Assess volume status
    ▪ Hemodynamically unstable/shock
      • Normal saline until stabilized
    ▪ Hypovolemic
      • ½ Normal saline (repletion rates vary depending on patients)
    ▪ Euvolemic
      • D5W (repletion rate vary depending on patient)
  ○ Ensure IV meds are given in D5W (not Normal saline, because this is on additional sodium load)

HYPERKALEMIA

– Serum potassium > 5.0

Differential Dx:
– Kidney failure
– Drugs (ACEI, ARB, k-sparing diuretics, bactrim, calcineurin inhibitors, heparin, beta-blockers)
– Hemolysis
– Tumor lysis syndrome
– Metabolic acidosis

Workup:
– Check EKG:
  ○ Peaked T waves
  ○ PR prolongation
  ○ QRS prolongation
  ○ Sine wave
  ○ PEA (Pulseless Electrical Activity)

Treatment:
- ○ Calcium gluconate—1 amp IVPB
  - ▪ Stabilizes cardiac membrane
- ○ Insulin—10 units
  - ▪ Shifts K intracellularly
  - ▪ Can repeat after labs are rechecked
  - ▪ Don't forget the D50!
- ○ B-agonist (albuterol nebulizer)
  - ▪ Shifts potassium intracellularly
  - ▪ Caution in patients with arrythmias
- ○ Sodium bicarbonate 50 mg (1 amp)
  - ▪ Shifts potassium intracellularly
  - ▪ Only effective if the patient is acidotic
- ○ Kayexalate start with 15 g × 1
  - ▪ Binds potassium in the gut
  - ▪ Ineffective if no colon
  - ▪ Can cause bowel necrosis if colonic motility problem (ileus, obstruction, post-op)

CHRONIC KIDNEY DISEASE

- • Stage 1: eGFR >90 with intrinsic damage (proteinuria, hematuria)
- • Stage 2: eGFR 60–89
- • Stage 3: eGFR 30–59
- • Stage 4: eGFR 15–29
- • Stage 5: eGFR < 15
  - ▪ Always consider referral to nephrology with CKD 3 or higher
- *AVOID*:
  - ○ Metformin
    - ▪ GFR < 30; or Cr > 1.6 (men), > 1.5 (women)
  - ○ NSAIDS
  - ○ Fleet enema/fleet phosphosoda
  - ○ Bisphosphonates if CKD 4 or 5 (discuss with nephrologist)
  - ○ IV contrast (if possible)
  - ○ Herbal supplements
  - ○ Aminoglycosides
  - ○ Discuss with nephrologist when ACEI/ARB is appropriate
  - ○ HCTZ (eGFR < 30)

Acute Kidney Injury:
- Abrupt loss of kidney function
- An increase in creatinine by
  - 0.5 mg/dL
  - 20 % if aseline Cr > 2.5 in less than 2 weeks
- *Oliguria:*
  - Urine output = 100–400 mL/24 h
- *Anuria:*
  - Urine output < 100 mL/24 h

Acute kidney injury is classified into 3 categories

1. Prerenal
- BUN/Cr > 20:1
- FENa < 1 %
- **Differential Dx**:
  - Urine sediment—bland
  - Decreased effective arterial volume (hypovolemia, CHF)
  - Renal vasoconstriction (NSAIDs, ACEI/ARB, hypercalcemia)
  - Hepatorenal syndrome
  - Large vessel disease (renal artery stenosis, fibromuscular dysplasia, thrombosis, embolism, dissection, vasculitis)
- **Treatment:**
  - Discontinue offending agents
  - Trial of volume resuscitation; start with NS 250–1,000 mL with volume and rate depending on volume status

2. Intrinsic
- BUN/Cr < 20:1
- FENa > 1 %
- Urine sediment
  - ATN—muddy brown casts
  - AIN—WBCs (eosinophils), WBC casts
  - GN—RBCs, RBC casts
- **Differential Dx**:
  - ATN (ischemia, toxins, IV contrast, rhabdomyolysis)
  - AIN (infectious, allergic, infiltrative)
  - Small vessel disease (cholesterol emboli; thrombotic microangiopathy—TTP/HUS, scleroderma, antiphospholipid Ab syndrome; glomerular diseases)
- **Treatment:**
  - Nephrology consult for dx and disease-specific recommendations

3. Postrenal
- BUN/Cr < 20:1
- FENa > 1 %
- Urine sediment
  - Typically bland, can have RBCs if GU pathology
- **Differential Dx**:
  - Bladder (BPH, neurogenic bladder, anticholinergic meds)
  - Ureteral (malignancy, LAD, retroperitoneal fibrosis, b/l stones)
- **Treatment:**
  - Foley catheter
  - GU tract imaging
  - Consider GU and nephrology consults

ALLERGIC REACTION

Presentation:
- Rash (urticaria)
- Bronchospasm
- Angioedema
- Nausea/vomiting
- Hypotension
- Eosinophilia

Treatment:
- Withdraw offending agent (medication, etc)
- If severe reaction occurs, constant monitoring of vital signs, including pulse oximetry, is essential
- If airway is compromised or angioedema is suspected:
  - Stat ENT consult for possible intubation
- *Epinephrine*
  - 0.3–0.5 mg IM in 5–15 min intervals prn
- *Glucocorticoids*
  - Solumedrol 1,000 mg IV qday
- *Antihistamines*
  - H1 antagonists:
    - Diphenhydramine 50 mg IV × 1
    - Hydroxyzine 50 mg po × 1
  - H2 antagonists
    - i.e., ranitidine 50 mg IVPB × 1
- *IVF*
  - If hypotensive, 250–1,000 mL of NS depending on volume status

References

1. Raschke RA, et al. The weight-based heparin dosing nomogram compared to a "standard care" nomogram. Ann Intern Med. 1993;119:874–81.
2. Yee WP, Norton LL. Optimal weight base for a weight-based heparin dosing protocol. Am J Health Syst Pharm. 1998;55(2):159S–62.
3. Hirsch J, Bauer K. Parenteral anticoagulants. The eighth ACCP conference on antithrombotic and thrombolytic therapy. Chest 2008; 141S–59.

Part III
Outpatient Clinical Care

Chapter 11
Musculoskeletal Medicine

Sagar S. Parikh, Naimish Baxi, and Sandia A. Padavan

Upper Extremity

GLENOHUMERAL OSTEOARTHRITIS (OA) (715.11)

- Shoulder cartilage destruction
- May predispose to shoulder impingement

Anatomy [1, 2]:
- Ball and socket joint allowing movement in all planes (flexion, extension, internal/external rotation, circumduction)
- Articular surface of glenoid is concave; hyaline cartilage covering glenoid is thicker toward the periphery and thinner in the center

Symptoms:
- Diffuse, deep pain at the shoulder (often at the posterior aspect)
- Pain worse with activity and weather changes
- Progressive stiffness, loss of motion
- Pain at night, based on position

S.S. Parikh, M.D. (✉) • N. Baxi, M.D. • S.A. Padavan, M.D.
Department of Rehabilitation Medicine, Mount Sinai Medical Center,
One Gustave Levy Place, Box 1240, New York, NY, USA

K.A. Sackheim (ed.), *Rehab Clinical Pocket Guide:*
Rehabilitation Medicine, DOI 10.1007/978-1-4614-5419-9_11,
© Springer Science+Business Media, LLC 2013

Physical exam:
- Inspection: May show generalized atrophy of shoulder muscles however rare.
- ROM: Can be limited in all planes especially with internal rotation.
- Crepitus can be felt on ROM
- Palpation: Tendenress to palpation along joint lines.
- MMT: Normal (unless pain limited)

Imaging:
- AP and Axillary X-ray: may show irregular joint surfaces, joint space narrowing, cystic/sclerotic changes, osteophytes, flattening of humeral head

Treatment:
- Heat, NSAIDs, relative rest during acute stages and activity modification
- Injection—steroid vs. viscosupplementation
- Severe cases may require surgical intervention with joint replacement or hemiarthroplasty

Rehabilitation Program [2]:
- Goal: Pain-free movement, increase ROM
- Modalities: TENs, heat
- ROM: pendulum exercises, shoulder extension exercises
- Stretching: gentle stretching to preserve motion
- Strengthening exercises: progressive resistive exercises with emphasis on rotator cuff, deltoid and subscapularis strengthening

BICEPS TENDONITIS (726.12)

- Often found concurrently with rotator cuff or labrum pathology
- Sometimes found concurrently with rotator cuff or labrum pathology, as the biceps tendon is often then overutilized leading to inflammation.

Anatomy:
- Short head of the biceps inserts at the coracoid process of the scapula
- Long head of the biceps passes through the bicipital groove of the humerus and inserts at the supraglenoid tubercle of scapula (most commonly affected)

Symptoms:
- Anterior shoulder pain worse with activity

Physical exam:
- Tenderness at the bicipital groove
- Provocative maneuvers include [3]
  - + *Speed's*—with elbow extended and forearm supinated, the examiner resists humeral forward flexion at 60°, positive when this causes pain over the biceps tendon
  - + *Yergason's*—with elbow flexed and forearm supinated, the examiner resists supination at the patient's wrist, positive when this causes pain over the biceps tendon

Imaging:
- Anterior/posterior/lateral/axillary view of shoulder normal
- MRI arthropathy with gadolinium may show increased signal within long head of biceps tendon

Treatment:
- Ice, NSAIDs, relative rest during acute stages and activity modification
- Injection: steroid injection into bicipital tendon sheath ideally under ultrasound guidance

Rehabilitation Program [2]:
- Goal: reduce inflammation, improve pain with movement, return to activity
- Modalities: Ice, TENs, U/S
- ROM: immobilization with posterior splint or sling for 2 weeks with passive elbow and shoulder ROM
- Stretching: pendulum stretch, biceps, and rotator cuff stretch
- Strengthening exercises: progressive resistive exercises for scapular stabilizer muscles, deltoid, rotator cuff, biceps strengthening

ROTATOR CUFF TEAR (726.10)

- **Function of rotator cuff muscles** [4]: stabilization, to depress the humeral head during overhead activities

- With weakness/absence of rotator cuff muscles, the humeral head is displaced superiorly during abduction due to unopposed action of deltoid
- Most commonly involves the Supraspinatus tendon/muscle close to the distal insertion (great tuberosity) as this region has decreased vascular supply
- Traumatic or degenerative
  - Traumatic in athletes or laborers
  - Degenerative tears in elderly
- **Categorization of tears [4]:**
  1. Full thickness
  2. Partial thickness type 1: tear on the superior surface into the subacromial space
  3. Partial thickness type 2: tear on the inferior surface on the articular side (can rapidly progress to full thickness)

Anatomy: (Table 11.1)
- 4 rotator cuff muscles: (**S.I.T.S.**)
  - **S**upraspinatus
  - **I**nfraspinatus
  - **T**eres minor
  - **S**ubscapularis

Symptoms:
- Pain in shoulder; can be referred to lateral triceps, dull and/or achy
- Difficulty with overhead activities
- Pain at night in side-lying position (on adducted shoulder of affected side as this decreases the blood supply of the muscle)

Table 11.1 Rotator cuff muscles, origins, insertions, innervations, and action

Muscle	Origin	Insertion	Innervation	Action
Supraspi- natus	Supraspinatus fossa (scapula)	Greater tuberosity of humerus (superior)	Suprascaular nerve (C5, C6)	Abduct (initiation of abduction to 15°)
Infraspi- natus	Infraspinatus fossa (scapula)	Greater tuberosity of humerus (middle)	Suprascaular nerve (C5, C6)	External rotation
Teres minor	Lateral Scapula	Greater tuberosity (inferior)	Axillary nerve (C5, C6)	External rotation
Subscap- ularis	Subscapular fossa (scapula)	Lesser tuberosity	Upper and Lower Subscapular nerve	Internal rotation, Adduction

Physical exam:
- May have decreased active ROM secondary to pain or weakness but passive ROM should be intact (unlike adhesive capsulitis)
  - It is important to check active *and* passive range of motion as this can be confused with adhesive capsulitis
- Rotator cuff weakness
  - Supraspinatus (most commonly affected)—Empty can test
  - Subscapularis—Gerber push off test
  - Infraspinatus—resisted ER with arm at side
- Provocative maneuvers—most commonly positive with full-thickness tears [3]
  - ***Drop arm test***—positive when patient unable to return the arm to the side slowly or has severe pain when attempting to do so after the shoulder is passively abducted to 90°
  - ***Empty can test***—positive when pain and/or weakness is elicited as patient's arm, fully internally rotated (emptying can) at 90° elevation in the scapula plane, resists downward pressure
  - ***Gerber or lift-off test***—patient is standing with hand behind the back with the dorsum of the hand raised off of the mid-lumbar spine, increasing both internal rotation and extension of the humerus; test is positive when patient is unable to move the dorsum of the hand off of the back, indicating subscapularis dysfunction
- Can also have positive impingement signs

Imaging:
- X-ray [2]
  - Upward migration of humeral head or subacromial or greater tuberosity sclerotic and/or cystic changes, avulsed fragments
  - Active 90° abduction films can show decreased acromiohumeral distance
  - Decreased acromiohumeral distance (<6 mm) may indicate rotator cuff tear
  - Distance >7 mm may indicate long-standing rotator cuff tear
- MRI: "gold standard": 100% sensitivity and 95% specificity for full-thickness rotator cuff tears
- Ultrasound [5]:
  - Hypoechoic or anechoic where fluid has replaced the area of torn tendon
  - Compression of area will show "sagging peribursal fat" sign

Treatment:
- Ice, NSAIDs, relative rest during acute stages, and activity modification
- Subacromial Injection: diagnostic and therapeutic
  - Posterolateral or Anterior approach [1]
  - 1½″ 22 gauge needle; inject Methylprednisolone or Triamcinolone: 40–80 mg with 3–5 ml of local anesthetic into the subacromial space directed towards the coracoid process
  - Injections should be done only for extreme pain as they can worsen the tendon pathology if done too frequently
- Consider surgical consultation if symptoms do not respond to conservative treatment or if patient has a disabling full-thickness tear

Rehabilitation Program [1, 2]:
- Goal: reduce inflammation, improve pain with movement, return to activity
- Modalities: Ice, TENs, Ultrasound to posterior capsule
- ROM: Active assisted with progression as tolerated
- Stretching
  - Posterior capsule stretching
  - Codman pendulum exercises
  - Wall walking
- Strengthening exercises: begin with Isometric exercises of:
  - Scapulothoracic stabilizers (shrugs, rowing, pushups)
  - Rotator cuff muscles
- Proprioception training:
  - Modified push-ups
  - Closed kinetic chain exercises progressing to open chain
- Postural biomechanics
- Task or sport-specific activities

SHOULDER IMPINGEMENT SYNDROME (726.11)

- **Rotator cuff tendonitis/tendonosis (726.10)**
- **Subacromial bursitis (726.19)**
- Rotator cuff tendons pass directly between the acromion/coracoacromial ligament and the humeral head

- The following can decrease the space through which the tendons pass:
  - Weakness of rotator cuff muscles can lead to rising of the humeral head
  - Edema of the tendon
  - Fluid accumulation within the subacromial bursa
  - Hooked or curved acromion
  - Subacromion osteophyte
  - Thickened ligaments
- Supraspinatus is the most commonly involved tendon/muscle
- **Neer's three stages [4]**
  1. Edema/hemorrhage (reversible)
  2. Fibrosis/tendonitis
  3. AC spur/rotator cuff tear

Symptoms:
- Gradual onset of anterolateral shoulder pain worse with overhead activity
- Difficulty sleeping on affected side
- Pain can radiate up towards the neck or down to the upper arm

Physical exam:
- Evaluation of cervical spine should be normal (can have referred symptoms from the shoulder)
- Tenderness may be illicited at the greater tuberosity or subacromial bursa
- Unlike rotator tears, strength should be normal but may be limited by pain
  - Weakness can be found with chronic symptoms
- Provocative maneuvers for impingement [3]
  - **+ Neer's**: Pain at shoulder with passive shoulder flexion with arm internally rotated
  - **+ Hawkin's**: Pain at shoulder with passive shoulder flexion to 90° with forceful internal rotation
- Detecting concomitant biceps tendon injury and/or underlying glenohumeral joint instability

Imaging:
- AP X-ray: may be normal but can show

- ○ Scerlosis of acromion undersurface, decreased acromiohumeral distance, osteophytes
- MRI:
- Ultrasound [5]
  - ○ Tendon hypoechogenicity or thickening with or without internal hypo or hyperechoic foci

Treatment:
- Ice, NSAIDs, relative rest during acute stages and activity modification
- Local modalities (cryotherapy, TENs, U/S)

Rehabilitation Program [1]
Phases of Rehab
- Acute (maximal protection):
  - ○ Goal: relieve pain, swelling, decrease inflammation, maintain flexibility
  - ○ Activity modification——eliminate exacerbating behavior (overhead throwing, reaching, lifting)
  - ○ Modalities: cryotherapy, TENS
  - ○ ROM exercises: Pendulum, AAROM (flexion, neutral external rotation), Grade 1 and 2 joint mobilization (inferior and posterior glides)
  - ○ Strengthening: submaximal isometric (external rotation, internal rotation, biceps, deltoids)
- Subacute:
  - ○ Goal: reestablish nonpainful ROM, retard muscular atrophy
  - ○ Modalities: cryotherapy, ultrasound
  - ○ ROM: flexion, abduction, external rotation and internal rotation in 45° of abduction, progress to 90° of abduction, Grade 2, 3, 4 joint mobilization (inferior, anterior, posterior glides)
  - ○ Strengthening: isometrics, scapulothoracic strengthening exercises, neuromuscular control exercises
- Intermediate strengthening
  - ○ Goal: normalize ROM, improve muscular performance
  - ○ ROM: AAROM, self-capsular stretching (anterior-posterior)
  - ○ Strengthening: side-lying neutral internal and external rotation, prone extension and horizontal abduction, standing flexion to 90°, serratus exercises (wall push-ups), tubing

progression in slight abduction for internal and external rotation strengthening, initiate arm ergometer for endurance
- Dynamic advanced strengthening
  - Goal: increases strength, endurance, power, neuromuscular control
  - "Thrower's Ten" Exercise program, plyometric exercises, isokinetics

ACROMIOCLAVICULAR (AC) JOINT PAIN (831.04)

- Direct impact to shoulder (football, biking)
- Treatment depends on the Grade of injury (Table 11.2)

Grades of AC Joint Injuries and Treatments

Relevant Anatomy:
- Joint between lateral end of clavicle and medial side of acromion (Table 11.2)
- Stabilized by acromio-clavicular ligaments (trapezoid, conoid, coracoacromial ligaments)

Symptoms:
- Anterior shoulder pain worsened by lifting the arm and overhead reaching

Table 11.2 Grades of AC joint injuries and treatments

Grade	AC ligament	CC ligament	Clavicle displacement	Treatment
I	Sprain	Intact	Mild superior	Conservative
II	Torn	Sprain	Definite superior	Conservative
III	Torn	Torn	25–100% increase in CC space	Conservative or surgical
IV	Torn	Torn	Posterior	Surgical
V	Torn	Torn	100–300% increase in CC space	Surgical
VI	Torn	Torn	Subacromial or subcoracoid location	Surgical

AC Acromioclavicular, *CC* coracoclavicular

- Can have radiation into the neck and down the arm
- Pain with ADLs that bring arm across chest (reaching into jacket pocket, tucking shirt in)

Physical Exam:
- Tender to palpation at AC joint
- Raised area at acromioclavicular joint caused by depression of scapula relative to clavicle
  - Noticeable deformity with Type III or greater
- Normal shoulder ROM—may be limited by pain
- Provocative maneuvers [3]:
  - ***Cross-body adduction test (Scarf test)***—positive when pain localized to AC joint while arm is maximally adducted with the arm in 90° of forward flexion
  - ***Active compression test (O'Brien)***—with arm in forward flexion to 90°, adducted to 10°, and internally rotated (thumb down), the patient resists the examiner's downward force; positive when pain produced by previous maneuver is alleviated with arm externally rotated (palm up)

Imaging:
- Radiographs: AP, lateral Y, axillary view
  - Weighted (10 lbs): widening of clavicular-coracoid area
- MRI: bone edema, detect extent of AC arthrosis
- Ultrasound: view joint space, soft tissue changes in arthritic AC joints, effusions

Treatment [1]: (based on grading; see chart above)
- Injection—1½″ 25 gauge needle; inject Methylprednisolone or Triamcinolone: 40 mg with 1 ml of anesthetic into the AC joint
- Type I and II—sling for comfort and ice for a few days, activities as tolerated, full activities at 4 weeks post-injury as long as tolerated
- Type III—may be treated conservatively, consider surgical repair if young and/or laborer
- Type IV to VI—surgical reduction and reconstruction

Rehabilitation Program: this is for general AC injury, can be specified further for specific severity of injury
- Goal: improve pain with range of motion
- Modalities: ice, u/s, phonophoresis
- ROM exercises [1]:

- ○ Initially—Active ROM for fingers, wrist and elbow throughout the day with gentle ROM of shoulder, simple ADLs (eating, dressing)
  - ○ Day 2–3—start Codman and pendulum
  - ○ 1–2 weeks post-injury—discontinue sling, slowly progress to gentle passive and A/AROM of motion at shoulder (flexion, abduction)
- Activity modification: No contact sports until pain resolved and full ROM achieved (2–6 weeks). Avoid heavy lifting, pushing, pulling, painful movements
- Strengthening: Shoulder girdle complex (weights or resistance bands), Scapula internal and external rotators (especially with scapula retractions and protractions)

ADHESIVE CAPSULITIS (726.0)

- AKA Frozen Shoulder
- Painful idiopathic loss of active *and* passive ROM
- More common with diabetes, thyroid disorders, inflammatory arthritis, and trauma
- **Three Stages** [4]
  1. Painful, freezing (3–6 months)
     (a) Synovitis that progresses to capsular thickening in anterior and inferior portions of the capsule with reduction in synovial fluid
  2. Progressive stiffness or adhesive (3–18 months)
     (a) Fibrosis of the capsule more pronounced and thickening of the rotator cuff tendons, glenohumeral joint space is decreased
  3. Thawing or resolution (3–6 months)
     (a) Chronic inflammation with resolution of joint space loss

Anatomy:
- Capsule encircles the glenohumeral joint and attaches to scapula, humerus, and long head of biceps
- Lined by thin synovial membrane

Symptoms:
- Pain, exacerbated by overhead activities, worse nocturnally
- Decreased motion at shoulder, inability to raise the arm

Physical exam:
- Diffuse tenderness to palpation
- Pain with movement
- Significant reduction in active *and* passive shoulder range of motion in all planes when compared to the unaffected side, especially in extremes of external rotation, abduction and adduction
- Loss of passive ROM helps to distinguish this from other shoulder pathology

Imaging:
- X-ray: normal, used to rule out other etiology
- MR Arthrograms: display contracted capsule, joint space narrowing
- MRI: thickening of coracohumeral ligament and subcoracoid space obliteration

Treatment:
- Ice, NSAIDs, moist heat
- Implement early aggressive therapy
  - Injections and analgesics may have to be used so patients can tolerate therapy
- Short trial of oral steroids
- Intra-articular injection [1]
  - 1½" 22 gauge needle; inject Methylprednisolone or Triamcinolone: 40–80 mg with 3–5 ml of local anesthetic into glenohumeral joint (subacromial space)
- May be 1–2 years before full ROM may possibly be restored

Rehabilitation Program:
- Goal: reduce pain and increase ROM at GH joint and scapula
- Modalities: pre-therapy—moist heating pad, TENS, ultrasound, iontophoresis; post-therapy—icing to control swelling
- ROM: aggressive mobilization with AAROM, AROM and PROM
- Stretching: stretch to limits with no restriction range, sustained stretch for 30 seconds at end range, external rotation passive stretch, overhead stretch, crossed adduction
- Strengthening: Once patient is progressing can add strengthening of rotator cuff muscles, closed chain isometric exercises and progress to open chain exercises with theraband

EPICONDYLITIS/OSIS (MEDIAL—726.31, LATERAL 726.32)

- Inflammation, pain, or tenderness in region of medial or lateral epicondyle of humerus
- Repetitive stress injury: poor throwing mechanics, repetitive lifting, etc.

Anatomy:
- **Lateral epicondyle**
  - Attachment site for the wrist extensors
    - Primarily affects extensor carpi radialis brevis (ECRB)
    - But also may include extensor carpi radialis longus (ECRL) and extensor digitorum communis (EDC)
  - Tennis elbow—overuse from a tennis backhand
- **Medial epicondyle**
  - Attachment site for the wrist flexors
    - Affects flexor carpi radialis (FCR), flexor carpi ulnaris (FCU), flexor digitorum superficialis (FDS), palmaris long (PL)
  - Golfer's elbow—repetitive wrist flexion in a golf swing

Symptoms:
- Pain in area of either lateral or medial epicondyles
- Pain may radiate proximally or distally
- Pain at elbow worsened by wrist movement

Physical Exam:
- Normal neurological exam (strength of wrist may be limited by pain)
- **Lateral epicondylitis** [3]
  - Tenderness over extensor (lateral) muscle origin
    - Located at or one fingerbreadth below lateral epicondyle
  - *Cozen's Test*—pain increased with resisted wrist extension (especially with elbow extending, forearm pronated, wrist radially deviated, hand in a fist)
  - *Mill's Test*—pain with full passive wrist flexion; this stretches the extensor tendons placing pressure at the epidcondyle
  - *Middle finger resistance test*—pain over lateral epicondyle with resisted extension of proximal interphalangeal joint
  - Evaluate for radial nerve entrapment—tenderness over course of nerve along radial head

- **Medial epicondylitis**
  - ○ Tenderness over flexor (medial) muscle origin
    - ▪ Located at or one fingerbreadth below medial epicondyle
  - ○ Pain with resisted wrist flexion
  - ○ Pain with full passive wrist extension

Imaging: used to rule out other pathology
- X-ray: used to rule out occult fractures, arthritis, osteochondral defects; rarely needed
- Ultrasonography: focal area of low echogenicity corresponding to areas of collagen degeneration and intratendinous fiber
- MRI: may be used to assess for inflammation, partial or complete tear or tendon, or tendon detachment; rarely needed

Treatment:
- Initial treatment: rest, avoidance of repetitive motions and activity modification, NSAIDs, thermal modalities (heat and ice)
  - ○ Lateral epicondylosis: tennis stroke and equipment modification (string tension, grip size)
  - ○ Medial epicondylosis: golf swing or baseball pitching modification to avoid excessive force on wrist flexors
- Forearm band (counterforce brace)—this is worn tightly distal to flexor or extensor muscle group, while not inhibiting bending of the elbow and not causing any paresthesias. This works to take the stress from the muscle insertion by creating a new stabilization point distally
- Neutral wrist immobilization splint
- Epicondyle Injection: into area of maximum tenderness
  - ○ 1 ½″ 25 gauge needle; inject Methylprednisolone or Triamcinolone: 20–40 mg with 1–2 ml of anesthetic at the affected epicondyle

Rehabilitation [1]:
- Modalities: ultrasound, electrical stimulation, phonophoresis, iontophoresis, heat, ice, massage
- Stretching: of wrist extensors or wrist flexors, posterior shoulder capsule
- Strengthening of wrist extensors or wrist flexors, concentric and eccentric; initially static (isometric) exercises advancing to progressive resistive exercise, also address proximal kinetic chain with scapular stabilization exercises

CARPAL TUNNEL SYNDROME (CTS) (354.0)

- AKA Median neuropathy at the wrist
- Compression of median nerve as it passes through the carpal tunnel
  - Idiopathic, repetitive stress or due to change in canal volume secondary to: thyroid disease, CHF, renal failure, mass, pregnancy, fracture, arthritis, rheumatoid tenosynovitis

Anatomy:
- Contents of carpal tunnel: Tendons of the FDS, FDP, FPL muscles, and the median nerve
- Bordered by the carpal bones inferiorly, transverse carpal ligament superiorly
- Median innervated muscles affected by CTS: first two lumbricals, opponens pollicis, abductor pollicis brevis, flexor pollicis brevis
- Dermatomes innervated by median nerve affected by CTS: palmar side of the first three digits and ½ of fourth digit

Symptoms:
- Paresthesias, numbness, pain, subjective swelling, and weakness in the hand (mostly the thumb, forefinger, and middle finger). Some patients will state it is the entire hand
- Exacerbated at night from compression during sleep
- Impaired ability to handle fine objects

Physical exam:
- Decreased light touch sensation at the above-mentioned region
- Weakness of intrinsic muscles of the hand, thumb abduction, flexion, and/or opposition
- In severe cases loss of thenar eminence due to muscle atrophy can be seen
- Provocative maneuvers: Phalen, Tinel's, reverse Phalen, Carpal compression test

Imaging:
- X-ray: if fracture or degenerative joint disease suspected
- Ultrasound: may show enlarged median nerve
- Electrodiagnostic testing: SNAP prolonged latency, decreased amplitude or absent; CMAP prolonged latency, decreased amplitude; abnormal spontaneous activity on EMG, see more details in EMG chapter

Treatment:
- Conservative management: wrist splinting in neutral position (0° of extension) for 3–4 weeks (during night and day to aide with acute flare)
- Ice, heat, NSAIDs, relative rest during acute stages and activity modification
- Oral steroids if pain is refractory
- Phonophoresis and iontophoresis
- Injection at the carpal tunnel [2]
  - 1½″ 25 gauge needle; inject Methylprednisolone or Triamcinolone: 20–40 mg with 1 ml of anesthetic into the carpal tunnel
- Surgery: carpal tunnel release in patient that do not respond to conservative measures or if the CTS is severe

Rehabilitation Program:
- Goal: decrease the compressive forces on the nerve, reduce inflammation, decrease pain
- Stretching: Flexion and extension stretching of wrist and forearm to promote tendon gliding
- Avoidance of aggressive strengthening

ULNAR NEUROPATHY (354.2)

- Locations of possible compression [4]:
  - Ulnar groove at the elbow (most common)
  - Proximal edge of flexor carpi ulnaris aponeurosis
  - Arcade of Struthers
  - Guyon's canal
    - Often secondary to cycling activity, wrist ganglionic cysts, or rheumatoid arthritis
  - Can occur months to years after distal humerus fracture (tardy ulnar palsy)

Anatomy:
- Ulnar nerve
  - Derived from C8 and T1 roots (lower trunk, medial cord of brachial plexus)
  - Course
    - Descends along medial head of triceps into Arcade of Struthers

- Continues posteriorly between medial epicondyle and olecranon (ulnar groove)
    - Continues distally in Cubital Tunnel and then through Guyon's Canal at the wrist (under the pisiform)
- Innervation [4]:
    - Flexor carpi ulnaris
    - Flexor digitorum profundus
    - Palmar ulnar cutaneous nerve—sensation over volar aspect of fourth and fifth digit
    - Dorsal ulnar cutaneous nerve—sensation of dorsal aspect of 4th and 5th digit
    - Dorsal digital nerves
    - Hypothenar Branch: opponens digiti quinti, abductor digiti quinti, flexor digiti quinti
    - Deep motor branch: palmaris brevis, four dorsal interossei, three palmar interossei, third and fourth lumbricals, adductor pollicis, deep head of flexor pollicis brevis

Symptoms:
- Numbness or paresthesias in dorsal and/or volar aspects of fifth and ulnar side of fourth digits
- Weakness in the hand
- Pain radiating proximally and/or distally exacerbated by elbow flexion as this places pressure on the nerve

Physical Exam [3]:
- Weakness with thumb adduction, hand grip, pincer grip
- Arcade of Struthers, Cubital Tunnel: injury here will demonstrate involvement of all ulnar nerve innervated muscles
    - Wrist flexion will deviate radially
    - Impaired sensation over volar and dorsal aspect of fourth and fifth digits
- *"Claw hand"*: at rest, unopposed pull of (extensor digitorum communis) EDC→extension of MCP→partial finger flexion of fourth and fifth PIP and DIP
- *Froment's Sign*: unable to hold piece of paper by thumb and index finger with thumb adduction, you will see the DIP of the thumb flex to compensate for weak adduction
- *Wartenberg's Sign*: inability to adduct fifth digit, the fifth digit lays in slight abduction due to unopposed insertion of the extensor digiti quinti

Table 11.3 Shea classification

Type 1	Involvement of hypothenar and deep ulnar branch
Type 2	Involvement of deep ulnar branch
Type 3	Involvement of superficial ulnar sensory branch

- Guyon's Canal: ulnar nerve trunk splits into deep and superficial branches
  - May involve all ulnar nerve innervated intrinsic hand muscles

Shea Classification (Table 11.3) [4]

Electrodiagnostics:
- Dependent on injury site, see EMG section for more detail
- NCS: abnormal SNAP and CMAP
- EMG: abnormal spontaneous activity in ulnar nerve innervated muscles

Treatment:
- Rest, protecting elbow with padding, NSAIDs, ice
- Surgery:
  - If conservative management fails, depends on location of injury:
    - Cubital tunnel release
    - Ulnar nerve transposition
    - Decompression at arcade of struthers
    - Subtotal medial epicondylectomy
    - Ulnar collateral ligament repair

Rehabilitation:
- Ergonomics: workstation modifications to decrease elbow flexion
- Strengthening: forearm pronator and flexor muscles; advanced strengthening with eccentric and dynamic joint stabilization exercises

DE QUERVAIN TENOSYNOVITIS (727.04)

- Inflammation or stenosis of the tendon sheath at the radial side of the wrist

- Overuse injury: related to household and recreational activities, involving fast repetitive pinching, grasping, pulling, and/or pushing
- Insidious onset, usually not associated with acute trauma
- Primarily affects middle-aged women (10:1)

Anatomy:
- Stenosing tenosynovitis of the synovial sheath of the tendons of:
  ○ Abductor pollicis longus
  ○ Extensor pollicis brevis

Symptoms:
- Pain in lateral/radial wrist, worse with thumb extension and grasping
- May be accompanied by stiffness in the region
- Paresthesias are rare

Physical Exam:
- Local swelling around radial wrist
- Tenderness at the radial wrist or around radial styloid
- Provocative maneuvers [3]
  ○ *Finkelstein test*: have the patient bend the thumb into the palm and bend the wrist into ulnar deviation, reproduction of pain at the radial wrist is a positive test [10]

Imaging:
- X-ray: rule out other wrist pathology such as distal radius or wrist fracture (especially scaphoid)
- Ultrasound: tenosynovitis characterized by distension in the tendon sheath with surrounding hypoechoic fluid

Treatment:
- Conservative treatment, including ice, NSAIDs, heat, splints, rest have shown limited benefit
- Thumb spica splint: immobilization; inhibits gliding of the tendon through the abnormal fibro-osseous canal, thumb remains immobilized in abduction and wrist in extension
- Corticosteroid injection into first extensor compartment
- Surgery: partially removing tendon sheath for decompression (83—92% cure rate)

Rehabilitation: Goal: decrease pain with range of motion, strengthen and regain range of motion at thumb, hand, wrist

- Modalities: ice, heat, electrical nerve stimulation, ultrasound, iontophoresis
- Activity modification

TRIGGER FINGER (727.03)

- Snapping or locking of a finger when it is flexed and extended due to nodular swelling or inflammation of flexor tendon sheath
- Arises from high pressures at the proximal edge of the A1 pulley, at the metacarpal head
- Most commonly affects middle-aged women, thumb, middle, and ring fingers
- Commonly found in patients with diabetes and rheumatoid arthritis

Symptoms:
- Pain at the proximal interphalangeal joint (not at metacarpophalangeal joint)
- Intermittent locking in flexion or extension of the digit, overcome by forceful active effort or passive assistance with the opposing hand
- Trigger thumb more often associated with pain than trigger finger

Physical Exam:
- Tender nodule over volar aspect of metacarpal head
- Pain with opening and closing of hand
- Joint contractures at interphalangeal joints (chronic)

Imaging:
- Not necessary; clinical diagnosis

Treatment:
- Splinting of metacarpophalangeal joint at 10–15° of flexion with proximal and distal interphalangeal joints free (up to 6 weeks) [1]
- Ice, NSAIDs
- Local corticosteroid injection with local anesthetic is often first line

- Use 27 gauge, 5/8 in. needle with 2–3 ml of steroid and anesthetic mixture (40 mg of methylprednisolone and 1 ml of 1% lidocaine)
- Injectate enters into the palm at the level of the distal palmar crease directly over the tendon
- Post-injection: avoidance of hand activities for 1 week, splint to protect area
- Often curative but may need to be repeated up to three times
- Surgery: A1 pulley release surgery (if conservative treatment fails)

Rehabilitation:
- Goal: to decrease pain and increase function
- Modalities: ice massage, contrast baths, ultrasound, iontophoresis with steroid
- Custom splinting

Lower Extremity

HIP OSTEOARTHRITIS (715.15)

- Degenerative joint disease of the femeroacetabular joint
- Wear and tear overuse injury causing gradual loss of articular cartilage in the synovial joint followed by hypertrophic reaction in subchondral bone and joint margins

Anatomy:
- *Hip joint*: ("femeroacetabular joint") comprised of the femoral head and the pelvic acetabulum (formed at the junction of the pubis, ilium, and ischium)
- *Capsule*: Fibrous capsule surrounding the joint and a portion of the femoral neck
- *Ligaments*: Triangular iliofemoral ligament (ASIS to intertrochanteric line), pubofemoral ligament (pubic portion of acetabular rim/pubic ramus to neck of femur), and ischiofemral ligament (ischial wall of acetabulum to neck of femur medial to greater trochanter)

Symptoms:
- Gradual onset of groin pain may be referred distally as far as the medial knee
- Joint stiffness

- Feeling of instability
- Worse with weight-bearing/rotational activity
- Difficulty arising from a chair, may need assistance of upper extremities or assistive device

Physical Exam:
- Inspection: Antalgic gait, favoring the affected side (patient will attempt to unload the affected hip when ambulating)
- ROM: Groin pain often felt with abduction and external rotation of lower extremity
- Examine other joints (knee, ankle, wrist, finger) for signs of OA
- MMT: Normal
- Reflexes: Normal
- Neurologically intact exam (unless there is concomitant muscle weakness along with the hip joint degeneration from a radiculopathy)
- Provocative Maneuvers
  - *FABER Test (Patrick Test)*—place ipsilateral heel on contralateral knee while the physicial applies force downward on ipsilateral knee (hip **F**lexed **AB**ducted, and **E**xternally **R**otated) when positive will produce groin pain

Imaging:
- AP X-ray of hip with measurements of minimal joint space (shortest distance between the femoral head margin and the acetabular edge) or Kellgren-Lawrence grading system (grading joint space narrowing along with other features including subcondral sclerosis, cysts, osteophytes). Cartilage breakdown, osteophyte overgrowth, joint space narrowing, bone sclerosis
- MRI: often not needed however useful if suspecting other diagnoses like labral tears or avascular necrosis

Treatment:
- Encourage weight loss
- Acetaminophen and NSAID (Naproxen 500 mg BID PO)
- Glucosamine (1 g daily) and chondroitin (1,200 mg daily) can be suggested however have not been scientifically proven to be joint protective.
- Hip Injections: posterior or anterior approach with fluoroscopic guidance using 4 ml of 1% Lidocaine or 0.25% Marcaine and 1 ml of Corticosteroid (specifics, such at 40 mg kenalog, methylprednisolone, dexamethasone, betamethasone, etc.) This can be therapeutic but is also done diagnostically prior to proceeding with hip surgery

Rehabilitation Program:
- Goal: Reduce Pain and regain proper biomechanics around to joint to limit abnormal joint alignment
- ROM: Specifically IR and ER of the hip; however, flexion and extension along with abduction and adduction can be emphasized. Allow AROM for mild symptoms and AAROM for moderate to severe symptoms.
- Stretching exercises: starting with gentle stretches and progressing to full stretches if painless (to prevent joint stiffness). Stretches for Hip flexor, adductor, iliotibial band, gastrocnemius and hamstring.
- Strengthening: Hip flexors and Abductors with standing leg raises and lateral leg raises, side-lying leg external rotation and abduction exercises, supine leg lifts with and without the use of a theraband. Will also allow a 30° mini squat exercise and gentle wall glides (closed-kinetic chain exercise).
- Ambulation training with straight cane (held in hand opposite of painful hip)
- Aqua-running where available

PIRIFORMIS SYNDROME (355.0)

- Piriformis muscle is compressing the sciatic nerve causing a sciatic neuropathy (either intrinsic muscle injury or compression at the pelvic outlet).

Relevant Anatomy:
- Piriformis and sciatic nerve both pass through the greater sciatic notch with variations on their anatomic relationship (sciatic nerve passing below the piriformis, passing through the muscle belly, as a divided nerve, and above the muscle belly).
- Piriformis originates in the anterior surface of the sacrum and inserts into the greater trochanter of the femur.

Symptoms:
- Buttock pain with/without radiation into the leg
- Occasional parasthesia in buttock and posterior thigh
- Pain with hip adduction and internal rotation
- Sitting on hard surfaces exacerbates symptoms

Physical Examination:
- Normal neurologic findings
- Tenderness to palpation from sacrum to greater trochanter with a taut palpable band
- Provocative Manuevers [3]:
  - *Freiberg sign*—pain with passive hip abduction and internal rotation
  - *A Pace Sign*—contraction of the piriformis with resistance to active hip external rotation and abduction

Treatment:
- NSAIDs and analgesic medications
- Heat to increased collagen distensibility
- Use of soft cushions for prolonged sitting
- Injection of piriformis: site is 1 cm caudal and 2 cm lateral to the lower border of the sacroiliac joint. 2 ml of 1% lidocaine with 1 ml of corticosteroid.

Rehabilitation Program:
- Goal: Reduce pain and increase stretch of piriformis muscle
- Modalities: ultrasound heat therapy for deep heating
- Stretching: Gentle piriformis stretch: hip internal rotation above 90° of hip flexion
- Strengthening Exercises: Strengthening of hip abductors with emphasis on gluteus medius
  - Sidewalking; theraband exercises

TROCHANTERIC BURSITIS (726.5)

- Peak incidence between the fourth and sixth decade of life
- Often due to repetitive microtrauma to the soft tissue structures around the greater trochanter; gluteal tendon degeneration and tears at the attachment induce inflammation in the bursae.
- Contributing factors: Hip abductor-external rotator weakness, hip osteoarthritis, lumbar spondylosis, leg-length discrepancies, and Iliotibial band syndrome
- Patients may often mistake lateral hip pain (greater tronchanter pain syndrome) as hip joint pain

Anatomy
- Bursa lies between the greater trochanter (bone) and the above ilio tibial tract and gluteus medius

Symptoms:
- Lateral hip/side pain
- Pain over the greater trochanter or just posterior to it with occasional radiation down the mid-lateral thigh
- Pain brought on by lying on that side when sleeping, or external rotation/abduction

Physical Exam:
- Localized area of tenderness found on palpation at the region of the greater trochanter (lateral thigh) with maximal tenderness at the attachment of the gluteus medius
- May have a Trendelenburg Gait
- Pain with resisted hip abduction when patient is lying on their side and at 45° of abduction
- Lumbosacral radiculolpathy should be ruled out with neurologic exam
- Examination for leg length discrepencies, or hip arthritis (FABER, FADIR, etc.)

Imaging:
- No specific imaging; however, calcifications may be seen in XR of the hip (either in the bursa or the tendinous attachment)

Treatment [1]:
- Ice, NSAIDs, Tylenol, activity modification (direct pressure should be avoided), topical ointments/patches
- Gentle stretching
- Weight loss
- Corticosteroid injection of the bursa—22 or 25 gauge needle containing 20–40 mg triamcinolone with 1% lidocaine (3–4 ml). Needle is advanced until contact is made with bone, then the needle is retracted slightly for the injection. New techniques involving Ultrasound may visualize the bursa as well as any inflammation.

Rehabilitation Program:
- Goal: Reduce Pain and restore proper biomechanics
- Modalities:
  - Initially: Ice massage, iontophoresis
  - After first week: Heat, phonophoresis, therapeutic ultrasound

- Stretching exercises gently in all planes (adduction, abduction, internal rotation, external rotation, flexion, extension). Stretching of the iliotibial band
- Strengthening focused on hip abductors, extensor, external rotators

LATERAL FEMORAL CUTANEOUS NERVE SYNDROME (355.1)

- Aka—Meralgia Paresthetica
- Seen in obese patients or those wearing tight compressive garments, belts, or straps. Can also occur due to scar tissue development or in pregnancy
- Compression or Entrapment of the lateral femoral cutaneous nerve as it exits the pelvis

Anatomy:
- Nerve fibers originate from the L2 to L3 roots
- Nerve travels lateral to psoas muscle anterior to the iliacus muscle and underneat the ilioinguinal ligament.

Symptoms:
- Burning (dysesthesia) pain and/or hypoesthesia over the anterolateral thigh
- Pain especially with hip extension
- No motor weakness

Physical Exam:
- Inspection: Look for signs of previous surgery/procedure with scar formation or indentation marks from tight clothing
- Palpation: Tenderness over the area just medial to the ASIS with reproduction of pain when palpated
- MMT: normal
- Sensation: Decreased in anterolateral thigh to light touch
- Reflexes: normal
- Hip extension may trigger the symptoms

Imaging:
- None necessary, although AP radiograph of pelvis can be done to rule out other abnormalities

Treatment [1]:
- Injection: done for acute pain, 4 ml Lidocaine only or 4 ml of Lidocaine with steroid as well (1-ml of 40 mg/ml Depo-Medrol or Kenalog) into the area of the nerve is both diagnostic (if it reduces the pain sensation) and therapeutic (2-cm medial and 2-cm inferior to the ASIS)
- Removal of tight clothing and weight loss
- Persistent and recurrent symptoms for 3–4 months may require surgical consult for nerve decompression

KNEE

ANTERIOR CRUCIATE LIGAMENT (ACL) TEAR (717.83)

- Main stabilizer of knee
- Primary function: resisting hyperextension and anterior tibial translation in flexion, some rotator control
- Tears result from rotational twisting, pivoting, valgus motion, or hyperextension force that overcomes strength of ligaments.
- Most commonly from a sudden deceleration during high-velocity movements in which a forceful contraction of the quadriceps is needed.
- Can also occur with tears of meniscus or medial collateral ligament.

Anatomy:
- Origin: anterior base of the tibia to the posterolateral corner of the intercondylar notch of the femur

Symptoms:
- Sudden pain and swelling
- Giving way of the knee, buckling, or locking
- Audible pop
- Instability of knee

Physical Exam:
- Inspection: acutely swollen (first 24 h)
- ROM: limited due to swelling and guarding
- Sensation: intact
- Provocative Maneuvers [3]

○ **Lachman test**—knee flexed at 25°; forward translation of tibia while femur stabilized. Increased motion of tibia with no solid endpoint indicates a tear of ACL

○ **Anterior Drawer test**—knee flexed 90°. Anterior translation of tibia on femur.

○ **Pivot-Shift test**—reproduce anterolateral instability by internally rotating the leg applying a valgus stress to the knee as it is flexed (looking for anterior migration of the tibia on the femur)

Imaging:
• Radiographs: AP, Lateral, Tunnel View
• MRI: most sensitive

Treatment:
• Initially rest, ice, compression, elevation, crutch walking
• Analgesic or anti-inflammatory (Naprosyn 500 mg po Bid × 5 days with food then prn afterwards)
• Sterile aspiration if knee effusion present
• Knee immobilizer or range-of-motion brace (ex. DonJoy Knee Braces)
• Surgery is the definitive treatment for younger patients (may not be needed in older patients who lead a more sedentary life). An ACL-deficient knee has a high incidence of instability in an active knee and can lead to further meniscal injury, articular injury, and degenerative changes if untreated.

Rehabilitation Program [1]:
Initial Phase
• Goals: Allow tissue healing, reduce pain/inflammation, increase ROM
• Modalities: cyrotherapy, E-stim
• Equipment: Knee stabilizing brace—Early weight-bearing attempts with brace
• ROM: AAROM flexion and extension while patient in sitting position , maintain ROM is important prior to surgery to avoid arthrofibrosis
• Strengthening: Static quadriceps and hamstrings exercises
• Bicycle/Pool exercises—general conditioning
• Start Neuromuscular and Proprioceptive retraining
• Crutch Ambulation

After (2–8 weeks)
- Goals: obtaining normal AROM, and muscle balance
- Modalities: Superficial heat, pulsed ultrasound, E-stim
- ROM, flexibility exercises
- Strengthening: Dynamic lower extremity strengthening
  ○ Closed kinetic chain exercises, multi-planar lower extremity joint exercises
- Gradual return to sports-specific training with functional bracing

After Reconstruction:
- Goal: Maintain ROM and strength
- Modalities: Cryotherapy, compression, and elevation to reduce swelling and pain
- ROM (most often patients lose more extension than flexion). AAROM in knee flexion and extension while patient is in sitting position
- Strengthening Exercises: Strength program including initial Isometric Quadricep and Hamstring exercises for first few days progressing to closed chain kinetic exercises followed by dynamic and open chain exercises weeks later
- Gradual return to sports-specific training

MENISCAL KNEE INJURIES

717.0 Internal derangement of knee
836.2 Other tear of cartilage or meniscus of knee, current
836.0 Tear of medial cartilage or meniscus of knee, current
717.1 Derangement of anterior horn of medial meniscus
717.2 Derangement of posterior horn of medial meniscus
717.4 Derangement of lateral meniscus
717.42 Derangement of anterior horn of lateral meniscus
- Menisci are thick and convex at the periphery (horns) and thin towards the center
- Axial load transmitted through a rotating flexed (or extended) knee.
- Due to its firm attachment to the joint capsule and collateral ligament, the medial meniscus is more often torn than the lateral. In

acute ACL tears usually occurring from a valgus blow to the patient's knee, the lateral meniscus is usually torn.
- Menisci distribute forces across knee and enhance stability.
- Five common types of meniscal tears: longitudinal, degenerative, flap tear, horizontal, and radial tear.
- Young patients often present with vertical–longitudinal tears (bucket-handle tear is most common) while older patients with degenerative joint disease suffer horizontal tears. Tears can also be full thickness or partial thickness. Bucket-handle tears usually in posterior two-thirds of meniscus and occur in athletes of 2030 years of age.

Anatomy [4]:
- Medial and Lateral menisci are connected to each other anteriorly, to the ACL, and to the femur, patella, and tibia via ligaments
- Only the periphery of the menisci receive adequate vascular supply (important implication for healing)

Symptoms:
- Reported "pop" or "snap"
- Deep knee bending is painful
- Mechanical locking
- Delayed swelling of knee

Physical Exam:
Inspection: Antalgic gait with decreased knee extension; knee effusion; posteriomedial or lateral knee tenderness on palpation
- Provocative Maneuvers [3]
- ***Bounce Home test***—pain or mechanical blocking when patient's knee is passively forced into extension
- ***McMurray's test***— the knee is held along joing line by one hand, and flexed to complete flexion while the foot is held by the sole with the other hand. Then a valgus stress is applied to the knee while the other hand rotates the leg externally while extending the knee. A positive test for a tear in the medial meniscus is indicated by a pain or a "click". The medial knee can then be stabilized in a fully flexed position and the leg internally rotated as the leg is extended during which pain or a "click" indicates a tear of the lateral meniscus.
- ***Apley Compression test***—axial load applied to a prone knee at 90° provides pain

Imaging:
- Weight-bearing AP X-rays only worthwhile in degenerative meniscal tears revealing degenerative changes in the joint
- MRI is most useful (sagittal and coronal planes)

Treatment:
- If knee is acutely locked, reduction should occur in 24 h
- Rest, Ice, and compression given initially
- Weight-bearing as tolerated
- Analgesics—Acetaminophen or opioids or NSAIDs
- Arthrocentesis—diagnostic and therapeutic for effusion
- Healing potential greatest for tears within the periphery of the menisci

Rehabilitation Program [1]:

Acute Phase
- Goal: decrease pain and swelling and increase ROM/strength (1 week)
- Modalities: cold for joint swelling
- ROM: Gentle ROM exercises of knee
- Ambulation training with crutch walking to off-load the limb progressed to ambulation independently as tolerated
- Strengthening Exercises:
  - Isometric close-chain strengthening exercises for quad strengthening without full knee extension, progressing to bicycle training
  - Strengthening of hip abductors, adductors, and extensors

Recovery Phase
- Goal: regain functional movement (2–8 weeks)
- Stretching: Hamstring/Quad stretching should continue
- Strengthening:
  - Open and closed chain kinetic chain exercises
  - Functional activities, resistive bands
- Proprioceptive and balance training
- Plyometric and sports exercises

Patient who have received surgical repair of their meniscus should start with nonaggressive, minimal shear exercises with a general advancement in weight-bearing status and increased range of motion and functional activities after 2–3 weeks

KNEE ARTHRITIS (715.96)

- Osteoarthritis is the most common form of knee arthritis
- Can involve all compartments of the knee (medial compartment, lateral compartment, patellofemoral joint)
- Most common involved in OA is medial compartment resulting in genu varum (bowleg)

Symptoms:
- Statistically affects older patients
- Insidious onset
- Buckling of knee due to bony areas impinging upon each other.
- Difficult climbing or descending stairs
- Stiffness and intermittent joint swelling can limit motion at extremes of flexion/extension

Physical Exam:
Inspection: may reveal angular deformity through the knee (varus or valgus), mild effusion

Palpation: tenderness along joint line extending into the medial hamstring tendon insertion and anteromedial tibia, thickening and osteophytes along the articular margin of the femur

Crepitus around patellofemoral joint

ROM: Loss of ROM—May note a decrease in range of motion of knee on subsequent visits

Imaging [4]:
- Weight-bearing AP radiographs with both knees in full extension—
  - Can also try weight-bearing AP radiographs with 40° of knee flexion to identifgy other areas of narrowing.
- Degenerative Arthritis—asymmetric joint space narrowing, bone sclerosis, periatricular cysts, osteophytes
- Inflammatory arthritis—symmetric joint space narrowing, disuse osteopenia, bony erosions at articular margins
- Lateral and patellofemoral views
- Intercondylar notch view or tunnel view can reveal osteophyte and osteochondral loose bodies

Treatment:
- Conservative management includes NSAIDS, and physical therapy including ice/heat modality
- Corticosteroids, Viscosupplementation (3 weekly injections)

- ○ 3 ml of 1% lidocaine with 40 mg of corticosteroid, 25 gauge needle
- Neoprene sleeve with elastic bandages
- Gravity eliminating exercises such as water aerobics and recumbent cycles
- Medial compartment narrowing—wear a lateral wedge in shoe
- Lateral compartment narrowing—wear a medial wedge in shoe
- Cane to offload the affected lower extremity

Rehabilitation Program:
- Goal: To alleviate pain and swelling and enhance functional capacity
- Modalities: If no swelling, then heat packs×10 min to warm up prior to exercise. If swelling present, use cold packs.
- Stretching: Stretching of hamstrings and quadriceps
- Strengthening:
  - ○ Progressive resistive exercises (weight training) in pain-free arcs of motion can improve endurance.
  - ○ Exercises geared toward the patient's desired function should be emphasized
- Ambulation training with cane in hand opposite the painful limb can help decrease pain.
- Postural alignment and joint positioning techniques

PATELLOFEMORAL SYNDROME (717.7)

- Affects women twice as often as men
- Most common theory is overuse injury from repetitive load of patellofemoral joint.
- Altered Biomechanics
- Improper patellar tracking
- No clear etiology

Symptoms:
- Diffuse, vague ache most likely in anterior knee
- Theater sign—pain with getting up after prolonged sitting with knee flexed
- Pain with ascending or descending stairs
- Occasional locking in extended position

Physical Exam:
- Inspection: Minimal effusion; Observe the tracking of the patella as the patient brings knee into extension

- Palpation: Pain along medial/lateral border of patella
- MMT: Normal
- Reflexes: Normal
- Observe the tracking of the patella as the patient brings knee into extension

Treatment:
- Patellar realignment with the use of a brace or tape may reduce improper positioning.

Rehabilitation Program:
- Goal: focus on deficiencies in strength, flexibility, and proprioception
- ROM: Full ROM of knee flexion/extension
- Strengthening:
  - Begin with closed kinetic chain exercises in range of 0–45° of knee flexion focusing on the quadriceps.
  - Home exercise program included "wall glides" or "lunges"
  - Selective strengthening of VMO and hip adduction

Ankle/Foot

ACHILLES TENDONITIS (845.09)

- Painful swollen tender area of Achilles tendon usually caused by repetitive eccentric contractions of the gastrosoleus complex causing inflammation and microtears of relatively inflexible Achilles tendon.
- Recurrent mechanical injury, inflammation and degeneration of the collage fibers in addition to a region of decreased vascularity of the tendon near the calcaneal insertion.
- Patients most often affected are middle-aged/elderly men who play sports and have relatively inflexible tendons. Likewise young athletes for particularly tight heel cords are predisposed as well.
- Increased risk of Achilles rupture
- Ask for history of Chronic quinolone exposure, steroid use, or smoking

Anatomy:
- Achilles tendon—calcaneal tendon insertion

Symptoms:
- Pain and tenderness in Achilles tendon in association with exercise especially motions involving a quick "push-off".
- A history of a traumatic event; hearing a "pop" should suggest Achilles tendon rupture.

Physical Exam:
- Subjective localization of pain and tenderness to palpation in Achilles tendon approximately 2.5 in. proximal to tendinous insertion
- Palpation: Tenderness to palpation along heel cord
- ROM: Limitation in ankle dorsiflexion
- Reflex: Achilles reflex normal
- Strength: Limited due to pain
- Sensation: intact
- Provocative Maneuvers [3]:
  - ***Thompson test***—to rule out rupture of the tendon (If tendon is intact—while patient is prone squeezing the calf should normally cause plantar flexion, If tendon has ruptured, no movement will occur)

Imaging:
- X-ray usually not needed and normal unless calcification of tendon suspected.
- MRI can be used to assess for partial rupture of the tendon only if suspected.
- Ultrasound is becoming a useful tool to look for inflammation/tears

Treatment:
- Goal: Decrease pain and reduce inflammation, activity modification which includes a gradual return to activity. Patient should initially halt incline running and interval burst training until pain and swelling subsides. Gradual return to activity can include swimming, aqua-running, bicycling, and walking initially with progression to jogging and eventual running.
- Rest or activity modification including initial icing—20 min three times a day—in the first couple weeks for edema reduction
- NSAIDs
- A Heel-life can provide some relief of pain
- Steroid injections contraindicated as it may weaken the structural integrity of the tendon.

Rehabilitation Program:
- Decrease swelling and pain, regain function and strength
- Modalities: iontophoresis, phonophoresis, ice over swollen tendon especially after therapy
- Consider small heel lift for severe tendinous pain
- ROM: AAROM of the ankle within the available range
- Stretching: Gentle stretching of the gastronemius, Achilles tendon, and hamstring for the first 3 weeks. For persistent tightness of the tendon, consider a night AFO dorsiflexion brace (5° of dorsiflexion) if patient is refractory to 6 weeks of treatment.
- Strengthening:
  - Isometric training to the gastroc/quadriceps/hamstring progress to PREs once patient is pain free. At about 2–3 weeks after rehabilitation has started, can begin eccentric exercises on the gastroc/Achilles tendon.
- HEP: teach runners stretching program to be done before and after training

ANKLE ARTHRITIS (715.97)

- Degeneration of the cartilage within the tibiotalar joint
- Posttraumatic degenerative joint disease (chronic)

Symptoms:
- Pain, swelling, stiffness, progressive deformity
- Pieces of cartilage break off forming a loose body
- Joint can "catch" in one position due to the loose body
- "giving way" or instability of joint due to muscle weakness or ligament laxity
- Stiff with initial weight-bearing but improves after walking
- Pain with walking prolonged distances

Physical Exam:
- Swelling, pain, and possibly increased temperature
- Pain along anterior talocrural joint line
- Possible reduced ROM
- Antalgic gait
- Rule out septic arthritis—acute, erythematous, swollen, severe pain

Imaging:
- X-ray—ap lateral weight-bearing

Treatment:
- Pain relief, minimize inflammation
- Nsaids or other analgesics
- Wrap-around ankle support for stability
- Injection (with 22 guage needle) of 3 ml of Lidocaine and 40 mg of corticosteroid. Needle insterted medial to anterior tibialis tendon and directed lateral and superior. Should not feel any resistance in the joint cavity.

Rehabilitation Program:
- Goal: reduce swelling and pain; regain stability
- Modalities: Cold packs for swollen ankle; Hydrotherapy
- Though a wrap-around ankle support (ankle stirrup) will do, one can order a custom-molded rigid AFO with rocker-bottom modification if needed.
- Instruction on cane-walking to reduce forces across ankle joint
- Mobilization, stretching techniques
- Strengthening: Strengthening of surrounding muscle groups for dorsiflexion, plantarflexion, inversion, and eversion (emphasis on everters)

LATERAL ANKLE SPRAIN (845.00)

- Most commonly the anterior talofibular ligament and calcaneofibular ligament
- Also on the differential are high ankle sprains (syndesmotic)—partial tear of distal anterior tibiofibular ligament—and medial (deltoid ligament) sprains
- Ligamentous Injury [4]:
  - Grade 1—partial tear of ATFL without laxity and only mild swelling with point tenderness but no instability
  - Grade 2—complete tear of the ATFL and partial tear of the CFL with mild laxity and moderate pain, tenderness, and instability

o Grade 3—complete rupture of ATFL and CFL resulting in considerable swelling, increased pain, significant laxity, and sometimes unstable joint
- The most common injury (due to excessive inversion) resulting in inversion of a plantar flexed foot causing ligamentous injury in the ankle

Symptoms:
- Pain/tenderness over injured ligaments
- Initial swelling around area of injury
- Decreased ROM
- Instability

Physical Examination:
- Inspection: edema and sometimes ecchymoses. Edema and swelling will cause a decreased ROM
- Palpate around the locations of the anterior and posterior talofibular ligaments, the calcaneofibular ligaments, the syndesmotic area, and the medial deltoid ligament.
- Palpate the distal fibula, medial malleolus, base of the fifth metatarsal, cuboid, lateral process of the talus, and epiphyseal areas for potential fractures
- Check for sensory changes in the distribution of the superficial and deep fibular nerves
- Strength testing for ankle dorsiflexion and eversion especially, however, plantarflexion and inversion should also be tested
- Special Tests [3]:
  o *Anterior drawer test*—plantar flex the ankle to 30° and apply an anterior force to the calcaneus while stabilizing the tibia with the other hand. Look for increased translation. If increased may indicate laxity ATFL.
  o *Talar Tilt test*—start with the ankle in the neutral position. Stabilize the tibia and cup the calcaneous. Apply valgus and varus translating forces and compare to unaffected side. A positive test produces a greater degree of translation of the calcaneous when compared to other side.
  o *Squeeze Test*—squeezing the proximal fibular and tibia at the midcalf. Pathology will produce pain in setting of a syndesmosis injury
  o Grading:
    ▪ Grade 1—negative talar tilt or anterior drawer sign

- Grade 2—positive anterior drawer sign
- Grade 3—positive anterior drawer sign and talar tilt test
  - ○ Complications—peroneal tendon injury

Imaging:
- X-ray with AP, lateral, oblique views. Look for avulsion fractures. Stress views of the ankle are rarely done and are usually achieved by imaging the ankle while in the end ranges of the anterior drawer and talar tilt test.

Treatment:
- Rest, ice, compresssion, and elevation
- Crutches can be used in the short run
- Grade 1 and 2:
  - ○ RICE, Nsaids, short duration of immobilization
  - ○ Physical Therapy
- Grade 3:
  - ○ Conservative vs. surgical consults
  - ○ Can try a 6-month trial of physical therapy

Rehabilitation Program:
- Goals: minimize swelling, decrease pain; increase ROM and strengthen
- Modalities: Ultrasound and Electrical stimulation are used as needed during rehabilitative phase to decrease pain and edema. Ice bags or cryocuff machine to decrease swelling.
- Protective Techniques: taping, cast boots for Grade 2 and 3 injuries
- ROM: AROM without resistance: dorsiflexion, inversion, foot circles, plantar flexion, eversion
- Stretching: Achilles stretching to avoid disuse contracture. Stretching only in dorsiflexion and plantar flexion to start.
- Weight-bearing permitted as symptoms allow. If not signs of abnormal gait, can try full weight-bearing exercises.
- Strengthening Exercises
  - ○ Dorsiflexion/eversion strengthening and static exercises to start
  - ○ Isometric exercises in pain-free range
  - ○ Toe strengthening—Toe Grab Exercises
  - ○ After 1–2 weeks can progress to exercises with more intensity including heel raises, toes raises, stairs, and quarter squats

- ○ Progress to concentric and eccentric exercises with tubing once there is pain-free weight-bearing. This includes inversion, eversion, plantar and dorsiflexion.
- Proprioception training in seated position and then in standing
  - ○ Seated Biochemical Ankle Platform System
  - ○ Wobble Board
- Elevation and ankle pumps for edema control
- After painless range and strengthening programs have peaked, can initiate in interval running and zig-zag aerobic exercises along with agility drills (back pedaling, side stepping).

HIGH ANKLE SPRAIN

- Disruption of the syndesmosis ligament complex (tibiofibular ligaments and interosseous membrane)
- Syndesmotic sprains have a longer recovery period (and more painful) than lateral sprains, however are more rare.
- Associated with deltoid ligament rupture or fibular fracture
- Difficult to bear any weight on affected ankle
- Can have Partial or Complete Tears
- Mechanism—pronation and eversion of the foot combined with internal rotation of the tibia on a fixed food (like being stepped on while lying prone)

Physical Exam:
- Point Tenderness and pain located primarily on the anterior aspect of the syndesmosis
- Unable to bear weight on ankle
- Provocative Maneuvers:
  - ○ Squeeze test [3]—squeezing the calf or lower leg along with slight rotational force produces pain in a high ankle sprain

Imaging:
- AP, Lateral and Mortise views of the ankle along with AP, lateral, and oblique views of the foot. Taken to rule out fractures of the malleoli, tallus, and base of 5th metatarsal that may also be painful after physical exam.

- Stress Radiographs taken with ankle in external rotation can display the diastasis (gap) between the tibia and the fibula.

Treatment:
- Partial syndesmosis tears—nonoperative treatment with removable cast for 6–8 weeks (partial weight-bearing with crutches)
- Complete syndesmosis rupture—treated by suture of the ligament and temporary screw fixation of the tibia and fibula as fibula is prone to misalignment. A walking boot is used for 6–8 weeks postoperatively. Full weight-bearing allowed at 6 weeks. Can allow active and passive ROM at day 7.

TARSAL TUNNEL SYNDROME (355.5)

- Entrapment or compression of the tibial nerve or any of its branches in the region beneath the flexor retinaculum in the medial aspect of the ankle.
- Most often idiopathic however compression of the nerve can occur from soft tissue masses (lipomas, neoplasms) or from tensile stretch of the tibial nerve from valgus deformity of the ankle or bony prominences.

Anatomy:
- Tarsal Tunnel—fibro-osseous structure that begins posterior to the medial malleolus. The laciniate ligament and the tensons of the PT, FDL, FHL provide the roof and floor.
- Nerve branches off Tibial nerve: medial plantar nerve, lateral plantar nerve, medial calcaneal nerve, and baxter nerve (branches off lateral plantar nerve)

Symptoms:
- Pain and paresthesias along with numbness over the sole of the foot
- Burning/aching pain
- Exacerbated by prolonged standing or walking
- Nocturnal pain worse
- Unilateral symptoms

Physical Exam:
- Tinel's sign over the tibial nerve or branches in the tarsal tunnel

- Valleix phenomenon—striking tibial nerve at the ankle that will elicit pain extending proximally
- Pain may also be reproduced on extension of the great toe and sustained passive eversion of the ankle.
- Decreased sensation to light touch or pinprick over the plantar aspect of the foot
- Muscle atrophy of intrinsic musculature may occur after long-standing compression
- Reflexes normal

Diagnostic Study:
- Electromyography
- MRI or ultrasound may be helpful to look for space occupying lesions

Treatment:
- Relative Rest
- NSAIDs (oral or topical), Neuropathic Pain Medication
- Medial arch for pronated foot or foot orthosis for a hindfoot valgus.
- Surgical Release in severe cases

Rehabilitation Program:
- Goal: to decrease painful sensation and increase function of foot
- Devices: Decreasing valgus ankle deformities, overpronated foot or hindfoot valgus with medial arch or foot orthosis
- Stretching protocol focusing on stretching the posterior elements of the distal leg (gastrocnemius, soleus) and the foot intrinsic. Stretching emphasized in a dorsiflexion posture.
- Strengthening: Heel and Toe walking exercises followed by exercises of the foot intrinsics (toe flexion, toe elevation, toe spreads, toe-pencil-grip)

PLANTAR FASCIITIS (728.71)

- Repetitive tensile stress of the soft tissue attachments to the plantar aspect of the heel
- Relative heel cord contracture (which often worsens during the night, since the heel is held in plantar flexion during sleep),
- Static support for the longitudinal arch of the foot, strain on longitudinal arch especially exerts medial aspect of plantar fascia

- Complication: Plantar Fascia Rupture (usually occurs with a history of a steroid injection to the plantar fascia)

Anatomy:
- Plantar fascia is a dense fibrous connective tissue structure originating from the medial tuberosity of the calcaneus. Shock absorber
- Divides into the medial, lateral, central band (aponuerosis)

Symptoms:
- Plantar aspect of foot or inferior aspect of heel pain
- Increased pain complaints in morning
- Difficulty with ambulation

Physical Exam:
- Inspection of lower extremity for pes cavus (high arch), pes planus (flat arch), leg length discrepancy, fat pad atrophy, arthritic changes.
- Inspect shoewear—look for shoewear with poor arch support or worn out soles.
  ○ Also important to ask the patient (as part of the history) if they switch between high heeled and flat shoes frequently.

Imaging:
- Generally not needed, however, can rule out calcaneal stress fracture with X-ray if suspected.

Treatment:
- Patient Education on stretching techniques
- Repetitive daily plantar and Achilles tendon stretches in the morning especially and throughout the day.
- Anti-inflammatories can be used but are often not needed and have variable results
- After 1 month without resolution or diminishing symptoms, can offer a Cam Book with foot in neutral position or slight dorsiflexion
- Cortisone Injection: only utilized after failure of initial rehabilitation program. Can be injected close to the region of the plantar fascia origin on the calcaneus however be cautious as it can cause weakening of the fascia
- In rare and most severe cases of refractory plantar fasciitis for over a year or 18 months, can suggest a surgical consult for fascial release

Rehabilitation Program:
- Goal: Reduce pain and swelling
- Teaching Home Stretching Program is most important

- Modalities: Ice to reduce inflammation, Iontophoresis, Ultrasound
- Stretching of plantar fascia and Achilles tendon
  - Seated plantar flexion stretches
  - Achilles tendon stretches/GastrocSoleus stretch
- Strengthening: Engage in stationary bike, swimming, and deep water running, can gradually progress to running on soft surfaces. Walking with heel inserts can be helpful in the short run. Progress to running on hard surfaces when pain free.
- Orthotic: 5° dorsiflexion night splint can be used

MORTON'S NEUROMA (355.6)

- Perineural fibrosis of a common digital nerve as it passes between the metatarsal heads
- Most commonly between toe digit 3 and 4
- 5:1 female-to-male ratio
- Repetitive Irritation or repetitive pressure

Symptoms:
- Plantar pain in the forefoot
- Burning sensation in affected toes with occasional numbness
- No increased likelihood of night time sensations

Physical Exam:
- Isolated pain in plantar aspect of webspace
- Applying direct pressure over the area in question and then squeezing the toes together with the examiner's other hand will reproduce pain
- Inspect each metatarsal through palpation and inspection

Imaging:
- Imaging not commonly used

Treatment:
- If tight-fit shoewear or heels are the culprit, suggest low-heeled, soft-soled shoe with a wide toebox.
- Metatarsal pads can be utilized to spread the metatarsal heads and reduce pressure on the nerve.

- Injection: using a 27 gauge needle of 1 in. or ½ in. length with 1 ml of lidocaine and 1 ml of corticosteroid injected proximal to metatarsal head
- If symptoms recur, surgical excision can be suggested in severe cases.

Rehabilitation Program:
- In addition to improving shoe-wear patients can receive therapy in the form of modalities including cryotherapy, ultrasound, phonophoresis, deep tissue massage, and stretching exercises
- Often times, a Home exercise program is all that is needed including Ice to reduce any associated inflammation.

AXIAL SPINE

Anatomy [4]
VERTEBRAE
- 7 Cervical vertebrae
  - C1 (Atlas); C2 (Axis); C3–C7
- 12 Thoracic vertebrae
- 5 Lumbar vertebrae
- 5 Sacral vertebrae—fused
- 2 Coccyx vertebrae

INTERVERTEBRAL DISCS
- Nucleus pulposus
  - Gelatinous, Type II collagen
- Annulus fibrosus
  - Radial-like structure made of type I collagen (lamellae) that encloses nucleus pulposus

LIGAMENTS
- Anterior longitudinal ligament (ALL)
  - Runs from base of skull to sacrum
  - Covers anterior aspect of each vertebral body and disc
  - Resists forward bending
- Posterior longitudinal ligament (PLL)
  - Runs from C2 to sacrum
  - Attaches to posterior rim of vertebral bodies
  - Tightens with forward bending

- Ligamentum flavum (LF)
  - Forms posterior aspect of spinal canal; laterally fuses with facet joint capsules
  - Attaches laminae to laminae by connecting adjacent vertebral arches longitudinally
  - Lengthens with flexion
- Interspinous ligament (ISL) and supraspinous liagaments (SSL)
  - Extends from spinous process to spinous process
  - Supraspinous—C7–L3

LUMBAR SPINE

SPONDYLOSIS (721)/SPONDYLOLYSIS (738.4)/ SPONDYLOLISTHESIS (756.12)

DEFINITIONS [4]:
- *Spondylosis*—degenerative osteoarthritis of the joints between vertebral bodies and neural foramina
- *Spondylolysis*—fracture of pars interarticularis
- *Spondylolisthesis*—displacement of vertebra in relation to vertebrae below, defect develops from small stress fractures

SPONDYLOLYSIS

- Most common location: L5 vertebra
- More common in males than females
- Usually due to stress fracture of pars
  - Seen in young adults who participate in sports with hyperextension forces
    - Gymnastics, wrestling, football, dance, swimming

Symptoms:
- Localized back pain
  - Worse with hyperextension, standing, laying prone

Physical Exam [6]:
- Inspection: Hyperlordosis; normal or antalgic gait

- Palpation: Usually non-tender to palpation; some discomfort can be illicited with percussion over midline lumbar region; tight lumbar paraspinals
- ROM: Full ROM, may be decreased if severe pain; tight hamstrings
- Reflexes: Normal unless a specific root is affected by the defect
- Strength: Normal unless a specific root is affected by the defect
- Sensation: Normal unless a specific root is affected by the defect

Imaging:
- X-ray—AP, lateral, and oblique views
  - AP view is usually normal
  - Oblique view to screen for fracture of the pars interarticularis
    - Appears as an area of hypolucency as the collar of the "Scotty dog"
- Bone Scan
  - To identify pars interarticularis stress fractures missed on oblique view
  - Positive at 5–7 days, up to 18 months
  - Negative bone scan, but positive radiograph → inactive spondylolytic defect or old unhealed fracture [6]
  - Differentiate acute vs. chronic fracture
    - Acute stress fractures are best identified with CT
- CT—More sensitive in identifying acute stress fractures, facet joint changes, disc herniations
  - Can classify as early vs. progressive vs. terminal stage
    - Early—Hairline crack in pars interarticularis
    - Progressive—Hairline crack in pars interarticularis becomes a gap
    - Terminal—Appears as a pseudoarthrosis, which is a nonunion which forms a false joint
- MRI—not as sensitive as CT for direct visualization of pars defect [6].

Treatment:
- Acetaminophen, NSAIDs, and analgesic medications

Rehabilitation Program:
- Goal: Reduce pain and promote healing of the pars defect
- Modalities: Bracing (until defect heals), TENS, acupuncture
  - Boston brace—to immobilize pelvis and prevent hyperextension
- Stretching: Hamstrings, lower back

- Strengthening Exercises: paraspinals, iliopsoas, internal oblique, transverse abdominis, lumbar multifidis
- ROM—hamstring stretching, lumbar flexibility motions [6]

SPONDYLOLISTHESIS [1]

- Displacement of vertebral body compared to the vertebral body below it
  - Anterolisthesis—anterior translocation of vertebral body
  - Retrolisthesis—posterior translocation of vertebral body
- **Five Types of Spondylolisthesis** (based on Wiltse classification system)
  1. *Degenerative*
     - Seen in elderly due to facet arthritis and facet remodeling
       - Causes a more sagittal orientation leading to slip
     - Degenerative spondylolisthesis with spinal stenosis
       - Most common indication for spinal surgery in elderly.
         - ♦ Clinical benefit with decompression and fusion vs. decompression alone
     - Most common location: L4-L5
  2. *Pathologic*
     - Very rare.
     - Damage to posterior elements from malignancy, infection, or metabolic bone disease
       - Examples: Paget's disease, tuberculosis, tumor metastases
  3. *Traumatic*
     - Very rare
     - Associated with acute fracture of inferior facets or pars interarticularis
  4. *Dysplastic*
  5. *Congenital*
     - Rare, but progresses rapidly
     - Associated with severe neurological deficits
     - Malformation of lumbosacral junction with small, incompetent facet joints

  - Difficult to treat due to posterior elements and transverse processes are poorly developed, leaving little surface area for a posterolateral fusion
6. *Isthmic/Spondylytic*
  - Otherwise known as spondylolytic spondylolisthesis
  - Acquired between age 6 and 16 years old
    - Prevalence of 5–7% in the U.S.
    - 90% of isthmic slips are low-grade(less than 50% slip)
    - 10% are high-grade (greater than 50% slip) [6]

Meyerding grading system:
- To asses severity of slip
- Measurements on lateral X-ray of distance from the posterior edge of the superior vertebral body to the posterior edge of the adjacent inferior vertebral body.
  - Distance is reported as a percentage of the total superior vertebral body length
    - Grade I: 5–25%
    - Grade II: 26–50%
    - Grade III: 51–75%
    - Grade IV: >75%
    - Over 100% is spondyloptosis
      - The vertebra completely falls off of the supporting vertebra [4].

Symptoms:
- May be asymptomatic
- If symptomatic, patient can have low back pain
  - Generalized dull, aching, buttocks pain that sometimes radiates to posterior thigh
    - Associated with intermittent shocks of shooting pain from buttocks down back of thigh and/or lower leg
    - Can have sciatica that extends below knee and into the feet
  - General stiffening of back, tightness of hamstrings with change in posture, gait
  - Slight lean forward due to lordosis
  - Waddling in severe cases due to increased pelvic rotation, decreased mobility in hamstrings
  - Atrophy of gluteal muscles due to disuse
  - Numbness and tingling sensation

- Difficulty moving from seated to standing position due to pain
- Exacerbation of pain with coughing, sneezing, days following activity (therefore, alleviated by rest)
- If associated with disc degeneration
  - Radiation of pain into lower extremity
  - Neurological symptoms in same distribution as the level of the affected disc
    - L4 nerve root—anterior thigh distribution
    - L5 nerve root—lateral thigh distribution
    - S1 nerve root—posterior thigh distribution

Physical Exam:
- Inspection: Usually normal, Severe cases: postural deformity
- Palpation: Tenderness of lumbar paraspinal muscles; If high-grade slip, you may find palpable step-off over spinous process at level of slip (due to forwards translated vertebra's posterior arch remaining in position)
- ROM: Limited lumbar flexion, hamstring tightness
- Reflexes: Symmetric bilaterally; hyper-reflexic or hypo-reflexic should be noted to rule out cord involvement, such as cauda equina or conus medullaris
  - Adductor reflex—L2, L3, L4—mostly L3
  - Patellar reflex—L2, L3, L4, mostly L4
  - Medial hamstring reflex—L5, S1—mostly L5
  - Strength: dermatomal weakness may be present if a radiculopathy or an element of stenosis is present—see *specific nerve root presentations* (Table 11.4).
- Sensation: Numbness/tingling in lower extremities. Saddle anesthesia should be noted to rule out cord spinal cord involvement.
- Provocative Maneuvers:
  - ***Unilateral extension test*** (aka Michelis' test)
    - Patient stands on one leg with contralateral hip and knee flexed while hyperextending the lumbar spine. The move is repeated with the contralateral leg. Pain ipsilateral to the planted foot indicates a positive test for spondylolysis [7].

Imaging:
- X-ray
  - Standing lateral view
    - To evaluate slippage of vertebrae; monitor progression

Table 11.4 Nerve root presentations (a)

Nerve root presentations [9]

T12-L3 Radiculopathy
- Sensation decreased: Inferior to umbilicus to medial aspect of knee
- Muscles affected most: Hip Flexion → Iliopsoas, Knee Extension → Quadriceps (Femoral N)
- Reflex decreased: None

L4 Radiculopathy
- Sensation decreased: Medial Malleolus and medial leg
- Muscles affected most: Foot Inversion → Tibialis Anterior (Deep Peroneal N)
- Reflex decreased: Patellar

L5 Radiculopathy
- Sensation decreased: First dorsal webspace and lateral leg
- Muscles affected most: Great Toe Extension → Extensor Hallucis Longus (Deep Peroneal N), Hip Abduction → Gluteus Medius (Superior Gluteal N)
- Reflex decreased: None

S1 Radiculopathy
- *Sensation decreased: lateral aspect of foot*
- Muscles affected most: Foot Eversion → Pernoneus longus and brevis (Superficial Peroneal N), Plantar Flexion → Gastrocnemius/Soleus (Tibial N)
- Hip Extension → Gluteus Maximus (Inferior Gluteal N)
- Reflex decreased: Achilles

- - Sagittal plane is emphasized (oblique orientation of lumbosacral intervertebral spaces)
  - Standing flexion/extension views
    - To evaluate instability of involved vertebrae
  - AP view
    - To reveal reverse Napoleon hat sign in severe slips
- L5 vertebra viewed end-on through the sacrum → gives appearance of upside-down Napoleon hat
  - Oblique view
    - To evaluate the integrity of the pars interarticularis
- Hypolucency on neck of Scotty dog (represents the collar).
- Bone scan
  - To evaluate acuteness of spondylotic lesion
  - Positive result with negative X-ray—recent injury (immobilization needed)
  - Negative result with positive X-ray—old injury that has not healed
- Single-photon emission computed tomography (SPECT) scanning

- ○ Sensitive in evaluating integrity of pars interarticularis
  - ▪ Abnormal with acute spondylosis
  - ▪ Normal once condition is chronic, even though healing has not occurred
- ○ Used to determine acuteness of slippage—help determine whether patient would benefit from spinal fusion
- CT scan
  - ○ Enhance bony details (beneficial for surgical evaluation)
  - ○ Size of pars defect can be measured
  - ○ Identify fibrocartilaginous tissue at the defect (can cause nerve root compression→radicular symptoms)
- MRI
  - ○ Enhance visualization of compression of dural sac, especially in degenerative cases
    - ▪ Posterior arch remains and increases compression from its advancement in slip [6]

Treatment:
- Pain control
  - ○ Acetaminophen, NSAIDs, and analgesic medications
    - ▪ If severe radicular component is present, a short course of oral steroids, such as Prednisone or Methylprednisolone.
- Grade I, II and III→Conservative treatment (especially if asymptomatic)
  - ○ Activity modification
  - ○ Pharmacological intervention
  - ○ Chiropractic treatment
  - ○ Physical therapy
  - ○ If increase in pain, consider TLSO bracing
  - ○ Avoid activities that exacerbate pain
- Epidural steroid injections
  - ○ Interlaminar or transforaminal
- Surgery
  - ○ Low grade
    - ▪ Considered after 6 weeks; after 6–12 months of failed conservative management
    - ▪ Postero-lateral fusion with decompression
  - ○ High grade
    - ▪ Posterior interlaminar fusion, in situ posterolateral fusion, in situ anterior fusion (ALIF), in situ circumferential fusion,

instrumented posterolateral fusion, and surgical reduction with instrumented posterolateral interbody fusion (PLIF).

Rehabilitation Program:
- Goal: Alleviate Pain; improve core stability
- Modalities: Thermal treatment, electrical stimulation and lumbar traction can help with reactive muscle spasm
- Stretching: Work on lower back, hamstring flexibility, and quadriceps stretching [1]
- Strengthening:
    - Spinal stabilizations exercises (flexion based)
        - Hip flexors, lumbar paraspinals, abdominals
    - Restrictions from contact sports for asymptomatic Grade 2 and 3

LUMBAR RADICULOPATHY (724.4)

- Most common causes:
    - Nerve root impingement
    - Disc herniation
    - Facet arthropathy

Symptoms:
- Pain at lumbar region and area of affected nerve root
    - Varies in severity and location
    - Severe, exacerbated by standing, sitting, coughing, sneezing
    - Location depends on nerve root affected
    - Starts in back, radiates down lower extremity
        - Can have both or just in buttocks or lower extremity
- Paresthesias
    - Dermatomal distribution of affected nerve root
- Weakness
    - Part of the limb

Physical Exam:
- Inspection: possible asymmetry in standing position, weight may be shifted over one side of pelvis to avoid pain
- Palpation: may have tenderness/spasm at lumbar region
- ROM: may have limited range or increased pain mostly with flexion
- Reflex: may be decreased at regions innervated by affected roots [8]

- ○ Patellar reflex—L2, L3, L4
- ○ Adductor reflex—L2, L3, L4
- ○ Medial hamstring reflex—L4, L5, S1, S2
- Strength:
  - ○ Weakness in distribution of affected disc
  - ○ Proximal weakness in nerve root distribution can differ between bilateral vs. peripheral neuropathy
- Sensation: may have decreased sensation at regions of affected roots [8]
  - ○ L1—oblique band on upper anterior portion of thigh (inferior to inguinal ligament)
  - ○ L2—inferior to L1, superior to L3 (see below)
  - ○ L3—oblique band on anterior thigh, superior to knee cap
  - ○ L4—medial aspect of leg
  - ○ L5—lateral aspect of leg and dorsum of foot
  - ○ S1—lateral malleolus and lateral aspect and plantar surface of foot [8]
- Provocative Maneuvers:
  - ○ ***Straight leg raise***—Patient sitting or supine, Leg raised straight up by examiner maintaining extension of the knee, Positive if pain is reproduced in lower extremity at 80–90°
  - ○ ***Slump test***—patient is seated, patient flexes neck to increase dural tension, Positive if pain s reproduced in lower extremity
  - ○ ***Seated root test***—patient seated on exam table, examiner lifts the affected leg into hip flexion and knee extension, positive if pain is reproduced at the affected lower extremity

Table 11.4—Nerve Root Presentations [9] (a)

Imaging:
- X-ray
  - ○ Typically unremarkable in radiculopathy secondary to herniated nucleus pulposus
  - ○ Used to rule out serious structural pathologic conditions
- MRI
  - ○ Study of choice for nerve root impingement
  - ○ Immediately ordered for progressive neurological deficits; suspected malignancy, inflammatory disease, infection
- EMG
  - ○ Used when diagnosis unclear (localization of pain to specific nerve root level)

- ○ Excludes other causes of sensory/motor impairments
- ○ Quantifies degree of axonal involvement

Treatment:
- Reduce inflammation
  - ○ Avoid bending and lifting (increases intradiscal pressure)
- Medications
  - ○ NSAIDs
  - ○ Opioids
  - ○ Anti-convulsants (gabapentin, lamotrigine), TCA (Doxepin, nortriptyline)
    - ▪ Peripheral neuropathy [5]
- Physical Therapy
- Epidural steroid injection
- Surgery
  - ○ Emergency—progressive neurological deficit (bowel/bladder incontinence)
  - ○ Single-root involvement has favorable outcome
  - ○ Concomintant stenosis

Rehabilitation Program:
- Goal: Alleviate pain; increase back/core stability
- Modalities: ice, heat, massage, TENS, electrical stimulation
- "Back school"
  - ○ Proper lifting, posture awareness
- Lumbar stabilization program
  - ○ Flexion/extension exercises (see below for biases)
- Strengthening
  - ○ Core strengthening (abdominals, paraspinals, gluteal)

Flexion Bias
- Commonly used with facet pathology
- Decreases facet joint compression
  - ○ Stretch lumbar muscles, ligaments
- Cardiovascular fitness program (exercises in slight lumbar flexion)
  - ○ Stationary bike
  - ○ Aquatic stabilization exercises [10]

Extension Bias
- Commonly used with discogenic pathology
- Decreases intradiscal pressure

- ○ Anterior migration of nucleus pulposus away from compression site
- May increase symptoms with large central disc herniation
- Concomitant cardiovascular fitness program to avoid exacerbation of symptoms during exercise [9]

LUMBAR SPINAL STENOSIS (724.02)

- Narrowing of spinal canal, nerve root vanacls, intervertebral foramina
- Combination of congenital and acquired stenosis is more common than congenital alone
- Acquired by degenerative changes
- Stenosis can affect various anatomic locations
  - ○ Central canal
  - ○ Lateral recess
  - ○ Foraminal/extramforaminal regions
- Adult canal
  - ○ AP diameter of lumbar spine15–27 mm
    - ▪ Stenosis when <12 mm

Pathophysiology:
- Acquired by degenerative changes; three stages:
  - ○ Disc dessication → loss of disc height
  - ○ Increased loading of facet joints → degeneration, osteophyte formation, narrowing of spinal canal
  - ○ Hypertrophy of ligamentum flavum, buckling with decreased disc height → further narrowing of spinal canal [4]

Symptoms:
- Back pain
  - ○ Axial (facet arthropathy)
  - ○ Chronic back pain with later development of leg pain
- Leg pain
  - ○ Radicular (nerve root compression)
  - ○ Unilateral/bilateral, monoradicular/polyradicular
- Buttock, thigh, and calf pain (neurogenic claudication)
  - ○ Discomfort: numbness, aches, pain (vascular claudication: cramping, tightness)

- ○ Downhill walking: Painful (vascular claudication: painless)
- ○ Uphill walking: Painless (vascular claudication: painful)
- ○ Alleviation: Flexed position, bending, sitting (vascular claudication: standing, resting, laying flat) [4]

Physical Exam:
- Inspection: wide-based gait (lack of balance due to involvement of posterior columns) ; Forward Lumbar flexed posture as this position may decrease pain
  - ○ size of canal increases in forward flexion by stretching ligamentum flavum out of the canal, reducing overriding laminae and facets, enlarging foramina
- Palpation: May have tenderness at paraspinal regions
- ROM: dependent on degree of pain, can range from limited to full PROM
- Reflex: possible diminished reflexes throughout; absent Achilles
- Strength: possible lower extremity weakness secondary to affected roots; strength may also be limited secondary to pain
- Sensation: Normal; can have sensory impairment in dermatome of affected nerve root [10]

Imaging:
- X-ray
  - ○ Flexion/extension views
  - ○ Disk space narrowing, instability, osteophytes, ligament calcification
- CT
  - ○ Coronal/sagittal views
  - ○ Central stenosis (<10 mm AP diameter)
  - ○ Lateral stenosis
  - ○ Foraminal stenosis [11]

Treatment:
- Acetaminophen, NSAIDs, mild opioids, non-benzodiazepine muscle relaxants
- Epidural steroid injections
- Surgical referral

Rehabilitation Program:
- Relative-rest
- Modalities (hot/cold packs, ultrasound iontophoresis, TENS)
- Flexion-based exercise program
  - ○ Williams Postural Exercises [10]

SI JOINT DYSFUNCTION (Congenital: 755.69; Acquired: 738.5)

SI joint is an L-shaped articulation between sacrum and ilium
- ○ Anteriorly: synovial joint
- ○ Posteriorly: syndesmosi
- SI joint dysfunction is uncommon and over-diagnosed
- Etiology is idiopathic; associated with following risk factors:
  - ○ Fall
  - ○ Leg-length discrepancy
  - ○ Prior lumbar fusion
  - ○ Pregnancy

Symptoms:
- Low back pain, typically below L5
  - ○ Infero-lateral to sacral sulcus
- Gluteal pain, typically below L5 extending to gluteal fold.
- Variations in pain referral; lower extremity pain (including foot)—excluding other etiologies
  - ○ Worse with prolonged sitting, standing, ascending stairs, running (large strides), extreme postures

Physical Exam—thorough exam of low back, hips, pelvis, to rule out other diagnoses.
- Inspection: Increased lumbar lordosis. Evaluate posterior superior iliac spine, anterior superior iliac spine, gluteal folds, pubic tubercules, ischial tuberosities, medial malleoli (to assess pelvic symmetry); muscle atrophy in gluteal muscles, distal extremities.
- Palpation: tenderness to affected SI joint
- ROM: dependent on degree of pain, can range from limited to full PROM
- Reflex: Normal
- Strength: Normal
- Sensation: Normal
- Measure leg-length
- Provocative Maneuvers:
  - ○ *Gaenslen Test*—Patient supine; laying close to edge of table
    - ▪ Knee is flexed
    - ▪ Contralateral leg (proximal to edge of table) is dropped off table causing hyperextension of hip
    - ▪ Pain is reproduced in SI joint dysfunction

- ○ **Sacral sulcus tenderness**
  - ▪ Apply pressrure to gluteal region
  - ▪ Reproduction of pain medial to posterior superior iliac spine is suggestive of SI joint disfunction
  - ▪ High rate of false positives (seen in axial pain, radicular pain, sacral fractures, facet syndroe, piriformis syndrome)
- ○ **Iliac Compression Test**
  - ▪ Patient in lateral decubitus position
  - ▪ Downward force applied to iliac crest
  - ▪ Pain is reproduced in SI joint dysfunction
- ○ **Patrick Test (FABER)**—Patient supine, knee is flexed on affected side and lateral malleolus is placed over patella of opposite leg. Downward pressure applied to flexed knee and opposite anterior superior iliac spine
  - ▪ Contralateral pain in hip/groin is reproduced in SI joint dysfunction [8]

Imaging:
- X-ray
  - ○ Ferguson views, AP views—to rule out seronegative arthropathies, which can present with sacroiliac erosions
- Bone Scan, CT
  - ○ Bone changes due to fracture, infection, tumor, arthritis
- MRI
  - ○ As above; soft tissue disease, marrow changes associated with sacroilitis
- Fluoroscopy
  - ○ Diagnostic and therapeutic SI injection—"Gold Standard"

Treatment:
- Relative rest
- Avoid provocative movements
- Hot/cold packs, topical analgesics
- Injections—diagnostic and therapeutic

Rehabilitation Program:
- Modalities: Ice, massage, heat, electrical stimulation
- Stretching of iliotibial band, hamstrings, external rotators, hip flexors.
- Strengthening of hip girdle and core muscles
  - ○ Gluteus maximus, gluteus medius, erector spinae, latissimus dorsi, biceps femoris, psoas, piriformis, oblique/transversus abdomius.

- Postural education exercises
- SI joints mobilization techniques
- Hip ROM [11]

CERVICAL SPINE

CERVICAL RADICULOPATHY (723.4)

- Most common causes:
  - Cervical disc herniation
  - Degenerative changes
    - Osteophyte formation, decreased disc height, degenerative changes of the anterior aspect of uncovertebral joint and posterior aspect of facets [7].
- Most affected nerve root: C7>C6>C5

Symptoms [12]:
- Neck pain radiating into shoulder, arm and/or hand
- May be associated with paresthesias at effected dermatome
  - Distribution depends on nerve root affected
- Worse with hyperextension, lateral bending and rotation to ipsilateral side
  - May improve with tilting head away from affected side
- Motor, sensory, or reflex changes—refer to *Specific Nerve Root Presentation* (Table 11.5)
  - Weakness; i.e. Pushing, pulling, grasping
- Myelopathy
  - Numbness, impaired fine motor skills

Physical Exam:
- Inspection: Normal or may see spasming muscles at cervical region in severe cases, patient may exhibit antalgic guarded movements
- Palpation: possible tenderness on ipsilateral cervical region
- ROM: Reduced range in extension, lateral bending, rotation towards affected side, but may be in all directions if severe, pain may be exacerbated with flexion
- Reflexes: Normal or decreased for reflexes innervated by affected roots
  - Biceps reflex: C5-C6
  - Brachioradialis reflex: C5, C6, C7

Table 11.5 Specific nerve root presentations (b)

Specific nerve root presentations [9]

C5 Radiculopathy
- Sensation decreased: lateral shoulder (Axillary N)
- Muscles affected most: Shoulder abduction→Deltoid (Axillary N), Suprapsinatus (Suprascapular N), Elbow Flexion→Biceps, Brachialis (both Musculocutaneous N)
- Reflex decreased: Biceps (Mostly C5, some C6)

C6 Radiculopathy
- Sensation decreased: lateral forearm, thumb, index finger and ½ middle finger (Musculocutaneous N)
- Muscles affected most: Radial Wrist Extensors→ECRL, ECRB (both Radial N)
- Reflex decreased: Brachioradialis

C7 Radiculopathy
- Sensation decreased: Middle finger
- Muscles affected most: Elbow Extenstion→Triceps (Radial N) Radial Wrist Flexor→FCR (Median N)
- Reflex decreased: Triceps

C8 Radiculopathy
- Sensation decreased: distal half of ulnar forearm, ring and little finger (Medial Antebrachial Cutaneous N)
- Muscles affected most: Ulnar Wrist Flexor→FCU (Ulnar N), Finger Flexors→FDS (Flexes PIP) all Median N, FDP (Flexes DIP), ½ Median N, ½ Ulnar N
- Reflex decreased: None

T1 Radiculopathy
- Sensation decreased: Medial upper ½ of forearm (Medial Brachial Cutaneous N)
- Muscles affected most: Finger Abduction→Dorsal Interosseii (Ulnar N)
- Reflex decreased: None

- ○ Triceps reflex: C6, C7, C8
- Strength: Weakness at muscles innervated by affected roots
- MMT—may have weakness of muscles innervated by affected roots
  - ○ C5—shoulder abduction (deltoid; rotator cuff)
  - ○ C6—elbow flexion (biceps); wrist extension (extensor carpi radialis longus and brevis)
  - ○ C7—elbow extension (triceps), finger extension (extensor digitorum communis)
  - ○ C8—thumb extension (extensor pollicis longus), ulnar deviation of the wrist (flexor and extensor carpi ulnaris)
  - ○ T1—adduction and abduction (hand intrinsics: interossei and lumbricals) [7]

- Sensation: Normal or decreased at areas innervated by affected roots [8]
  - C5—lateral arm
  - C6—lateral forearm, thumb, 1st/index finger, half of 3rd/middle finger
  - C7—3rd/middle finger
  - C8—4th/ring and 5th/middle fingers, medial forearm
  - T1—medial arm
- UMN signs:
  - Hoffmans reflex—tapping or flicking the nail of the terminal phalanx of the middle/3rd finger
    - Positive result: flexion of terminal phalanx of the thumb
  - Babinski sign—rubbing the lateral aspect of the sole of the foot from a lateral to medial direction up the arch with a blunt instrument
    - Positive result: Dorsiflexion of the hallux
  - Spasticity—velocity dependent resistance to stretch across a joint, resulting in hyperexcitability of the stretch reflex [4]
    - Positive result: lack of inhibition results in excessive contraction of the muscles, leading to hyperflexia (overly flexed joints)
- Provocative Maneuvers:
  - **+ *Spurling sign***—radicular pain reproduced when head extended and rotated toward involved extremity with axial loading

Imaging:
- X-ray
  - May be negative
  - Can show disc-space narrowing, subchondral sclerosis, osteophyte formation
  - Oblique view
    - Foraminal stenosis at level of suspected radiculopathy
  - Open-mouth view
    - To rule out atlantoaxial joint injury
- Atlantodens interval (ADI)—from posterior aspect of anterior C1 arch to odontoid process
- Distance should be < 3 mm in adults, < 4 mm children
  - Increase in distance suggests instability
- CT
  - To evaluate bony elements, rule out fracture
  - Myelography—preferred over plain CT to rule out spinal cord compression and underlying atrophy

- MRI
  - To evaluate soft-tissues
    - Ligament and disc disruption
  - To evaluate amount of cerebrospinal fluid surround cord in stenotic region [11]

Treatment:
- Mild cases can be treated with topical medications, Tylenol and NSAIDS
- If refractory can consider opiates, muscle relaxers
- Medrol dose pack or epidural injections may provide relief

Obtain surgical referral if:
- Severe or progressive weakness or numbness
- Myelopathy—UMN signs
- Intractable pain

Rehabilitation Program:
- Goal: Alleviate Pain, increase function, increase pain-free ROM
- Modalities: Ice, heat, massage, TENS, electrical stimulation
- Progressive stretching in full ROM of neck
- Strengthening of cervical paraspinals, shoulder girdle, back muscles [10]
- Ergonomics
  - Top of screen should be at eye level
  - Bifocals should not be worn while using computer (causes excessive hyperextension of neck)
  - One pillow use at night
  - No reading/watching tv in bed
  - Do not hold phone in nape of neck
  - Turn the entire body, rather than the head alone to prevent laterally rotated positions for prolonged periods of time

CERVICAL SPINAL STENOSIS (723.0)

- Pathologic narrowing of the spinal canal
- Congenital or acquired
  - Congenital due to short pedicles
  - Acquired due to degenerative, hypertrophic changes affecting discs, facet joints, uncovertebral joints, ligamentum flavum
- Compression of spina cord common at C5-7, otherwise known as "cervical myelopathy"

- Adult canal
  - ○ AP diameter of cervical spine 12–14 mm
    - ▪ Stenosis when <10 mm

Symptoms:
- Axial neck pain
  - ○ Due to intervertebral disc degeneration, zygopophaseal joint arthritis
- Radicular arm pain, paresthesias, numbness, weakness of upper extremity
  - ○ Due to foraminal stenosis
- Myelopathic symptoms of upper extremities, neurogenic bladder and bowel, sexual dysfunction, unsteady gait, weakness, paresthesias, numbness
  - ○ Due to central foraminal stenosis

Physical Exam: Depends on location of lesions. Typically LMN in upper extremity; UMN in lower extremity.

- Inspection: Cervical lordosis; look for UMN or LMN findings, including muscle atrophy in supraspinatus, infraspinatus, deltoid, triceps, and first dorsal interosseus muscles.
- Palpation: Tenderness lateral to neck in supraclavicular fossa
- ROM: Limited secondary to stiffness, pain
- Reflex: hyporeflexia in upper extremities; hyperreflexia in lower extremities
- Strength: weakness in upper extremities
- Sensation: diminished in upper extremities
- Neuro: decreased tone in upper extremities; increased tone in lower extremities
- Provocative Maneuvers [3]:
  - ○ *Spurling sign*—radicular pain when head extended and rotated toward involved extremity with axial loading
  - ○ *Lhermitte sign*—electric-like sensation down back when neck flexed

Imaging:
- X-ray C-spine
  - ○ Facet and uncovertebral joint arthropathy
  - ○ Intervertebral disc space narrowing
  - ○ Neuroforaminal narrowing
  - ○ Spondylolisthesis (with flexion and extension views to evaluate for instability)

- CT
  - Can assess degree of bone disease
  - Dynamic views of of neuroal compression with flexion/extension
- MRI
  - Osseous/soft tissue disease
  - Can assess degree of spinal cord/nerve root compression [6]

Treatment:
- Conservative for pain, but no myelopathic symptoms
- Surgical referral—if cervical myelopathy suspected
- Soft neck collar for a few days/alternating periods of collar removal for severe radicular pain
- Ice, heat, TENS
- NSAIDs, Tylenol at regular intervals, short-course of opioids, muscle relaxants
- High-dose steroids (for functionally limiting pain) with 7–10 day taper
- Neuropathic pain agents for persistent radicular pain
  - Gabapentin, pregabalin, TCAs, clonazepam—for persistent radicular pain
- Epidural steroid injections
- Patient education
  - Worsening gait, bowel/bladder incontinence
  - Fall precautions and prevention in elderly
  - Avoid aggravating activity in severe cervical stenosis.
    - Horseback riding, motorcycle riding, climbing ladders, contact sports [4]

Rehabilitation Program:
- Modalities: ice, heat, massage, TENS, electrical stimulation
- Patient education
  - Keeping active
  - Avoiding activities that can cause injury
    - Extremes of cervical flexion/extension
- Stretching, isometric exercises in painful phase
- Strengthening, isotonic exercises once pain-free ROM achieved
- HEP
- Work-site evaluation, restrictions (ergonomics)
- Cognitive behavioral therapy, biofeedback, relaxation therapy [10]

SCOLIOSIS (737.43)/KYPHOSIS (737.10)

Scoliosis: deformity of the spine causing lateral and vertebral rotation
- Causes:
  - (1) Congenital
  - (2) Degenerative
  - (3) Neuromuscular (poor muscle control due to cerebral palsy, muscular dystrophy, spina bifida, polio)
  - (4) Idiopathic

Symptoms—correlate with degree of curvature (>20°)
- Pain/paresthesias/hyperesthesia
  - ○ Adults
  - ○ Children usually pain free
- Shortness of breath (restrictive lung disease)
- Limited activity tolerance

Physical Exam:
- Inspection: thoracic/lumbar curvature of spine; asymmetry of back noted with forward flexion; breast, waist fold contour, iliac crest and/or shoulder height asymmetry
  - ○ Deformities—Humping of the back, Asymmetric shoulders/hips/breast size
- Palpation: Non-tender to palpation
- ROM: Can range from limited to full PROM
- Reflex: Normal, unless curvature > 40°
- Strength: Normal
- Sensation: Normal, unless curvature > 40°
- Special:
  - ○ Drop plumb line from occiput/C7 spinous process
    - ▪ Inspect for lateral deviations from the line
  - ○ Measure leg-length [4]

Kyphosis: sagittal deviation in spinal aligment
- Normal kyphosis: 20–40°
- Pathologic kyphosis due to:
  - ○ Osteoporotic compression fractures
  - ○ Tumors
  - ○ Juvenile kyphosis
  - ○ Post-radiation therapy

Symptoms—correlate with degree of and location of kyphosis
- Pain and stiffness
  - Intermittent
  - Located at apex of curve
  - Lower back pain (due to compensatory lumbar lordosis)
- Cardiopulmonary compromise (rare)

Physical Exam:
- Inspection: Forward displacement of head/neck which cause compensatory lumbar lordosis; rounding of back (not corrected in prone position)
- Palpation: Reproduction of pain of palpation of spinous processes
- ROM: loss of ROM in all cervical and lumbar planes; restricted trunk extension (d/t deformity and/or pain); tightness in pectoralis/hamstring muscles
- Reflex: Normal. Hyperreflexia should be noted and consider cord involvement.
- Strength: Normal
- Sensation: Normal

Imaging:
- X-ray (Scoliosis series).
  - Erect AP/lateral views of entire spine (occiput to sacrum)
  - Lateral view (evaluate for spondylolysis/spondylolisthesis)

Treatment:
- Goal: To identify progressive curvature of spine
  - Serial assessment—if scoliotic curve <20°, kyphotic curve <40°
  - Bracing/surgery—if scoliotic curve >20°, kyphotic curve >40°
    - Night-time orthoses
- Pain: NSAIDs, TENS [2]

Rehabilitation Program:
- Exercise—improves posture
- AAROM of the spine in all planes within the available range
  - Cervico-thoracic extension exercise (kyphosis)
  - Pelvic tilt (to treat compensatory lordosis)
- Stretching/strengthening pectoralis, hamstrings, and hip flexors
- Bracing: body jacket thoracolumbosacral orthosis (night-time use)
- HEP

RED FLAGS IN SPINAL PAIN

The following signs indicate more serious causes of back pain which are potentially life threatening and require further workup.

Suspect **cauda equina** with the following:
- Urinary incontinence
- Saddle anesthesia
- Decrease anal sphincter tone/fecal incontinence
- Bilateral lower extremity weakness/numbness
- Progressive neurologic deficit

Suspect **cancer** with the following:
- History of cancer
- Unexplained weight loss
- Pain at night or at rest

Suspect **infection** with the following:
- Persistent fever
- Severe pain
- History of intravenous drug abuse
- Lumbar spine surgery within past year
- Recent bacterial infection
  - UTI
  - Pyelonephritis
  - Cellulitis
  - Pneumonia
  - Wound
- Immunocompromised

Workup
- CBC with differential
- Comprehensive metabolic panel
- Blood cultures
- ESR
- CRP
- XR
- CT scan
- MRI

References

1. Brotzman B, Wilk K. Clinical orthopedic rehabilitation. Philadelphia: Mosby; 2003.
2. Frontera W. Essentials of physical medicine and rehabilitation. Philadelphia: Saunders Elsevier; 2008.
3. Malanga G. Musculoskeletal physical exam: an evidence-based approach. Philadelphia: Mosby. Elsevier; 2006.
4. Cuccurullo S. Physical medicine and rehabilitation board review. New York: Demos Medical Publishing; 2010.
5. Jacobson J. Fundamentals of musculoskeletal ultrasound. Philadelphia, Pennsylvania: Saunders; 2007.
6. Litao A. Emedicine. [Online] December 14, 2011. http://emedicine.medscape.com/article/95691-clinical#showall. Accessed 11 June 2012.
7. Krabak B. Passor musculoskeletal physical examination competencies list. PASSOR Task Force on Musculoskeletal Education; 2001.
8. Hoppenfeld S. Physical exam of the spine extremities. Saddle River, NJ: Prentice Hall; 1976.
9. Hoppenfeld S. Orthopedic neurology. Sydney Australia: J.B. Lippincott Company; 1977.
10. Greene B. Essentials of musculoskeletal care. Columbia, Missouri: American Academy of Orthopaedic Surgeons; 2001.
11. Wheeless C. Wheeless online. [Online] April 12, 2012. http://www.wheelesonline.com/ortho/lumbar_stenosis. Accessed 11 June 2012.
12. Malanga G. Emedicine. [Online] December 14, 2011. http://emedicine.medscape.com/article/94118-workup#showall. Accessed 12 June 2012.

Chapter 12
Interventional Pain Management

Houman Danesh and Jennifer Sayanlar

Clinical Pearls [1]

- If a patient has diabetes or significant comorbidities, use lower dose of steroids (ex. 40–60mg of Kenalog).
- If patient experiences severe pain on injection of medication **confirm needle placement** first. If incorrect placement, re-place needle under imaged guidance. If correct needle placement, give pauses between injecting the medication. The increased pressure from the volume of medication on the inflamed nerve root can increase their pain and most commonly dissipates in seconds. On the other hand if pain is severe you may consider aborting the procedure.
- If you meet resistance during injecting, do not inject or force the medication into the region.
- Always aspirate for possible intravascular placement of needle. Aspirating for intravascular placement may not always result in back flow of blood. Negative aspiration of blood does not mean you are not intravascular.

H. Danesh, M.D. (✉)
Department of Anesthesiology, The Mount Sinai Hospital,
1 Gustave Levy Lane, Box 1192, New York, NY 10029, USA
houman.danesh@mountsinai.org

J. Sayanlar, D.O.
Pain Management and Palliative Care, Pain and Wellness Center,
Englewood Hospital, Englewood, NJ, USA

K.A. Sackheim (ed.), *Rehab Clinical Pocket Guide:*
Rehabilitation Medicine, DOI 10.1007/978-1-4614-5419-9_12,
© Springer Science+Business Media, LLC 2013

- Even if an office staff already asked the patient about antico-agulants, ASK AGAIN to verify. This can be very helpful to prevent bleeding complications.
- Although there is no evidence to support a maximal steroid dose allotted per year, most clinicians adhere to 3–4 injections per 6–12 months. Caution is always given when administering steroids and patients overall health and comorbidities should be considered prior to each injection.

Contraindications to Injection Therapy [2]

- ○ Current Infection (UTI, URI, Dermatologic, etc)
- ○ Bleeding diathesis, history of coagulopathy
- ○ Possible pregnancy
- ○ Current use of anticoagulants

Medications to Consider Stopping Prior to a Procedure

- If a patient is on an anticoagulant for example Coumadin or Plavix for treatment/prevention of a medical condition such as stroke, myocardial infarction, DVT etc., then permission from the prescribing physician should be obtained prior to stopping the medication before the procedure.
- There are cases where the risk of anticoagulation outweighs the benefit of this procedure and physicians are unable to proceed.
- Anticoagulants can be stopped for an average of 7–10 days prior to procedures. Each medications has specific recommen-dations that should be followed accordingly. Below are some examples but recommendations of prescribing physician should be followed. If not safe to proceed with injection, the injection should be avoided.
  - **NSAIDS:** some studies have shown no increase in risk for spinal hematoma unless there is concurrent use of another anticoagulation or multiple NSAIDs

       ◦ Can consider holding for 3–5 days prior
- **Aspirin:** some studies have shown no increase in risk for spinal hematoma with low dose baby aspirin. More caution is always used with higher doses and cervical procedures. If conservative can consider stopping aspirin products 5–7 days prior to procedure. This should only be done with permission from the prescribing physician.
  - For lumbar procedure low dose aspirin alone may be ok depending on physician preference
- **Lovenox and Xarelto:** stop for 24 hours *only if you have permission from the prescribing physician*
- **Plavix:** stop for 7–10 days *only if you have permission from the prescribing physician*
- **Coumadin:** stop for 5 days *only if you have permission from the prescribing physician, you will need to have the patient's INR checked the day of or the day prior to the procedure*
  - INR should be < 1.5 or lower prior to proceeding
  - Can also stop for 10 days with no repeat INR
- **Pradaxa:** stop for 2 days if normal kidney function, for 3 to 5 days if kidney impairment *only if you have permission from the prescribing physician*
- **Herbal medications and vitamins that also may be associated with bleeding:** Garlic, grapeseed extract, vitamin E, vitamin C, Ginkgo biloba, Panax ginseng, omega 3 vitamin tablets, fish oil

Steroid Medications

Naturally occurring corticosteroids are classified into three functional groups: *mineralocorticoids, glucocorticoids, and adrenal androgens.* Glucocorticoids, originally named for their role in glucose metabolism, are the corticosteroid most commonly used for interventional pain procedures.

Several therapeutic mechanisms of action for corticosteroids have been proposed:
1. Anti-inflammatory effects
2. Neural membrane stabilization
3. Neuromodulation

As a general rule, the anti-inflammatory efficacy and duration of activity are greater with less soluble corticosteroid preparations. For many years the type of corticosteroid selected is usually based on the duration of action and anti-inflammatory potency. However, recently, the steroid particulate size relative to a red blood cell and aggregation is emerging as a major determinant of corticosteroid selection.

Serious adverse events have been increasingly reported in patients undergoing transforaminal epidural injections with particulate corticosteroid solutions. For example, inadvertent injection of a steroid particulate into the artery of Adamkiewicz during thoracic or lumbar transforaminal epidural steroid injection (left side more commonly than right side) has theoretically resulted in spinal cord ischemia. Therefore, non-particulate steroids such as betamethasone should be used for cervical and transforaminals injections as they are less likely to cause ischemia and complications.

Steroid medication	Equivalent dose	Epidural dose (mg)
Kenalog (Triamcinolone)	4	40–80
Celestone (Betamethasone)	0.6	6–12
Decadron (Dexamethasone)	0.75	8–16

Steroid Equivalent Dosing (i—Data adapted and modified from Interventional Techniques in Chronic Spinal Pain, Manchikanti and Singh)

Billing for Interventional Pain Procedures

Medication Codes

These codes are subject to change and should be verified prior to using.

Medication code	1 Unit equivalent
J1030	Depomedrol 40 mg
J1040	Depomedrol 80 mg
J1100	Dexamethasone 1 mg
J3301	Kenalog 10 mg
J0702	Celestone 3 mg
J3490	Lidocaine/Marcaine (1 unit only)
J1885	Toradol 15 mg
Q9965	Omnipaque (1 unit only)

Table 12.1 Properties of steroids used in spinal injections

Agent	Biological half-life (h)	Anti-inflammatory potency	Salt-retaining potency	Particulate size (aggregation)
Hydrocortisone (Hydrocortone)	8–12	1	1	
Triamcinolone (Kenalog 40)	12–36	5	0	RBC size to 133 (extensive, densely packed)
Methylprednisolone (Depo-Medrol)	12–36	5	0.5	RBC size (few, densely packed)
Dexamethasone (Decadron)	36–72	25	0	RBC size (none)
Betamethasone (Celestone, Soluspan)	36–72	25	0	Varied size (extensive, densely packed)

Properties of Steroids Used in Spinal Injections (Table 12.1)

(ii—Information adapted and modified from Essentials of Pain Management, Benzon)

Pre-procedure medications if needed:

Medications should be taken 30 min prior to procedure; repeated dose can be given if not fully effective after 30 min
Vitals should be monitored when premedications given and patient should always have a companion to safely escort them home

- Xanax 0.5 mg–2 mg p.o. or sublingual × 1–2 doses depending on patient tolerability
- Valium 5–10 mg p.o. if needed

Some physicians choose to perform their procedures with sedation. In this case, no oral medications would be needed.

LUMBO-SACRAL INJECTIONS

Lumbar Interlaminar Epidural Steroid Injection (IL LESI) [3]

- **Indications**
  - ○ Lumbar radicular pain secondary to:
    - Herniated disc
    - Ligamentum hypertrophy
    - Stenosis—central or neuroforaminal
    - Spondylolisthesis
  - ○ Internal Disc Disruption (IDD)
- **Target on fluoroscopy**
  - ○ Identify the space between the lamina of the vertebrae at the desired level
  - ○ If the desired level has a very narrow entrance point, consider proceeding with injection at the level above or below to facilitate needle entry.
  - ○ For post-surgical patients, they should have an interlaminar injection above or below the operative sites. Needle placement through the operative site may increase the chances of a wet tap as the anatomy has changed and scar tissue is present. Transforaminal or caudal approach can also be used instead to avoid this issue.
- **Needle insertion**
  - ○ **Fluoroscopy view:** align the vertebral bodies so that the end plates are lined up—this is done by head or foot tilt. This

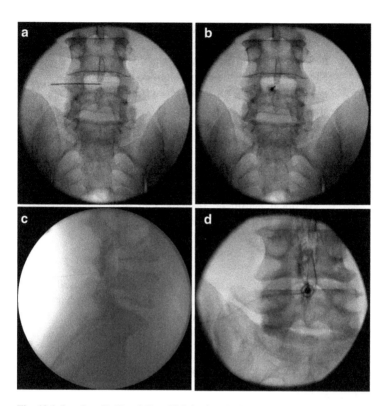

Fig. 12.1 Lumbar Epidural Steroid Injection (**a**) Fluoroscopy picture indicating the start position and location to anesthetize when starting procedure (**b**) AP fluoroscopy view of the tuohy needle in place (**c**) Lateral fluoroscopy view showing the contrast spread. (**d**) AP fluoroscopy view indicating LESI contrast spread

will show as a single solid line on the end plates rather than two separate lines. You can also try to align the view so it opens the interlaminar space to facilitate needle entry.

○ **Entry Point:** slightly lateral to the spinous process or in center if the space is large (Fig. 12.1a). If the patient's pain is only in one leg you can enter slightly towards the side of the pain.

○ Anesthetize the skin with 1% Lidocaine parallel to the beam of the X-ray.

○ Start approaching towards the epidural space with the tuohy needle (Fig. 12.1b) with the obturator in place—this is done on AP view to ensure midline placement of needle.

- ○ Once you feel the resistance of the ligamentum flavum, switch to loss of resistance with air or saline technique under lateral X-ray to ensure proper depth.
- ○ **Final position:** Needle tip should be just beyond the posterior border of the posterior bony column in the epidural space.
- ○ Confirm needle placement with 0.5 ml of contrast on AP and/or lateral views under live fluoroscopy (Fig. 12.1c and d).
- ○ **Medication injected:**
  - ▪ Total Volume: 5–6 ml
  - ▪ Mixture of: 40–120 mg Kenalog (usually 80 mg), 1–2 ml of local anesthetic (usually 1 ml of 0.25% of bupivacaine), and 2–3 ml of preservative free normal saline
- • **Billing Codes**
  - ○ 62311 (includes contrast)
  - ○ 77003 (fluoroscopy)
  - ○ Include appropriate medication codes and units used
  - ○ 724.4 Lumbar radiculopathy or 724.02 for lumbar spinal stenosis are some commonly used diagnosis codes

Lumbar Transforaminal Epidural Steroid Injection (TFESI) [4]

- • **Indications**
  - ○ Lumbar radicular pain secondary to:
    - ▪ Herniated disc
    - ▪ Ligamentum hypertrophy
    - ▪ Stenosis-central or neuroforaminal
    - ▪ Spondylolisthesis
  - ○ Transforaminal or caudal approach is preferred when dealing with postsurgical patients who suffer from continued radicular pain as it can avoid accidental wet tap because of surgically altered anatomy
- • **Target on fluoroscopy**
  - ▪ *On AP View*: below the pedicle (approaching the neck of the scotty dog)
  - ▪ *On Lateral View*: Dorsal to the dorsal root ganglion in upper third of intervertebral foramen

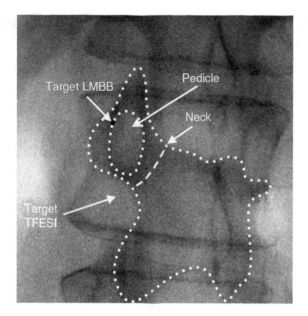

Fig. 12.2 Fluoroscopy picture outlining the Scotty dog on oblique view outlined in white. This view is used when determining target positions for Lumbar Medial Branch Block and Transforaminal Epidural Steroid Injection

- **Needle insertion**
  - **Fluoroscopy view:** use foot or head tilt to align the end plates of the appropriate level, oblique 10–20° towards the affected side, goal is to see the scotty dog
  - **Entry Point:** slightly lateral and below the pedicle
  - Anesthetize the skin slightly at the entry point with 1% Fig. 12.3a Lidocaine parallel to the beam of the X-ray
  - Curved spinal needle inserted
  - Advance the needle, this can mostly be done on an AP view to ensure proper needle placement (Fig. 12.3b). If at any time you are unsure of depth check a lateral view.
    - Make sure your depth is appropriate without going too far medial on your approach
    - Goal is to keep the tip of the needle just below the pedicle
    - *If you find yourself getting too medial but not deep enough, you can turn the curve of the needle laterally and advance, this can help redirect the needle to stay at optimal location below the pedicle*

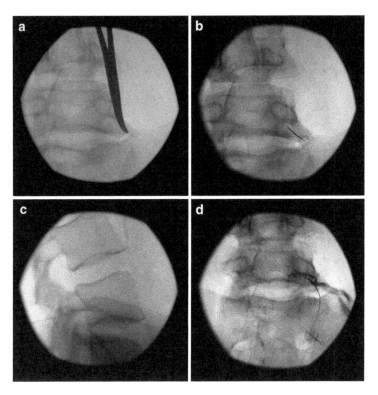

Fig. 12.3 Lumbar Transforaminal Steroid Injection (**a**) AP Fluoroscopy picture indicating the start position and location to anesthetize. (**b**) AP fluoroscopy view of the quincke spinal needle in place. (**c**) Lateral fluoroscopy view of the quincke spinal needle in place. (**d**) AP fluoroscopy picture indicating proper contrast spread

- ○ Advance the needle till you feel slight resistance of the ligament surrounding the neural foramen
- ○ **Target:** Confirm on lateral view (Fig. 12.3c)
  - ▪ Needle tip needle placement should be about to penetrate the neural foramen
- ○ Advance the needle till it is inside the upper 1/3 of the neural foraminal space
- ○ Confirm proper needle placement with 0.5 ml of contrast injected on AP or lateral view under live fluoroscopy Fig. 12.3d
- ○ **Medication injected:**
  - ▪ Total Volume: 5–6 ml

- Each level: 1-3 ml, 20-40mg of Kenalog or equivalent dose of non-particulate steroid
- Mixture of: 20-120mg Kenalog (usually 20-40mg per level), 1-2 ml of local anesthetic (usually 1ml of 0.25% of bupivacaine), and 2-3ml of preservative free normal saline
- Consider non-particulate steroid such as betamethasone to avoid complications
- **Billing Codes**
  - 64483 (first level) this code includes fluoroscopy and contrast
  - 64484 (additional ipsilateral level) this code includes fluoroscopy and contrast
  - Include appropriate medication codes and units used
  - If doing bilateral procedure shoulder bill 64483 with a modifier 50 (signifying 1 level done bilaterally)
  - 724.4 Lumbar radiculopathy is a commonly used diagnosis code

Lumbar Medial Branch Blocks (LMBB) [6]

The facet joints are innervated by the medial branches of the lumbar dorsal rami.
- **Indications**
  - Low back pain
  - Lumbar Facet Arthropathy
  - Lumbar Spondylosis
  - Diagnostic injection to diagnose facet arthropathy
  - Therapeutic injection for symptomatic treatment of facet arthropathy
- **Target on fluoroscopy**
  - In the oblique view, target is slightly above or at the "eye" of the scotty dog or the junction of the superior articulating process (SAP) and the transverse process (TP) which the target nerve crosses, midway between the superior border of the transverse process and the mamilloaccessory notch.
    - *If the joint is on the right,* you are targeting the **1 o'clock** position on the eye of the scotty dog

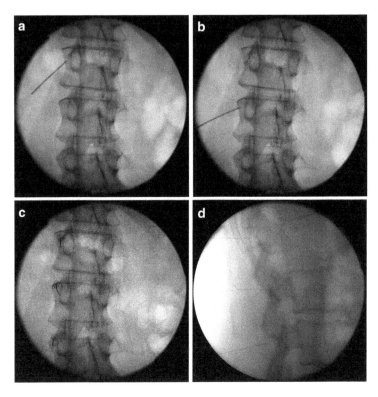

Fig. 12.4 Lumbar Medial Branch Block (**a**) Fluoroscopy picture indicating the start position and location to anesthetize. (**b**) Fluoroscopy picture showing the first needle inserted and the starting location for the second. (**c**) AP fluoroscopy picture with quincke spinal needles in proper location at 3 lower lumbar levels. (**d**) Lateral fluoroscopy picture with 3 quincke spinal needles in place at the lumbar medial branch locations

- ▪ *If the joint is on the left*, you are targeting the **11 o' clock** position on the eye of the scotty dog
- **Needle insertion**
  - ○ **Fluoroscopy view:** AP to the appropriate level, oblique 10–20° towards the affected side
  - ○ **Entry Point:** slightly lateral and above the pedicle (Fig. 12.4a and b)
  - ○ Anesthetize the skin at the entry point with 1% Lidocaine parallel to the beam of the X-ray
  - ○ Insert the curved spinal needle
  - ○ Advance the need towards the target point

- *If you are too medial you may need to pull back on the needle and advance with the curved tip pointing laterally to gain depth*
  - After the needle hits bone, the needle is not advanced further
  - **Final position:** (Fig. 12.4c) On AP view, the end point should be at the junction of the SAP and the TP or the eye of the scotty dog. Fig. 12.4d shows positioning on lateral view
  - **Medication injected:**
    - Total Volume: depends on amount of levels injected
      - 3–6ml if 3 levels unilaterally
      - 6–12ml if 3 levels bilaterally
    - Each level: 1–2 ml total per level
    - Mixture of: 20–120 mg Kenalog (usually 20–40 mg per level), 1–2 ml of local anesthetic (usually 1 ml of 0.25% of bupivacaine), and 2–3 ml of preservative free normal saline
- **Billing Codes**
  - 64493 (first level) this code includes fluoroscopy
  - 64494 (second level) this code includes fluoroscopy
  - 64495 (third level) this code includes fluoroscopy
  - Include appropriate medication codes and units used
  - 721.3 Lumbar Spondylosis w/o Myelopathy is a commonly used diagnosis code
  - If procedure is done bilaterally a modifier 50 should be used on each level done bilaterally

Lumbar Radiofrequency Ablation (RF) [7]

- **Indications**
  - Lumbar facet arthropathy/Spondylosis
    - Only if 1 or more successful medial branch blocks have been done previously
- **Types of Radiofrequency**
  - *Pulsed:*
    - Controversial—May not be covered by patient's insurance
    - Creates a pin point pulsed burn causing stunning of the nerve
    - This is done between 40 to 70°C for 240 pulses

- ○ *Thermal*
  - ▪ *Creates a football like sphere burn*
  - ▪ This is done at 80 °C for 90 s in the lumbar region
  - ▪ Causes wallerian degeneration of medial branch that starts about 3 weeks after the procedure
- **Target on fluoroscopy**
  - ○ On oblique view, target is above and the "eye" of the "scotty" dog at the junction of the SAP and the TP which the target nerve crosses, midway between the superior border of the transverse process and the mamillo-accessory notch
    - ▪ *If the joint is on the right*, you are targeting the **1 o' clock** position on the eye of the scotty dog
    - ▪ *If the joint is on the left*, you are targeting the **11 o' clock** position on the eye of the scotty dog
  - ○ *Pulse:* needle can be perpendicular to the nerve, this is accomplished with the superior aproach
  - ○ *Thermal:* needle should be parallel to the nerve to achieve the largest lesion, this is accomplished with the inferior approach
- **Needle insertion**
  - ○ Confirm placement of grounding patch on patient, this should be on the extremity opposite the side of the injection
  - ○ **Fluoroscopy view:** AP of the appropriate level, oblique 10–20° towards the affected side
    Entry point:
    - ▪ Sup*erior approach*- slightly lateral and above the pedicle to be perpendicular for pulse
    - ▪ *Inferior approach*- if aiming to be parallel for thermal start slightly inferior and lateral to target point
  - ○ Anesthetize the skin at entry point with 1% Lidocaine parallel to the beam of the X-ray (Fig. 12.5a)
  - ○ Curved RF needle with exposed lesioning tip is inserted
  - ○ Advance the needle towards the target point
    - ▪ After the needle hits bone, the needle is not advanced further Fig. 12.5b and c
  - ○ **Testing:**
    - ▪ *Sensor*y: starting at 0 up to 1Hz to confirm proper needle placement. The patient should feel pressure or sensation below 1 Hz. Ideal placement will have stimulation below 0.5 Hz

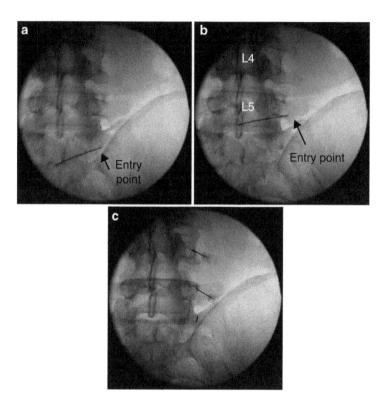

Fig. 12.5 Lumbar Radio Frequency (Inferior approach)—(**a**) Fluoroscopy picture indicating the start position and location to anesthetize for needle placement at sacral ala. (**b**) Fluoroscopy picture indicating Lumbar RF needle started at ala, start position for L5. (**c**) Fluoroscopy picture indicating Lumbar RF needles in place at L4, L5, and Ala

- *Motor:* starting at 0 up to 2. You should see the contracting of the multifidus muscles. You do not want to see or have the patient feel any stimulation or movement at the extremity. Lower extremity muscle movement, severe pain, or sensations in the leg requires needle repositioning
○ Do not inject local anesthetic until needle placement has been confirmed by testing as this can disrupt testing and lead to complications. Once placement is confirmed by sensory and motor testing, 0.5 cc of 1% or 2% lidocaine is injected at each site to anesthetize prior to lesioning
- Lesioning can begin 30 s to 1 min after injecting the anesthetic

- ○ If severe pain down the leg during lesioning, stop lesioning immediately and re-check needle position
- ○ After lesioning has completed, a mixture of steroids and local anesthetic are used to prevent post-lesioning inflammation
- **Billing Codes**
  - ○ 64635 (first level) this code includes fluoroscopy
  - ○ 64636 (each additional level) this code includes fluoroscopy
  - ○ Include appropriate medication codes and units used
  - ○ 721.3 Lumbar Spondylosis w/o Myelopathy is a commonly used diagnosis code

Sacral Transforaminal Epidural Steroid Injection (S1 TFESI) [8]

- **Indications**
  - ○ Sacral radicular pain secondary to:
    - ▪ Herniated disc
    - ▪ Ligamentum hypertrophy
    - ▪ Stenosis—central or neuroforaminal
    - ▪ Spondylolisthesis

Transfoaminal approach is recommended for postsurgical sacral spine with continued radicular as this can avoid accidental wet tap because of surgically altered anatomy

- **Target on fluoroscopy**
  - ○ Target points
    - ▪ *On AP V*iew: into the desired sacral foramen
    - ▪ *On Lateral View*: at the level of the intended sacral foramen, at appropriate disc space
- **Needle insertion**
  - ○ **Fluoroscopy view:** AP of the appropriate level, this may require some head or foot tilt to properly visualize the appropriate sacral foramen. S1 appears as a circle while S2-4 are more oval in shape.
  - ○ **Entry Point:** slightly lateral and below the neural foramen opening
    - ▪ *If the joint is on the right*, start at **5 o'clock** and move towards **11 o'clock** to enter the foramen

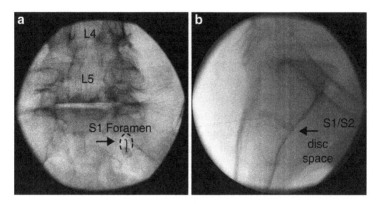

Fig. 12.6 S1 Transfoaminal Steroid Injection—(**a**) AP fluoroscopy view of quincke spinal needle in the S1 foramen. (**b**) lateral view of needle in S1 foramen

- *If* the joint is on the left, start at **8 o'clock** and move towards **1 o'clock** to enter the foramen
  - Anesthetize the skin slightly at the entry point with 1% Lidocaine parallel to the beam of the X-ray
  - Insert curved spinal needle
  - Figure 12.6a advance the needle till you feel the bone surrounding the foramen, you can then gently move the needle against the bone until it drop it into the neural foramen. If you choose to go directly into the foramen, be careful not to move too deeply. Obtain a lateral view to ensure proper depth (Fig. 12.6b). In the latter case, the needle may not come in contact with the surround foraminal bone, so be careful about depth as not to cause complications.
    - Goal is to keep the tip of the needle within the foramen opening
  - Once you feel bone or as if the needle slipping into the foramen obtain a lateral view
  - Confirm proper needle placement with 0.2–0.5 ml of contrast medium injected under live fluoroscopy on AP and/or lateral view
  - **Medication injected:**
    - Total volume: 2–3ml per level
    - Mixture of: 20–80mg Kenalog (usually 20–40 mg per level), 1–2 ml of local anesthetic (usually 1ml of 0.25% of bupivacaine), and 2–3 ml of preservative free normal saline

- ▪ Consider using non-particulate steroid to avoid complications
- **Billing Codes**
  - ○ 64483 (first level) this code includes fluoroscopy and contrast
  - ○ 64484 (additional ipsilateral level) this code includes fluoroscopy and contrast
  - ○ If bilateral procedure use code 64483 with modifier 50
  - ○ Include appropriate medication codes and units used
  - ○ 724.4 Lumbosacral Radiculopathy is a commonly used diagnosis code

Sacroiliac Joint Injection (SIJ) [9]

- **Indications**
  - ○ Sacroiliitis as a diagnostic or therapeutic injection
  - ○ Low back pain radiating to the lower extremity, usually stopping at the knee
- **Target on fluoroscopy**
  - ○ Bottom 1/3 of the SI joint
- **Needle insertion**
  - ○ **Fluoroscopy view:** Start with AP view of the affected joint, then oblique away from the affected side till you fully line up the anterior and posterior joint lines. This allows you to see the maximum opening space in the SI joint.
  - ○ **Entry Point:** Start just laterally to the bottom 1/3 of the joint line.
  - ○ Anesthetize the skin at entry point with 1% Lidocaine parallel to the beam of the X-ray.
  - ○ Advance the curved spinal needle until you hit bone. The tip should be just lateral to the joint line. You may want to inject a small amount of anesthetic at this point to avoid discomfort. The bony areas maybe more sensitive when approached with the needle. You can advance the needle medially on the bone until you feel the needle drop into the joint space.
  - ○ Confirm proper needle placement with 0.2–0.5 ml of contrast medium injected under live fluoroscopy on AP or lateral view. Fig. 12.7.
  - ○ **Medications injected:**
    - ▪ Total volume 2ml

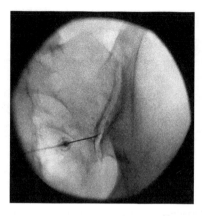

Fig. 12.7 Sacroiliac injection—Fluoroscopy picture indicating Sacroiliac injection—oblique view with needle in inferior portion of joint

- ▪ Mixture of: 20–40mg Kenalog or equivalent steroid plus 1–2 ml of local anesthetic (0.25% bupivacaine)
- **Billing Codes**
  - ○ 27096 (Sacroiliac Joint Injection)
  - ○ 77003 (fluoroscopy)
  - ○ Include appropriate medication codes and units used. You are able to bill separately for contrast with this procedure
  - ○ 720.2 Sacroiliitis is a commonly used diagnosis code
  - ○ Modifier 50 can be used if procedure is done bilaterally

CERVICAL INJECTIONS

Cervical Interlaminar Epidural Steroid Injection (CESI) [10]

- **Indications**
  - ○ Cervical radicular pain
  - ○ Cervical stenosis
  - ○ Acute herniated disc
  - ○ Cervical spondylolisthesis
  - ○ Post surgical cervical spine with continued radiculopathy- in this case would go below surgical region

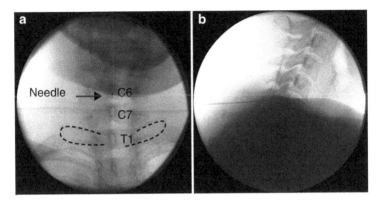

Fig. 12.8 Cervical Epidural Steroid Injection—(**a**) AP fluoroscopy view showing needle placement. (**b**) Fluoroscopy picture indicating CESI Lateral with contrast

- **Target on fluoroscopy**
  - Identify the space between the lamina of the vertebrae of the desired level
  - C7/T1 is the safest level and is most commonly used
- **Needle insertion**
  - **Fluoroscopy view:** Start with AP view of appropraite level. Can use head of foot tilt to open the interlaminal space and align the endplates. This will show as a single solid line on the end plates rather than two separate lines.
  - **Entry Point:** slightly lateral to the spinous process, goal is to stay midline.
  - Anesthetize the skin parallel to the beam of the X-ray
  - Advance the tuohy needle carefully till you feel the slight resistance of the ligamentum flavum (Fig. 12.8a)
    - If while advancing you are unsure of your depth you can always check a lateral view to ensure you are not progressing too deeply. Some physicians proceed with entire injection on lateral view to ensure proper depth and increased safety.
  - Once you feel the resistance of the ligamentum flavum, switch to loss of air or saline technique under lateral X-ray.
  - Needle tip should be just beyond the posterior border of the base of the spinous process.
    - Not every patient has a full ligamentum at the cervical region, so always advance cautiously as you may not

always feel resistance. Always proceed with extra caution in the cervical spine.
- ○ Confirm needle placement with 0.5 ml of contrast under live fluoroscopy on AP and lateral view. Fig. 12.8b.
- ○ **Medication Injected:**
  - ▪ Total Volume: 4ml
  - ▪ Mixture of: 1-2ml of non-particulate steroid and 2ml of preservative free normal saline
  - ▪ Some practitioners avoid using local anesthetic in the cervical region to avoid complications
- • **Billing Codes**
  - ○ 62310 (includes contrast)
  - ○ 77003 (fluoroscopy)
  - ○ Include appropriate medication codes and units used
  - ○ 723.4 Cervical Radiculopathy is a commonly used diagnosis code

Cervical Medial Branch Blocks (CMBB) [11]

- • **Indications**
  - ○ Cervical facet arthropathy
  - ○ Cervical spondylosis
  - ○ Dignostic or therapeutic injection
- • **Target on fluoroscopy**
  - ○ On AP view → the waist of the vertebral body Fig. 12.9a
  - ○ On Lateral view → the center of the trapezoid at desired level. Fig. 12.9b
  - ○ C3–C6, center of the articular pillar with the same segmental number as the target nerve
  - ○ C7, high on the apex of the superior articular process of C7
- • **Needle insertion**
  - ○ Start with an AP view. Can use head or foot tilt to align the end plates of the desired level.
  - ○ **Fluoroscopy view:** Using a curved tip spinal needle, the needle is advanced slowly into skin in line with the fluoroscopy, with target point at the waist of the vertebral body
  - ○ Needle is advanced towards the waist line while keeping the curve of the needle facing medially towards the midline of the patient

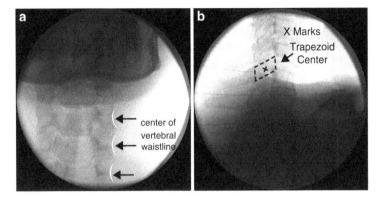

Fig. 12.9 Cervical Medial Branch Block—(**a**) AP fluoroscopy view with cervical vertebrae waist outlined in white and the target position indicated with an arrow. (**b**) Lateral fluoroscopy view showing needle placement at center of trapezoid

- After the needle touches bone, turn the needle curve facing laterally
- Change to a lateral view
- When you turn the curve of the needle laterally the needle will slip over the edge of the bone
- Then, advance the needle to the center of the trapezoid
- Confirm needle placement with 0.2–0.5 ml of contrast, with live fluoroscopy on AP and lateral view
- **Medications injected:**
- Total Volume: depends on amount of levels injected
    3ml if 3 levels unilaterally
    6ml if 3 levels bilaterally
- Each level: 1ml total per level
- Mixture of: 1–2ml of non-particulate steroid, 1–4ml of local anesthetic(usually 1ml of bupivacaine) to equal desired total of volume
- **Billing Codes**
    - 64490 (first level) this code includes fluoroscopy
    - 64491 (second level) this code includes fluoroscopy
    - 64492 (third level) this code includes fluoroscopy
    - Include appropriate medication codes and units used
    - 721.0 Cervical Spondylosis w/o Myelopathy is a commonly used diagnosis code

Cervical Radiofrequency Ablation (Cervical RF) [12]

- **Indications**
  - ○ Cervical facet arthropathy
  - ○ Cervical spondylosis
  - ○ Radiofrequency is only indicated if the patient had a successful response with 1 or more medial branch blocks.
- **Types**
  - ○ *Pulsed:*
    - ▪ Controversial—May not be covered by patient's insurance
    - ▪ Creates a pin point pulsed burn causing stunning of the nerve
    - ▪ This is done between 40 to 70 °C for 240 pulses
  - ○ *Thermal:*
    - ▪ Creates a Football like sphere burn
    - ▪ This is done at 80 °C for 60 s
    - ▪ Causes wallerian degeneration of medial branch that starts about 3 weeks after the procedure
- **Target on fluoroscopy**
  - ○ On AP view → The waist of the vertebral body
  - ○ On Lateral view → the center of the trapezoid at desired level
  - ○ C3–C6, center of the articular pillar with the same segmental number as the target nerve
  - ○ C7, high on the apex of the superior articular process of C7
- **Needle insertion**
  - ○ Start with an AP view of appropriate level, can use head or foot tilt to align end plates
  - ○ **Fluoroscopy view:** Using a curved tip needle, the needle is advanced slowly into skin in line with the fluoroscopy, with target point at the waist of the vertebral body
  - ○ Needle is advanced towards the waist line while keeping the curve of the needle facing medially towards the midline of the patient
  - ○ After the needle hits bone, turn the needle curve facing away from midline
  - ○ Change to a lateral view
  - ○ When you turn the curve the needle should just slip over the edge of bone
  - ○ Then, advance the needle to the center of the trapezoid

- o Placement is verified with AP and lateral view on fluoroscopy
- o Testing:
- o Sensory: starting at 0 up to 1 Hz. Proper needle placement the patient will feel pressure or sensation below 1 Hz
- o Motor: starting at 0 going up to 2. You should see the contracting of the multifidus muscles. You do not want to see or have the patient feel any stimulation or movement at the extremity. Muscle movement or severe pain requires need repositioning
- o Do not inject local anesthetic until needle placement has been confirmed by testing as this can disrupt testing and lead to complications.
- o Once placement is confirmed by sensory and motor testing, 0.5 cc of 1% or 2% lidocaine is injected at each site to anesthetize prior to
- o Lesioning can begin 30 s to 1 min after injecting the anesthetic
- o After lesioning has completed, Confirm needle placement with 0.2–0.5 ml of contrast, also make sure nonvascular placement
- o Then, a mixture of steroids and local anesthetic are used to prevent post-lesioning inflammation at the root
- o If needle properly placed, a combination of anesthetic (0.25% bupivicaine) and steroid (safest in the cervical region are Celestone—nonparticulate, Kenalog—particulate but water soluble or Dexamethasone—non particulate but lipid soluble), 0.5–1 ml at each level
- **Billing Codes**
  - o 64633 (first level) this code includes fluoroscopy
  - o 64634 (each additional level) this code includes fluoroscopy
  - o Include appropriate medication codes and units used
  - o 721.0 Cervical Spondylosis w/o Myelopathy is a commonly used diagnosis code

OTHER PAIN INTERVENTIONS

Spinal Cord Stimulator (SCS) Trial [13]

- **Indications**
  - o Failed back syndrome
  - o Chronic neuropathic intractable pain of the trunk and/or limbs

- ○ Chronic regional pain syndrome (CRPS)
- ○ Peripheral Neuropathy
- ○ Post-laminectomy syndrome
- ○ Lumbar radiculitis
- **Premedication for SCS trial**
  - ○ Antibiotics: Can use IV or PO antibiotics
    - • Loading dose 45 min prior to procedure
    - • Depending on allergy
      - ○ Ancef 2g OR Clindamycin 600 mg IV
      - ○ Keflex 2,000 mg OR Clindamycin 900 mg PO
  - ○ If not being done under sedation can consider PO sedatives
    - • Valium 30 min prior to procedure
    - • Xanax 0.5–2mg mg #2 tabs, this is for during the procedure if patient needs
  - ○ You do not want the patient to be over sedated as they need to be alert for the stimulation portion of this procedure to determine proper coverage
- **Target on fluoroscopy**
  - ○ Identify the space between the lamina of the vertebrae at the desired level, most commonly L1/2
- **Needle insertion**
  - ○ **Fluoroscopy view:** Start with AP view of level below. Use head or foot tile to align endplates and open interlaminal space
  - ○ **Entry Point**: (Paramedian Approach) – Just medial to the pedicle of the vertebral body one level below desired level
  - ○ Anesthetize the skin parallel to the beam of the X-ray
  - ○ Using an 11 blade, create a small opening for the metal tuohy to advance through
  - ○ Advance the needle at a shallow angle to the skin <45° advancing towards the interlaminar space
    - • The shallow angle is to ensure proper passage of the lead when threaded
    - • You do not want to thread a lead with the needle at 90° to the skin as this can cause sheering and breakage
  - ○ You can aim the needle towards the lamina to ensure depth
  - ○ If at any point you are unsure of your depth check a lateral view as early as you need
  - ○ Once you hit bone obtain a lateral view
  - ○ Then, you can place the loss of resistance syringe on and slowly advance off of the bone till you feel the loss

- You may need to steepen the needle angle to 30–45° and engage into the ligament
○ Once you have successfully reached the epidural space change to an AP view. Remove the obturator and start to thread the lead into position
  - If at first the lead does not thread smoothly, you may not be at the epidural space yet. Do not force the lead into the space, it should advance easily.
○ Thread the lead slowly while steering towards midline of the desired level (usually top of T8 but depends on patients location of pain)
○ At any time you can check a lateral view to make sure the lead is posterior
  - At times the leads can advance anteriorly which can cause sensations at the abdomen and chest during stimulation. If anterior placement is a concern check a lateral view
○ Once the leads are properly placed, the device representative will start testing to confirm proper placement
○ After you have obtained proper stimulation coverage, the leads can be sutured or secured with steri-strips or stayfix to avoid lead migration. Then the entire area is properly bandaged with large tegaderms.
○ **Post-procedure medications:**
  - If not allergic, Keflex 500 mg BID-q6 for 10 days (or duration of the trial)
  - If allergic then use, Clindmycin 300 mg tid/qid for 10 days
  - If done in the office, patient must fill the prescription prior to the procedure and bring his pills the day of the procedure
○ **Post-procedure instructions:**
  - No twisting, bending, heavy lifting
○ Patient is to return in 1 week to have the leads removed
- **Billing Codes**
  ○ 63650: Percutaneous lead implantation of neurostimulator (includes fluoroscopy)
  ○ If doing bilateral procedure use 63650 again with a Modifier 51
  ○ L8680: denotes the number of contacts 4,8,16
  ○ 95972: Complex programming
  ○ Use appropriate diagnoses such as:

- o Lumbar radiculopathy (724.2), CRPS (upper limb 337.21, lower limb337.22), peripheral neuropathy (356.8), failed back or post-laminectomy syndrome (lumbar 722.83, thoracic 722.82, cervical 722.81)

INJECTION COMPLICATIONS [2, 14, 15]

Some of the complications that can occur with spinal injections are discussed in this section. This however, does not include all possible complications.

- o Vasovagal response
- o Intravascular or intrathecal uptake of medication
- o Injection of the nerve root and subsequent pain
- o Infection—skin, abcess, diskitis, arachnoiditis, meningitis etc.
- o Allergic reaction to medications
- o Bleeding
- o Epidural Hematoma
- o Spinal cord injury or transient neurological symptoms

Prior Allergy to Contrast

If known allergy you can use omniscan or magnevist instead of contrast, but these may be difficult to see on fluoroscopy.

If you are doing a case that requires contrast, you can premedicate patient with steroids and benadryl prior to avoid reaction to the medication. Use caution when deciding to proceed [2]

12 h prior to contrast exposure
- Prednisone 20–50 mg p.o.
- Ranitidine 50 mg p.o.
- Diphenhydramine 25–50 mg p.o.

2 h prior to contrast exposure
- Prednisone 20–50 mg p.o.
- Ranitidine 50 mg p.o.
- Diphenhydramine 25–50 mg p.o.

Just prior to injection
- Diphenhydramine 25 mg i.v.

Information adapted and modified from Essentials of Pain [2] Management, Benzon

Post Dural Puncture Headache

Definition: headache that occurs due to dural puncture, symptoms are more likely in young individuals, worse when standing or sitting, improves with laying down.

Treatment: lay patient down, increase PO fluids or start IVF, can use fioricet for symptomatic treatment, increase caffeine intake. In severe cases may need to do an epidural blood patch.

Vasovagal Response

Definition: prodrome of sypmtoms which include light headedness, nausea, ringing in ears, weakness, and visual changes which in severe cases, may lead to a loss of consciousness.

Treatment: place patient in trendelenburg position and give bolus of IVF or encourage PO intake (if mild symptoms). Make sure patient and vitals are monitored to prevent fall.

Intravascular Uptake of Medication

3D digital subtraction can help to recognize intravascular spread but this cannot always be prevented.

Treatment:

If there is **anesthetic** injected intravasculary abort, injection. If signs of lidocaine toxicity give intralipids IV

Intravascular **contrast** may be cleared in patients with normal renal function without event

Particulate **steroid** in the artery of Ademkowitz may lead to paraplegia at the L3 level. Particularly for TFESI which are done on the left side, as the descending loop of the artery of Ademkowitz may come down to the L3 level

Transient Neurological Symptoms

Definition: increased pain or dysesthesia
Presents within 24 h following procedure
Possibly secondary to intrathechal lidocaine
May take 72 h to fully wear off

Make sure patient is safe when standing from procedure table to avoid falls
Treatment: rest, muscle relaxers, analgesics, nsaids

Epidural Hematoma

Definition: bleeding at epidural space
Presents within 0–2 days following procedure
Symptoms: pain, sensory and/or motor changes, bowel or bladder changes
May occur from bleeding of prominent epidural venous plexus
Medical emergency—can lead to spinal cord compression and severe neurological deficits
Diagnosis: Emergent MRI
Treatment: Surgical laminectomy and evacuation of hematoma
Best to have surgery within 8 h of onset of symptoms

Superficial Abcess

Definition: involves skin and surrounding tissues
Present with possible fever, localized tissue swelling, erythema, and/or drainage
Rarely have neurologic sequelae
Treatment: may require antibiotics, drainage, and appropriate dressing

Epidural Abcess

Definition: abcess located at epidural space
Can lead to spinal cord compression
Related most commonly to hematogenous spread of infections from other regions of body
Most commonly caused by Staph Aureus
Presents days to weeks after injection
Risk Factors: Diabetes, IVDA, RF, Alcoholism, Trauma, Malignancy
Symptoms: increased back pain, often severe, changes in sensory, motor and bowel or bladder disturbances

Diagnosis: CBC with leukocytosis, Blood cultures, emergent MRI
Treatment: Emergent laminectomy and decompression, evacuation of pus
IV antibiotics for 1 month followed by PO for 2 months

Post-Radiofrequency Neuritis

Definition: inflammation at the medial branches post-RF
Symptoms: Severely increased pain after RF
Treatment: Although not currently supported by literature, medrol dose pack and muscle relaxers to aide with the increased pain (ex. Flexeril or valium)

Acute Allergic Reaction to Medications

If severe can be treated with immediate Epipen injection
Otherwise can use Benadryl IM, IV and IVF infusion for symptomatic support (see Medical Complications and Emergency chapter for more details)

Arachnoiditis

Definition: acute local inflammatory response with fibrosis and adhesion formation
Presents in days to months following procedure
Very rare
Can result from infections or blood in epidural space or inthrathecal injection of medications
Symptoms: gradual onset of motor and sensory changes that progress
Diagnosis: MRI
Treatment: IV methylprednisolone, nsaids

If your patient answers all of these questions before each procedure it may help you avoid certain issues

PRE-PROCEDURE CHECKLIST

DATE:_____

PATIENT NAME: _____

HAVE YOU TAKEN ANY BLOOD THINNING MEDICATIONS IN THE PAST 10 DAYS?
YES   NO

INCLUDING BUT NOT LIMITED TO:

ASPIRIN	YES	NO	**ADVIL**	YES	NO
ALEVE	YES	NO	**IBUPROFEN**	YES	NO
NAPROSYN	YES	NO	**CELEBREX**	YES	NO
MOBIC	YES	NO	**COUMADIN**	YES	NO
PLAVIX	YES	NO	**HEPARIN**	YES	NO
MOTRIN	YES	NO	**RELAFEN**	YES	NO

DO YOU HAVE ANY ALLERGIES TO:

CONTRAST	YES	NO
IODINE	YES	NO
SHELLFISH	YES	NO

HAVE YOU HAD CONTRAST BEFORE?
YES   NO

HAVE YOU HAD ANY RECENT INFECTIONS/ILLNESSES?

URINARY TRACT INFECTION	YES	NO
RESPIRATORY ISSUES	YES	NO
SKIN INFECTIONS	YES	NO
OTHER INFECTION	YES	NO

DO YOU HAVE DIABETES?   YES   NO

HAVE YOU EVER HAD ANY ISSUES WITH STEROIDS? YES   NO

Females Only:

IS THERE ANY CHANCE YOU COULD BE PREGNANT? YES   NO

PATIENT SIGANTURE_____

Office use only:
Pre- Procedure Vitals
BP: /   HR: _____   O2 sat:_____% on RA Glucose_____

Patient has companion to escort them home?   YES   NO

Pre-medication given____mg Xanax _____mg Valium

Post- Procedure Vitals
BP: /   HR: _____   O2 sat:_____% on RA

Table 12.2 Fluoroscopy-guided injections: summary chart

		Technique [1, 2]	Notes
MBB/ dorsal rami	L1–4 MBB	Patient prone, image ipsilateral **oblique** to view the "scotty dog."	Nomenclature: Identity of joint is numerically identical to TP onto which needle is placed, but names of nerves one segment less[XVI]
		Target: above and behind "eye" of "scotty dog." Stop when needle tip hits bone. Then confirm with AP view, the target **is junction of the superior articular process (SAP) and the transverse process (TP)**. This point is midway between the mamillo-accessory notch (Man) and the superior border of TP.	That is: L4–5 jt innervated by MB of L3,L4 which cross L4 and L5 TP respectively
		Ideal contrast dye pattern: smooth medial border against lateral surface of SAP base.	For each Z-joint, treat 2 nerves
		Anatomy: MB enters posterior compartment of back by curving around concavity of ventral edge of neck of SAP, turns medially under mamillo-accessory ligament.	1 ml Bupivicaine 0.25% per nerve 3.5–5 in., 25 gauge spinal needle Give pain diary
	L5 DR MBB	Patient prone, image AP, occasionally with 15–20° of ipsilateral obliquity to visualize behind the S1 SAP.	Dreyfuss in Spine 1997—target specific Kaplan Spine 1998—valid test
		Target: at the superior junction of the **sacral ala and the SAP of the sacrum**. The L5 DR lies in a **notch** between these two bones.	Billing per lumbar/sacral paravertebral facet joint level, second level, etc.
		Ideal contrast dye pattern: smooth margin medially around base of sacral SAP.	Bilateral—use modifier 50
		Anatomy: L5-S1 joint innervated by MB L4 DR (crosses L5 TP) and DR of L5 (crosses sacral ala).	Coding: lumbago, lumbar strain/sprain, lumbar spondylosis

TF ESI	Lumbar TFESI		
		Subpedicular: Patient prone. Start with oblique view: *Target:* **superior, lateral, and anterior aspect of neural foramen of exiting nerve root** = most inferior aspect of pedicle which forms superior margin of intervertebral foramen. (**chin of scotty dog**) The apex of the SAP should bisect 1/4–1/3 of the vertebral body when the obliquity is adequate. A cephalad or caudal tilt can maximize the foramen opening. This also correlates with the 6 o'clock position of the pedicle. Note: 6 o'clock position of pedicle is not visualized on oblique view because it is a radiographic observation uniquely associated with AP views. Needle approach should start slightly below and/or lateral to target point. Stop when once needle has "purchase," switch to AP and lateral views to confirm needle tip at back of VB (remember it is concave) and not past 6 o' clock on AP. Final view AP: Target: superior, lateral, and anterior aspect of neural foramen of exiting nerve root. (Correlates with **"6 o'clock"** position of **pedicle** which forms superior margin of intervertebral foramen). Contrast pattern: outlines spinal nerve and dorsal root ganglion, passes rostrally around inferior and medial aspects of pedicle into the intervertebral foramen above.	"Safe" triangle 4 ml 1% lidocaine for local anesthesia 40 mg triamcinolone (or 1 ml of a depot (or long acting)) steroid preparation + 2 ml 0.25% bupivicaine or normal saline per level Billing: injection, single level lumbar TF epidural, each additional level, if bilateral modifier 50 (fluoroscopy included) Coding: thoraco-lumbar radicultis/neuritis, displacement of intervertebral disc lumbar/thoracic, spinal stenosis, lumbar stenosis Names to know: Lutz APMR 1998 Seiner and Fraser J Bone Joint Surg 1997 Vad Spine 2002

(continued)

Table 12.2 (continued)

	Technique [1, 2]	Notes
S1 TFESI	Patient is positioned prone. Rotate image intensifier cephalad and slightly ipsilateral oblique, superimposing anterior and posterior S1 foramen. *Target*: **superior lateral aspect of S1 neural foramen**. May visualize the silhouette of S1 pedicle immediately cephalad to the target. Puncture point lateral margin of S1 posterior sacral foramen, aim towards dorsal surface of sacrum immediately opposite lateral margin of S1 posterior sacral foramen. Stop once needle has "purchase," then switch to lateral view to confirm depth, Should be 1/3–1/2 way in the sacral canal at the level of the S1–S2 disc space. Contrast dye pattern: spread medially along S1 spinal nerve sleeve.	
Lumbar IL ESI	Patient positioned prone. Image AP with caudal tilt to open up IL space with approx 10° ipsilateral oblique. *Target*: inferior interlaminar space on symptomatic side at level of pathology or one segmental level below. (Higher risk of intrathecal puncture at the level of central stenosis or large disc herniation, more room below and medicine tends to flow upward). Alternatively, radiographic anatomy may dictate optimum placement site.	Billing: inj, single level lumbar epidural **Fluoro guidance** Coding: thoraco-lumbar radicultis/neuritis, displacement of intervertebral disc lumbar/thoracic, spinal stenosis, lumbar

MBB		
Cervical MBB	Can be done prone or side lying. If side lying, must achieve a true **lateral** view of the cervical spine: see superimposed silhouettes of the **articular** pillars (formed by articular processes and interarticular pars) (see Netter) of ipsilateral and contralateral sides. Confirm this by tilting the X-ray beam slightly to temporarily **separate** the superimposed silhouettes[[xvi]]	Failure to confirm a true lateral view hazards directing a needle towards the contralateral side of the neck
		Stay within: for C3–C7: middle half of area of articular pillar where target nerve courses
C3–C6 MBB	Lateral: *Target point:* **centroid** of **articular pillar** with **same segmental number as target nerve branch**. (centroid: at intersection of two diagonals of diamond-shaped articular pillar) [[xvi]]	Stay within for C7. Triangular silhouette of C7 SAP
	AP: needle rests on concave lateral surface of articular pillar	Error zone for TON: rectangular area bounded by C3 SAP anterior edge, upper and lower lines perpendicular to this edge passing posteriorly from apex of SAP and from bottom of C2–C3 intervertebral foramen, and posterior line approx through posterior edge of C2 inferior articular process[[xvi]]
	Contrast pattern: fills concavity of articular pillar spreading rostrodorsally	
C7 MBB	Lateral:	
	Target point: **high on apex of C7 SAP.** (Nerve branch is here since base of C7 TP occupies most of C7 articular pillar's lateral aspect, thus forcing C7 MB to reside higher than other cervical MB; Also C7 TP not easily seen on lateral views, so must confirm with AP/PA view—needle tip should be against lateral margin of SAP).	Bupivicaine 0.25%,
	May have variations in innervation, so may repeat block 1–2 additional sites.[[xvi]]	
	With patient prone:	
	Caudal tilt, get the "waist and pillar" view, and aim for the waist, confirm with lateral that the needle is at the centroid of the articular pillar or slightly superior.	

(continued)

Table 12.2 (continued)

	Technique [1, 2]	Notes
TON	Lateral view: **3 target points** used (TON has variable location relative to C2–C3 Z-joint, and is thicker than caudal MB). *Target points:* on a vertical line which bisects C2–C3 joint. **High** target point: opposite level of the apex of C3 SAP. **Low** target point: opposite bottom of C2–C3 intervertebral foramen. **Middle** target point: midway between these aforementioned points, usually at the level of the C2–C3 joint space. Needle inserted to target middle of 3 target points and progressively advanced until rests on target point, withdraw slightly, inject 0.3 ml LA, then readjusted for other target points. Repeat. Want an extracapsular injection, not intra-articular. Contrast pattern should show this.	administer 1.5–3 in. 25 gauge needle Billing: per cervical paravertebral facet joint level, second level, bilateral—use modifier 50 Coding: cervicalgia, cervical sprain/strain, cervical spondylosis Names to know : Bogduk, Barnsley, Lord,
Cervical IL ESI	Similar to lumbar, start AP, ipsilateral oblique approx 10°, caudal tilt to open interlaminar space. Approach through interlaminar space between C7 and T1 due to larger opening, drive under lateral to minimize spinal cord puncture, feel for a loss of resistance, inject dye, look for an epidural fat pattern.	2 ml betamethasone, 2 ml normal saline or bupivicaine 0.25% Billing: injection, epidural, fluoro guidance Coding: cervical radiculopathy, cervical HNP, spinal stenosis (cervical)
RFA	Must place electrode in groove aka "neck" of SAP parallel to target nerve. Approach from below target zone. Must be done with patient prone, obtain "waist and pillar" view, aim for the waist of the articular pillar, needle tip advanced until just posterior to the foramen. Recommend an AP and an oblique pass to confirm placement.	Billing now by joint, not nerve Coding: cervicalgia, cervical sprain/strain, spondylosis

SI Joint	Patient prone. AP to contralateral oblique view. The **medial joint silhouette** represents the **posterior** joint plane and the **lateral joint silhouette** the **anterior** joint plane. Attempt to radiographically "separate" the anterior and posterior joint planes. Next, optimally visualize the medial silhouette (this occurs when the inferior aspect of the medial cortical line is maximally defined).	"Deceptively difficult"
		Bupivicaine or lidocaine
		Contrast 0.3–0.5 ml
	Target: within inferior 2.0 cm aspect of medial joint silhouette. Stop when needle hits sacrum, then withdraw slightly and redirect towards joint space.… Entry into joint known by loss of bony resistance as tip slips between sacrum and ilium. Check lateral view.	22–25 gauge, 3.5 in. needle
	Contrast: outlines joint space	Billing: (code for injection procedure for SIJ , fluoro is included) actual code #, for bilateral use modifier 50
	If the above technique fails, an alternative target is the hyperlucent zone formed where the caudal aspects of the medial and lateral joint silhouettes cross with rotation of the C-arm.	Coding: lumbago, lumbar sprain/strain, sprain/strain of sacroiliac region. Can also use ankylosing spondylitis, sacroilitis not elsewhere classified, disorders of sacrum, lumbosacral sprain—unspecified site of sacroiliac region sprain
	Anatomy:	
	Innervation:	
	Posterior: DR (L4) L5, S1-3, (S4)	
	Anterior: VR L5-S2	

Target, approach, billing and coding ([XVI] and [XVII]—Information gathered from ISIS Guidelines and Atlas of Image-Guided Spinal Procedures)

All injections should be done with contrast unless otherwise contraindicated

Dosages of medications are given as an example. Actual medications, dosages, needle choices, and target approaches may vary

Table made and provided by Emerald Lin, M.D. and Jonathan Kirschner, M.D.

Post-procedure Instructions

1. After the procedure you should rest. You may resume your normal daily routine the next day. However, be careful to avoid strenuous activity or any activities that cause pain or discomfort.
2. Your injection included Lidocaine or Marcaine (numbing medication) and Celestone, Kenalog, Dexamethasone, or Depo-medrol (steroid medication). The numbing medication will last for the next 3–5 h, 24 h at most. The steroid will begin working within 2 days to 1 week (for some patients it may take 2 weeks to start working).
3. Immediately following the procedure, your legs may feel shaky or weak. These sensations are temporary and common.
4. Temporary typical side effects include stomach upset, flushing, headaches, increased energy level, increased appetite, rapid heartbeat, abnormal menstrual cycle, and irritability.
5. Refrain from the following for 24–48 h after your procedure:
   ° Do not take a bath, swim, or sit in a hot tub. Showers are okay.
   ° Do not sit for more than 1–2 h in any one spot.
   ° Do not exercise unsupervised.
6. Tenderness at the site of the injection is normal and can last for a few days. To dull the pain, use ice packs over the injection site for 15–20 min, only once per hour for the first 24 h.
7. Headaches are another possible side effect, but they occur only in less than 1% of all patients. Lying down for 24–36 h with your head no higher than one pillow and resting are the best treatments. If you experience a headache following a procedure that is extreme please call your physician.
8. You should take any prescribed pain medications.
9. Eat a well-balanced diet and try to avoid fatty and high-sugar foods. Supplement your meal with a multivitamin and 200 mg of vitamin C to help your body cope with the stress pain.

If you have any questions regarding your procedure, please call physician's office. If you have any emergencies and the office is closed please ask for the answering service and page your doctor or call 911 or go to local emergency room.

Information adapted from Dr. Joseph E. Herrera

Acknowledgment All fluoroscopic images were collected by Dr. Kimberly Sackheim. A special thanks to Dr. Jan Slomba and Dr. Halland Chen for their collaboration in obtaining and formatting these images.

References

1. Interventional Techniques in Chronic Spinal Pain Manchikanti, Laxmaiah and Singh, Vijay ASIPP publishing.
2. Benzon H, et al. Essentials of pain management. New York: Elsevier; 2011.
3. Manchikanti L, Boswell MV, Singh V, Benyamin RM, Fellows B, Abdi S. Epidural injections in the management of chronic low back pain. Pain Physician. 2009;12:109–35.
4. Wybier M. Lumbar epidural and foraminal injections: update. J Radiol. 2010;91:1079–85.
5. Botwin K, Natalicchio J, Brown LA. Epidurography contrast patterns with fluoroscopic guided lumbar transforaminal epidural injections: a prospective evaluation. Pain Physician. 2004;7:211–5.
6. Schwarzer AC, Aprill CN, Derby R, et al. The relative contributions of the disc and zygapophysial joint in chronic low back pain. Spine. 1994;19(7):801–6.
7. Kline MT. Stereotactic radiofrequency lesions as part of the management of chronic pain. Orlando, FL: Faul M Deutsh; 1992.
8. Furman M, Thomas L. Contrast flow selectivity during transforaminal lumbosacral epidural steroid injections. Pain Physician. 2008;11:855–61.
9. Maigne J, Aivaliklis A, Pfefer F. Results of sacroiliac joint double block and value of sacroiliac pain provocation tests in 54 patients with low back pain. Spine. 1996;21(16):1889–92.
10. Bradly G, Pentalcorin J, Mallempati S. Optimizing patient positioning and fluoroscopic imaging for the performance of Cervical Interlaminal Epidural Steroid Injections. PM&R. 2010;2(8):783–6.
11. Bogduk N. Aprill C: on the nature of neck pain, discography and cervical zygapophysial joint blocks. Pain. 1993;54:213–7.
12. Lord SM, Barnsley L, Wallis BJ, et al. Percutaneous radio-frequency neurotomy for chronic cervical zygapophysial-joint pain. N Engl J Med. 1996;335(23):1721–6.
13. Kumar K, Nath RK. Toth c: Spinal cord stimulation is effective in the management of reflex sympathetic dystrophy. Neurosurgery. 1997;40:503–8.
14. Karaman H, Kavak GO, Tüfek A, Yldrm ZB. The complications of transforaminal lumbar epidural steroid injections. Spine (Phila Pa 1976). 2011;36:E819–24.
15. Akkaya T, Sayin M. Transforaminal epidural steroid injection and its complications. Agri. 2005;17:27–39.

Chapter 13
Musculoskeletal Pelvic Pain and Pelvic Floor Dysfunction

Jaclyn Bonder, John-Ross Rizzo, Nayeema Chowdhury, and Samia Sayegh

- Causes of pelvic pain in women are often difficult to diagnose and manage [1].
- Researchers estimate that 12–20 % of women have chronic pelvic pain, and up to 1/3 of all women will have pelvic pain and/or pelvic floor disorders during their lifetime [2].
- Pelvic floor muscles play an important role in supporting the abdominal and pelvic viscera, controlling bladder and bowel function, and in sexual activity [3]. Thus, dysfunction affecting any of these muscles or the pelvic joints and ligaments can produce a diverse range of signs and symptoms [4].

Pelvic Anatomy and Support:
The pelvic organs in females are supported by a dynamic system of muscles, ligaments, and connective tissue attachments to the bony pelvis.
- **Levator Ani Muscle Complex**:
  - Comprised of three muscles: the pubococcygeus, puborectalis, and iliococcygeus muscles

---

J. Bonder, M.D. (✉) • J. Rizzo, M.D. • N. Chowdhury, D.O. • S. Sayegh, D.O.
Department of Rehabilitation Medicine, NYU Langone Medical Center,
240 E 38th St, 15th Floor, New York, NY 10016, USA
e-mail: jaclyn.bonder@nyumc.org; nchowd01@nyit.edu; ssayegh@nyit.edu

K.A. Sackheim (ed.), *Rehab Clinical Pocket Guide:*
Rehabilitation Medicine, DOI 10.1007/978-1-4614-5419-9_13,
© Springer Science+Business Media, LLC 2013

- This complex and the coccygeus muscle provide the primary support of the pelvis.
- **Pelvic Floor Muscles** can be divided into three layers [5]:
  - <u>Layer 1</u> is superficial
    - Includes: the superficial perineal muscle, bulb-cavernosus/spongiosus, ischiocavernosus, perineal body, and the external anal sphincter
  - <u>Layer 2</u> makes up the Urogenital Diaphram
    - Includes: the perineal membrane, sphincter urethra, and the deep transverse perineal muscle
  - <u>Layer 3</u> makes up the Pelvic Triangle/Diaphragm
    - Includes: the levator ani muscle(LAM) and the coccygeus muscle, the arcus tendineus (which blends with the endopelvic fascia and the obturator internus fascia), and the urogenital hiatus (which is the opening for the urethra and vagina where prolapse can occur)
    - Other muscles in this layer include obturator internus(OI) and piriformis (Fig. 13.1)
- **Bony Landmarks**:
  - Urogenital Triangle—formed by the pubic symphysis/arch, ischiopubic ramus, and the ischial tuberosity
  - Anal triangle—formed by the ischial tuberosity, sacrotuberous ligament, coccyx, and ischial spine
- **Joints:**
  - Sacroiliac
  - Hip
  - Pubic symphysis
  - Lumbar spine
- **Ligaments**:
  - Sacrotuberous (ST) ligament, sacrospinous (SS) ligament, and the long dorsal sacroiliac ligament provide the majority of support and stability for the pelvis
    - ST and SS ligaments are important because they are contained in the pelvic floor
    - Long dorsal sacroiliac ligament helps maintain pelvic stability at the SIJ
    - Defect in any of these ligaments can lead to pelvic floor dysfunctions and posterior pelvic pain

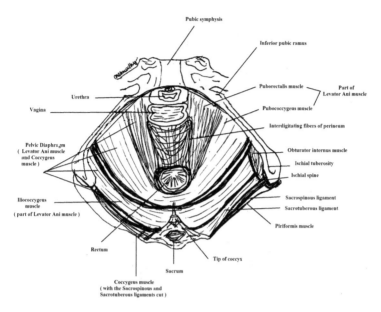

Fig. 13.1 Inferior view of pelvic floor

      – Entrapment of nerve in area of ST or SS ligament may be a source of pain
- **Endopelvic fasica**:
  ○ Comprised of the uterosacral and cardinal ligaments
  ○ Responsible for stabilization of the pelvic organs allowing the pelvic musculature to provide optimal support of the pelvis
- **Innervation**:
  ○ Pelvic organs and pelvic floor muscles: innervated by S2, S3, and S4 segments of the spinal cord
  ○ Sacral segments fuse to form the pudendal nerve which innervates the urinary and external anal sphincter and is important for sexual function
  ○ Levator ani, coccygeus muscles, and the urogenital diaphragm, although poorly understood, appear to be innervated by a direct connection of S2, S3, and S4 nerve fibers

○ Pudendal nerve is susceptible to entrapment at many locations in the pelvic floor along its course

Pelvic Floor Function:

Arnold H. Kegal was a gynecologist who invented the Kegel Perneometer and Kegel exercises, published in 1948. Since Kegel, many individuals have proven that pelvic floor musculature is critical for support of pelvic organs. These muscles function as a sling to hold pelvic contents, they resist an increase in intra-abdominal pressure, and they exist at baseline in a state of continuous contractions to keep the urogenital hiatus closed in order to maintain continence. A maximum voluntary contraction causes the pubocoggyeous and puborectalis to further compress the urethra, vagina, and rectum against the pubic bone.

• Types of Muscle Activity/Inactivity:
  ○ <u>Voluntary Contraction:</u> pelvis moves ventrally and cranially
  ○ <u>Voluntary Relaxation:</u> patient is capable of relaxing on demand. The pelvis descends from the ventral position
  ○ <u>Involuntary Contraction:</u> occurs before an increase in abdominal pressure (e.g., cough)
  ○ <u>Involuntary Relaxation:</u> occurs with straining (e.g., with defecation)

Sacroiliac Joint:

Posterior pelvic pain related to the sacroiliac (SI) joint is a common cause of low back pain in young females [6]. Risk factors that contribute to SI joint pain include increased parity, previous low back pain, emotional stress, obesity, young maternal age, a low educational level, and physically demanding stress on the lower back [7]. SI joint pain due to pregnancy is usually described as stabbing in nature and located in the buttock [8], with radiation as far down as the knee [9]. The pain may worsen during weight bearing and patients may experience pain-free periods [10].

Sacroiliac Joint Anatomy:

The SI joints are

• Two bicondylar joints that are formed between the articular surfaces of the sacrum and the ilium bones with approximately 2–18° of movement. The joints are covered with two types of cartilage:
  ○ Sacral surface with hyaline cartilage
  ○ Ilial surface with fibrocartilage

- There are no muscles that act directly on the joint and as such its stability is due to strong ligamentous connections.
- Ligaments:
  - <u>Anterior SI Ligament</u>: is in most cases a slight thickening of the anterior joint capsule that contributes to stability of the joint
  - <u>Posterior SI Ligaments</u>: can be divided into short (intrinsic) and long (extrinsic) portions
    - Short functions to keep the SIJ from distracting
    - Long (AKA long dorsal ligament) connects the sacrum and the PSIS
  - <u>Interosseous SI Ligament:</u> keeps the sacrum and ilium together and prevents distraction of SIJ
  - <u>Sacrospinous and Sacrotuberous ligaments</u>: restricts posterior rotation of the ilia
- Innervation (poorly understood):
  - Anterior portion of the SIJ is innervated by the dorsal rami of L1-S2
  - Posterior portion of the SIJ is innervated by the dorsal rami of L4-S3
  - Joint capsule receives proprioceptive and pressure fibers

History to Evaluate For Causes of Pelvic Floor Dysfunction:
- Pain characteristics:
  - Quality, intensity, onset, location, parasthesias, aggravation/relief, radiation, progression
  - Timing (detailed, i.e., longer or shorter episodes, length of symptom free periods, and velocity of symptom onset and offset)
  - Constitutional symptoms and red flags
- Associations:
  - With menstrual cycle, urination, defecation, and/or physical activity
- Medications:
  - Type, quantity, frequency, duration, effect, combination
- Nonmedicinal interventions:
  - PT, aerobic exercise, yoga, acupuncture, CAM
- Previous testing:
  - Inquire about any previous diagnostic tests or treatment for pain

- Additional history:
  - Obtain a menstrual, sexual, gynecologic, obstetric, and contraceptive history
  - Past medical and surgical history with attention to previous pelvic trauma or surgery
  - Family history of relevant clinical conditions (i.e., uterine cancer)
- Social history:
  - Assess the possibility of domestic violence and sexual or physical abuse
  - Comprehensive review of systems
    - Should include detailed questions about urinary and/or fecal incontinence, urinary frequency, urinary urgency, dysuria, constipation, and dyspareunia
- Caveats:
  - Pay particular attention to symptoms that may lead you to a diagnosis of endometriosis, pelvic inflammatory disease, gastrointestinal disease, urinary disease, musculoskeletal disease, and psychiatric illness

Physical Exam to Evaluate Causes of Pelvic Floor Dysfunction:
- Lower extremity neurologic exam:
  - Muscle strength testing, sensory testing, reflexes, and balance
- Lower extremity musculoskeletal exam:
  - Gait, posture, and pelvic symmetry
  - Palpate torso, lower back, gluteal muscles, and bony elements
  - Assess range of motion at lumbar spine and hips
- Conduct special tests of the SIJ, pubic symphysis, hip, and L-S spine
- Assess the pelvic floor by performing vaginal and rectal examinations:
  - Pelvic Floor External assessment:
    - Inspect the labia, perineum, and introitus
    - Palpate pubic symphysis, labia, and perineum
    - Observe PFM contraction and relaxation
    - Assess for prolapse and involuntary relaxation of PFM

- Check for an anal wink
- Perform sensory testing

○ Pelvic Floor Internal assessment: (Vaginal)
- Inspect and perform Q-tip test.
- Palpate the ischial spine and check for Tinel's sign (pudendal nerve paresthesia).
- Palpate the pelvic muscles and compare the left vs right sides. Check for pain, bulk, and tone. Assess the levator ani, obturator internus, and piriformis muscles.
- Assess long hold contractions for 5 s.
- Assess 5–10 quick flick contractions.

○ Pelvic Floor Internal assessment: (Rectal)
- External: Inspect for hemorrhoids or lesions, perform sensory testing, check for anal wink reflex, and palpate the coccyx externally.
- Internal: Examine the internal anal sphincter(IAS) and external anal sphincter(EAS). Check for resting tone and contraction of the IAS and EAS. Examine coccyx position, mobility, and tenderness.
- Examine the coccygeus m.,OI, LAM, and piriformis.
- Conduct special tests of the SIJ, pubic symphysis, hip, and L-S spine.

- **Potential Findings** include:
  ○ Pelvic instability, bone and joint pain
  ○ Muscle tightness, muscle spasm, muscle weakness
  ○ Trigger points, neuropathic pain, and referred pain (from the L-S spine, gluteal region, and hips)

Pelvic Pain and Pelvic Floor Disorders

Chronic pelvic pain (CPP) is defined by ACOG as noncyclic pain of 6 or more months' duration that localizes to the anatomic pelvis, anterior abdominal wall at or below the umbilicus, the lumbosacral back, or the buttocks and is of sufficient severity to cause functional disability or lead to medical care [11].

Musculoskeletal conditions and pelvic floor dysfunction (PFD) are common causes of chronic pelvic pain [12]. PFD can be due to a wide range of issues that occur when the muscles that make up the pelvic floor are weak, too tight, or strained. Pathology affecting the pubic symphysis, sacroiliac (SI) joint, low back, coccyx, and/or hip joint are also potential etiologies of CPP. Such problems are also commonly related to lumbopelvic or SI dysfunction (restriction or instability). CPP can also arise from poor posture related to chronic low back pain, SI dysfunction, pregnancy, childbirth, trauma such as a bad fall, previous surgery, or even infections. When evaluating women who have pelvic pain, practitioners must ask questions about history of surgery, trauma, urinary or fecal incontinence, constipation, dyspareunia, and pelvic pain associated with certain activities and with menses. If left undiagnosed, musculoskeletal pelvic floor disorders can affect normal bowel and bladder function, intimacy, and can severely impact quality of life [13].

Musculoskeletal causes of pelvic pain and pelvic floor dysfunction:

- **Pelvic Girdle Pain (PGP)**
  - ○ Specific form of low back pain experienced between the iliac crest and the gluteal fold, commonly in the area of the sacroiliac joints
  - ○ Usually due to dysfunction in the coordination of the ligaments, muscles, and joints in the posterior part of the pelvis
  - ○ Pain may radiate to the posterior thigh and may or may not be associated with pubic symphysis pain
  - ○ Standing, walking, and sitting endurance capacity may be reduced
  - ○ PGP does not present with sensory changes or weakness, which helps differentiate it from lumbar radiculopathy
- **Pregnancy-related PGP**
  - ○ Common cause of PGP due to increased biomechanical strain on the entire pelvis
  - ○ Physiologic changes in pregnancy-related hormones (such as relaxin) are thought to cause hypermobility and laxity of pelvic ligaments
  - ○ Changes in spine posture related to the anterior movement of the center of gravity during pregnancy is usually

> manifested as increased lordosis of lumbar spine and can put strain on pelvic floor, low back, and hip muscles
> ○ Back pain before pregnancy increases risk for back pain during pregnancy

- **Posture**
  - ○ Muscle imbalance due to improper posture can involve the abdominal muscles, thoracolumbar fascia, lumbar extensors or hip flexors, and abductors leading to local or referred pelvic pain
- **SI Joint Dysfunction**
  - ○ Impaired mobility or restriction of the sacroiliac joint can inhibit the normal function of the pelvic floor muscles
  - ○ Joint malalignment can occur if the soft tissue surrounding the sacroiliac joint has caused one of the iliac bones to rotate
- **Viscero-somatic response**
  - ○ Sensory receptors from pelvic visceral structures send afferent impulses to the spinal cord at the same level as somatic structures in this region. Impulses are then sent back which lead to sensory and motor changes in the muscle, skin, and fascia of the trunk and pelvic floor [14].
  - ○ Persistent contraction of PFM due to noxious stimuli such as endometriosis, painful bladder syndrome, fibroids, and irritable bowel syndrome will lead to pain and abnormal function.
  - ○ As a result, the body recruits other muscles (such as the iliopsoas) to compensate for abnormal function. This can lead to pelvic floor, posterior pelvic, and LBP.
- **Hip Pathology/Injury**
  - ○ Hip pain can originate from soft tissue or bone
  - ○ Soft tissue causes include tendonitis, bursitis, nerve entrapment/compression and muscle strains
  - ○ Bony causes include stress fractures, avulsion injuries, acetabular labral tears, FAI, and AVN
  - ○ Pathology of the hip can result in decreased range of motion and eventually cause tightening, shortening, and imbalance of the surrounding pelvic floor muscles which lead to pelvic floor pain
  - ○ Pain from the hip may radiate to the pelvic floor

- **Myofascial Pelvic Pain Syndrome**
  - ◦ Persistent irritation of the pelvic floor muscles can eventually lead to trigger points associated with myofascial pelvic pain syndrome.
  - ◦ Overuse injuries, trauma, postural/joint abnormalities, pelvic asymmetry, and visceral pathology can lead to the development of trigger points [15].
  - ◦ Muscles with trigger points can experience increased tightening and shortening of the muscle over time. This can create more pain, weakness, and musculoskeletal imbalance and lead to the development of additional trigger points.
  - ◦ Pain is usually aching, diffuse, persistent, and can vary in intensity.
  - ◦ Pain may be felt in the pelvis, vagina, vulva, rectum, or bladder and can refer into the thighs, buttocks, or lower abdomen.
  - ◦ MPPS of the PFM can lead to other symptoms such as urinary frequency, dysuria, constipation, or dyspareunia.
  - ◦ Treatment options include medications, stretching exercises, physical therapy, OMT, and trigger point injections [16].
- **Fibromyalgia (FM)**
  - ◦ Commonly found in women from 20 to 65 years of age and associated with chronic and widespread pain for more than 3 months.
  - ◦ Other associated conditions and symptoms include fatigue, headaches, IBS, sleep disturbances, and mood disturbances.
  - ◦ Increasing number of patients with FM have experienced pelvic pain.
  - ◦ Upon examination, 11/18 tender points must be present to diagnose FM. However, FM can be diagnosed with fewer tender points if the history is consistent and the major differentials have been excluded.
  - ◦ FM does not cause any abnormalities in laboratory testing or imaging.

- Although difficult to treat, several medications can be used including anti-depressants, anti-inflammatory drugs, analgesics, and anticonvulsants.
- **Pelvic Floor Tension**
  - Caused by involuntary spasm of the pelvic floor muscles (e.g., piriformis, levator ani, iliopsoas, obturator internus)
  - Causes include pelvic surgery, pregnancy, trauma, and disorders that lead to inflammation
  - Symptoms can include dyspareunia and aching pelvic pain, which is aggravated by sitting for prolonged periods and relieved by heat and lying down with the hips flexed
- **Myalgia**
  - Muscle pain commonly due to overuse or injury to a muscle/group of muscles
  - Can also be associated with various diseases or disorders such as Systemic Lupus Erythematosus, Polymyalgia Rheumatica, Polymyositis, Dermatomyositis, and Multiple Sclerosis
  - Other common causes include viruses, infections, medications such as statins and ACE inhibitors, cocaine, and severe potassium deficiency
- **Coccydynia**
  - A common disorder involving localized pain in the coccyx (tailbone)
  - Usually caused by direct external trauma from a fall backwards into a sitting position
  - Other causes include repetitive minor trauma (i.e., air or car travel, bicycle riding), injury in childbirth, and degenerative joint changes [17]
  - Pain with direct pressure on the coccyx during a rectal examination without signs of inflammation is usually diagnostic
  - Pain associated with sitting (especially leaning back), pain upon rising, prolonged standing, and occasional pain with defecation and sexual intercourse
  - Symptoms usually resolve over weeks to months and should be managed conservatively for at least two months before resorting to more invasive management [18]

- Conservative options include analgesics, protection with donut or wedge pillows, and heat or cold modalities
- Intractable symptoms can be managed with a series of coccygeal injections using local anesthetic with or without glucocorticoids
- Coccygectomy is a last resort [19]

- **Levator Ani Syndrome**
  - Refers to chronic or recurrent rectal pain with episodes that can last 20 min or longer in the absence of organic disease
  - Root cause is pelvic floor muscle tension or myalgia
  - Patients may present with deep, dull, aching pain in the rectum or vagina, referred pain to the thigh and buttock, sensation of "sitting on a ball," pain with sexual intercourse and urinary frequency and urgency
  - Initial treatment includes conservative management with hot baths, analgesics, muscle relaxants, levator muscle massage, biofeedback, and TENS electrical stimulation

- **Piriformis Syndrome**
  - Can cause impingement of sciatic nerve as it passes through the piriformis muscle
  - Can lead to inhibited gluteus medius and overload of obturator internus from abduction function
  - Underlying causes include prolonged sitting, hip/lower back torsional injury, fibrosis due to trauma, hyperlordosis, muscle anomalies with hypertrophy, and partial or total nerve anatomical abnormalities
  - Other less common causes include pseudoaneurysms of the inferior gluteal artery adjacent to the piriformis, cerebral palsy, total hip arthroplasty, fibrodysplasia ossificans progressive, and vigorous physical activity
  - Patients may present with pain and weakness as seen with a L5-S1 radiculopathy and may report difficulty sitting due to intolerance of weight bearing on buttock
  - Shortening of the affected lower extremity may be seen
  - Treatment options include conservative management with heat modalities, stretching and steroid injections if symptoms persist

Other potential causes of musculoskeletal pelvic pain
- Vulvar conditions: Vulvodynia and/or vestibulities

- Vaginismus
- Vulvar vestibulitis syndrome
- Infiltration of gynecologic metastases/benign growths
- Sexual assault
- Referred pain from lumbar spine

Other Conditions Associated with Pelvic Floor Dysfunction

Pelvic Organ Prolapse

Pelvic organ prolapse (POP) is the herniation of the pelvic organs to or beyond the vaginal walls and is a common condition that affects women [20]. It is estimated that 3–11 % of women suffer from symptomatic POP [21].

- Prolapse type
  - ○ Cystocele and/or urethrocele: hernia of the anterior vaginal wall usually associated with the descent of the bladder and/or urethra
  - ○ Rectocele: hernia of the posterior vaginal segment usually associated with descent of the rectum
  - ○ Enterocele: hernia of the intestines to or through the vaginal wall
  - ○ Apical compartment prolapse: descent of the uterus and cervix, cervix alone, or vaginal vault into the lower vagina, to the hymen, or beyond the vaginal introitus. Enteroceles are often associated with apical prolapses
- **Risk factors**
  - ○ Vaginal birth
  - ○ Increasing parity, advancing age, obesity, hysterectomy, frequent valsalva maneuvers (such as with chronic constipation), and jobs that involve heavy lifting
- **Symptoms**
  - ○ Sensation of pelvic or vaginal fullness, pressure, or protrusion of tissue from the vagina.

- Patients frequently describe this as "feeling a bulge" or like something is "falling out of the vagina" (especially at times of straining or coughing)
- May have other pelvic floor disorders including urinary frequency and/or incontinence, bowel dysfunction, and sexual complaints

- **Treatment**
  - Symptomatic prolapse can be managed expectantly with conservative or surgical therapy.
  - Treatment is generally not indicated for women with asymptomatic prolapse
  - Conservative treatment options for women with POP include vaginal pessaries, pelvic floor muscle exercises, biofeedback, and behavioral therapy
  - Surgical candidates include women with symptomatic prolapse who have failed or declined conservative management of their prolapse

There are numerous surgeries for prolapse, including vaginal and abdominal approaches with and without graft materials

Urinary Incontinence:

Defined as involuntary loss of leakage. Major types of urinary incontinence include:

- **Urge incontinence**
  - Leakage with sudden urgency due to uninhibited bladder contractions (called detrusor overactivity)
  - "Key in door" phenomenon: frequently experienced when close to a bathroom
  - Treatment options include anticholinergics, TCAs, and behavioral training (biofeedback) [22]
- **Stress incontinence**
  - Leakage with maneuvers that increase intra-abdominal pressure due to loss of bladder and urethra support and/or problems with the urethrae sphincter function
  - Is the most common cause of urinary incontinence in younger women and is the second most common cause in older women; often associated with POP
  - Treatment options include Kegel exercises, pessaries, and vaginal vault suspension surgery
- **Mixed incontinence**
  - Most common type of urinary incontinence in women

- ○ Combination of urge and stress incontinence
- ○ Treatment based upon which type of incontinence (stress or urge) is predominant
- **Overflow incontinence** (incomplete bladder emptying)
  - ○ Dribbling and/or continuous leakage due to impaired detrusor contractility and/or bladder outlet obstruction
  - ○ Symptoms include weak urinary stream, dribbling, intermittency, hesitancy, and frequency
  - ○ An elevated postvoid residual volume can result in nocturia
  - ○ May occur due to obstructions from anti-incontinence surgery scars or POP
  - ○ Suprasacral spinal cord injury patients can develop neurological obstruction from detrusor-sphincter dyssynergia, in which interruption of spinal pathways leads to uncoordinated urethral sphincter contraction and bladder contraction; high risk of hydronephrosis in these patients
  - ○ Treatment options in acute setting include urethral catheter and timed voiding
- **"Neurogenic bladder"**
  - ○ Malfunctioning urinary bladder due to neurologic dysfunction or insult emanating from internal or external trauma, disease, or injury
  - ○ Symptoms range from detrusor underactivity to overactivity, depending on the site of neurologic insult
  - ○ Urinary sphincter may also be affected, resulting in sphincter underactivity or overactivity and loss of coordination with bladder function
- Urinary incontinence may also be due to ***reversible medical factors,*** particularly in older patients (e.g., UTI and decreased mobility)

Painful bladder syndrome (PBS) (also known as Interstitial Cystitis (IC))

- Recurring pain or discomfort in the bladder and the surrounding pelvic region.

- Signs and symptoms may include pain before, during, or after urination, urinary urgency, frequency, or hesitancy, dyspareunia, pain in the back, suprapubic area, and/or abdomen, nocturia
- PBS is often associated with PFD; the pelvic muscles can become hypertonic and constricted as a response to guarding against bladder pain which ultimately increases the symptoms

Fecal Incontinence:

Fecal incontinence is associated with the unintentional loss of stool and possibly flatus as well. Pelvic floor muscles are influential in coordinating bowel movements and controlling the contraction and relaxation of the anal sphincter. A dysfunction in the pelvic floor muscles, anal sphincters, decreased rectal sensation, or a combination of any of these dysfunctions can lead to fecal incontinence.

- **Etiology**
    - Anal sphincter tears or trauma to the pudendal nerve from vaginal deliveries or surgical trauma
    - Impaired rectal sensation due neurological disorders such as diabetes, spinal cord injuries, or pudendal neuropathy
- **Treatment**
    - Conservative measures include avoiding foods (e.g., caffeine) or activities (e.g., exercise after eating) which are known to worsen symptoms
    - Bowel regimen training and improving perianal skin hygiene
    - Specific treatments (pharmacologic, biofeedback, implants, and surgery) may each have a role in individual settings

PM&R Treatment Options

Pelvic pain may be classified as acute or chronic. After a thorough examination and obtaining a history including symptoms, the degree of episodes, and frequency of exacerbations, a variety of interventions may be used. Overall, a comprehensive multidisciplinary treatment plan and patient education is the key to pain relief and a successful outcome.

Pelvic Pain Modalities:

Physical therapy and rehabilitation treatment can help improve PFM function and general mobility by treating them, as well as their synergists, in the trunk and hip. PT can help localize the cause of dysfunction and can help treat pain through different modalities.

- Treatments include:
  - Manual therapy to improve restrictions in movement
  - Pelvic floor muscle exercise
  - Lengthening and strengthening exercises to create muscle balance
  - Myofascial release
  - Soft tissue mobilization (to treat adhesions, trigger points, and promote desensitization)
  - Muscle energy techniques
  - Strain-counterstrain
  - Joint mobilization
  - Ultrasound therapy and ice
- Pharmacologic Agents for Pelvic Pain:
  - Medication regimens include NSAIDs, antidepressants, muscle relaxants, anti-seizure medications (carbamazepine, pregabalin, tiagabine, topiramate, valproic acid, and lamotrigene), oral local anesthetics (mexiletine, tocainide, flecainide), and long-acting opioids [23].
- Additional Interventions:
  - Biofeedback Therapy
    - A painless, noninvasive means of cognitively treating patients with urinary incontinence, fecal incontinence and other symptoms of pelvic floor dysfunction [24]
    - Electromyographic surface electrodes and an abdominal wall surface electrode are used to help patients improve control of pelvic floor and abdominal wall musculature [25]
    - Surface electrodes on a probe can be inserted either vaginally or anally [26]
    - Probe/electrodes are connected to a computer or audio monitor and patients are able to use the visual and/or audio patterns that are seen/felt to learn which muscles are being affected by their pelvic floor dysfunction [27]
    - Patients can then use this information to learn how to consciously contract and relax these areas of dysfunction [28]

- Use of biofeedback has been recommended by the American Gastroenterological Association for patients with fecal incontinence associated with structurally intact sphincter rings [29]
- May improve fecal incontinence by three general mechanisms: assisting striated muscles of the pelvic floor to contract more efficiently, enabling patients to better perceive rectal distension, and improving sensory and strength coordination required for continence
- Has also been proven to be effective in preventing and reversing fecal incontinence due to pregnancy for the first year after delivery
○ Transcutaneous Electrical Nerve Stimulation (TENS unit):
  - TENS unit is a battery powered device that is worn externally
  - Delivers low levels of electrical stimulation through the skin and to the affected muscles
  - Used to manage chronic pain via the gate-control theory and is used in cases where pelvic floor muscles are damaged or constricted
  - In PFD and pelvic pain, the TENS unit is usually applied to the lower back or hip joints to help increase blood flow to that area, strengthen/heal damaged muscles, and to block pain
○ Sacral nerve stimulation:
  - For patients with structurally intact muscles, sacral nerve root electrical stimulation can restore continence
  - Sacral stimulation is particularly effective in patients with neurologic disorders
  - Implanted stimulator is placed into the S3 sacral foramen via an electrode which provides low-grade stimulation
  - The sacral nerve stimulator was FDA approved in April 2011 for treatment of chronic fecal incontinence in patients who have failed conservative treatments

References

1. Lukacz ES, Lawrence JM, Contreras R, et al. Parity, mode of delivery, and pelvic floor disorders. Obstet Gynecol. 2006;107:1253.
2. Varma MG, Brown JS, Creasman JM, et al. Fecal incontinence in females older than aged 40 years: who is at risk? Dis Colon Rectum. 2006;49:841.
3. Boreham MK, Richter HE, Kenton KS, et al. Anal incontinence in women presenting for gynecologic care: prevalence, risk factors, and impact upon quality of life. Am J Obstet Gynecol. 2005;192:1637.
4. Fultz NH, Burgio K, Diokno AC, et al. Burden of stress urinary incontinence for community-dwelling women. Am J Obstet Gynecol. 2003;189:1275.
5. Netter, Frank H. "The Netter Collection of Medical Illustrations—Images for Scientific, Pharmaceutical, and Legal Professionals." The Netter Collection of Medical Illustrations—Images for Scientific, Pharmaceutical, and Legal Professionals. Saunders Elsevier. Web. 4 June 2012. http://www.netterimages.com/.
6. MacEvilly M, Buggy D. Back pain and pregnancy: a review. Pain. 1996;64:405.
7. Colliton J. Managing back pain during pregnancy. Medscape Womens Health. 1997;2:2.
8. Fast A, Shapiro D, Ducommun EJ, et al. Low-back pain in pregnancy. Spine (Phila Pa 1976). 1987;12:368.
9. Wang SM, Dezinno P, Maranets I, et al. Low back pain during pregnancy: prevalence, risk factors, and outcomes. Obstet Gynecol. 2004;104:65.
10. Ostgaard HC, Andersson GB. Previous back pain and risk of developing back pain in a future pregnancy. Spine (Phila Pa 1976). 1991;16:432.
11. Reiter RC. A profile of women with chronic pelvic pain. Clin Obstet Gynecol. 1990;33:130.
12. Farquhar CM, Steiner CA. Hysterectomy rates in the United States 1990–1997. Obstet Gynecol. 2002;99:229.
13. Howard FM. The role of laparoscopy in chronic pelvic pain: promise and pitfalls. Obstet Gynecol Surv. 1993;48:357.
14. Cervero F, Laird JM. Visceral pain. Lancet. 1999;353:2145.
15. Scott NA, Guo B, Barton PM, Gerwin RD. Trigger point injections for chronic non-malignant musculoskeletal pain: a systematic review. Pain Med. 2009;10:54.
16. Hong CZ. Lidocaine injection versus dry needling to myofascial trigger point. The importance of the local twitch response. Am J Phys Med Rehabil. 1994;73:256.
17. Fogel GR, Cunningham 3rd PY, Esses SI. Coccygodynia: evaluation and management. J Am Acad Orthop Surg. 2004;12:49.
18. Nathan ST, Fisher BE, Roberts CS. Coccydynia: a review of pathoanatomy, aetiology, treatment and outcome. J Bone Joint Surg Br. 2010;92:1622.
19. Balain B, Eisenstein SM, Alo GO, et al. Coccygectomy for coccydynia: case series and review of literature. Spine (Phila Pa 1976). 2006;31:E414.
20. Oliphant SS, Jones KA, Wang L, et al. Trends over time with commonly performed obstetric and gynecologic inpatient procedures. Obstet Gynecol. 2010;116:926.

21. Wu JM, Hundley AF, Fulton RG, Myers ER. Forecasting the prevalence of pelvic floor disorders in U.S. Women: 2010 to 2050. Obstet Gynecol. 2009;114:1278.
22. Nygaard I. Clinical practice. Idiopathic urgency urinary incontinence. N Engl J Med. 2010;363:1156.
23. Steege JE, Metzger DA, Levy BS. Chronic pelvic pain: an integrated approach. Philadelphia, PA: WB Saunders; 1998.
24. Ko CY, Tong J, Lehman RE, et al. Biofeedback is effective therapy for fecal incontinence and constipation. Arch Surg. 1997;132:829.
25. Ryn AK, Morren GL, Hallböök O, Sjödahl R. Long-term results of electromyographic biofeedback training for fecal incontinence. Dis Colon Rectum. 2000;43:1262.
26. Guillemot F, Bouche B, Gower-Rousseau C, et al. Biofeedback for the treatment of fecal incontinence. Long-term clinical results. Dis Colon Rectum. 1995;38:393.
27. MacLeod JH. Management of anal incontinence by biofeedback. Gastroenterology. 1987;93:291.
28. Byrne CM, Solomon MJ, Young JM, et al. Biofeedback for fecal incontinence: short-term outcomes of 513 consecutive patients and predictors of successful treatment. Dis Colon Rectum. 2007;50:417.
29. Madoff RD, Parker SC, Varma MG, Lowry AC. Faecal incontinence in adults. Lancet. 2004;364:621.

Chapter 14
Rheumatology

Richard G. Chang, Aziza Kamani, Anureet Brar, and David N. Bressler

Osteoarthritis

Pathophysiology: Noninflammatory joint disorder characterized by articular cartilage deterioration, resulting in decreased joint space and new bony spur formation (osteophyte) along joint surfaces and margins.

R.G. Chang, M.D., M.P.H. (✉) • A. Kamani, M.D. • A. Brar, D.O.
Department of Rehabilitation Medicine, Mount Sinai Medical Center,
One Gustave Levy Place, Box 1240, New York, NY 10029, USA
e-mail: richard.chang@mountsinai.org

D.N. Bressler, M.D.
Department of Rehabilitation Medicine, Elmhurst Hospital Center,
7901 Broadway, Elmhurst, NY 11373, USA

K.A. Sackheim (ed.), *Rehab Clinical Pocket Guide:*
Rehabilitation Medicine, DOI 10.1007/978-1-4614-5419-9_14,
© Springer Science+Business Media, LLC 2013

Classification: [1]

Primary/Idiopathic

a. Localized: primarily targets the knees, MTP, DIP, CMC, hips, spine

b. Generalized: involves three or more joint sites

   Secondary: factors which may increase risk for osteoarthritis (OA)

   - Trauma
   - Pseudogout-Calcium pyrophospate dihydrate (CPPD) deposition disease
   - Congenital or developmental disorder osteonecrosis
   - Rheumatoid arthritis
   - Gouty arthritis
   - Septic arthritis
   - Paget disease of bone
   - Diabetes mellitus
   - Acromegaly
   - Hypothyroidism
   - Neuropathic (Charcot) arthropathy
   - Frostbite

Symptoms:

- Dull and achy pain
- Localized tenderness, stiffness that lasts <½h
- Generally worse after activity or at the end of the day
- Locking of joint or audible crepitus during activity

Physical Exam:

- Asymmetrical joint involvement
- Crepitus with passive/active ROM
- Joint enlargement secondary to chronic wear and tear of cartilage and joint surfaces
- Joint effusions
- Heberden's nodes (DIP joint osteophyte formation)
- Bouchard's nodes (PIP joint osteophyte formation)

Diagnosis:

Clinical impression based upon the patient's age and history and physical exam, along with radiographic findings. Patients may complain of pain in one joint, but be sure to examine joint above and below and look for signs/symptoms of pain, decreased ROM, or abnormal positioning or alignment (e.g., femoral retro/anterversion, genu varum/valgum, pronated feet) Radiographic findings do not necessarily correlate with degree of pain or findings on exam.

Imaging:

One can obtain X-ray (XR) of affected regions. Commonly affected regions include: First MTP joint, CMC joint, Acromioclavicular joint, Hips, Knees, and Cervical (Luschka joints of C3-5) and Lumbar spine. For hip and/or knee, standing films are preferable to assess normal weight-bearing load on joint space.

X-ray findings:

- Asymmetric joint space narrowing (knees-medial joint; hip-superior lateral joint)
- Subchondral sclerosis, Subchondral cysts, Osteophyte formation
- Heberden's nodes (DIP), Bouchard's nodes (PIP)

Labs: may be done to rule out other causes of similarly presenting joint pain [2]

- Erythrocyte sedimentation rate (ESR), C-reactive protein (CRP) used as markers of inflammation, not entirely specific, but differential includes Rheumatoid arthritis (RA), Reiter's syndrome, septic arthritis, systemic lupus erythematosus (SLE), ankylosing spondylitis (AS). ESR >30 mm/h and/or CRP >80 mg/L minimally increases likelihood of infectious and or inflammatory etiologies such as septic arthritis or rheumatoid arthritis, respectively [2–4].
- Rheumatoid factor (RF) with/without ACPA (Anti-citrullinated peptide antibody) to rule out RA
- Arthrocentesis, synovial fluid analysis if any suspicion for infection or inflammatory process
- Lyme ELISA/Western Blot to rule out Lyme disease (low on differential unless history of exposure to ticks or travel to area where Lyme disease is endemic) (Table 14.1)

Treatment:
Nonpharmacologic [6–9]

- Weight loss (if overweight/obese)
- Orthotics: Lateral-wedged insoles (for genu varum, medial compartment knee pain) or viscoelastic shoe inserts to provide shock absorption for knee/ankle/ft.
- Bracing (medial/lateral offloading brace for non-obese patients)
- Joint protection, e.g., patellar taping
- Acupuncture

Table 14.1 Classes of Synovial Fluid. From pages 26–27, Chapter 3: Arthrocentesis and Synovial Fluid Analysis. Pocket primer on the rheumatic diseases, 2nd ed. Klippel, John H. Arthritis Foundation, 2010. [5]

Measure	Group I (Noninflammatory)	Group I (Inflammatory)	Group III (Septic)	Group IV (Hemorrhagic)
Color	Yellow	Yellow/white	Yellow/white	Red
Clarity	Transparent	Transparent/opque	Opaque	Opaque
Viscosity	High	Variable	Low	Not applicable
Mucin clot	Firm	Variable	Friable	Not applicable
WBC	2,000	2,000–100,000	> 100,000	Not applicable
PMNs	< 25%	>50%	> 95%	Not applicable
Culture	Negative	Negative	Positive	Variable

PMNs (polymorphoclear cells)

Medications [10, 11]
Mild to moderate pain:

- Acetaminophen extra strength 500 mg 1–2 tabs every 8 h as needed for pain, doses of up to 3–4 g/day (>2 g/day increases risk for GI/Liver complications)
- *Topicals*: Capsacian cream, lidoderm, flector patch, voltaren (diclofenac) gel, pennsaid. Can be used as monotherapy or adjuvant therapy

  ○ Capsaicin cream should be applied to the symptomatic joint three to four times daily; a local burning sensation is common, recommended to be applied with gloves and patients should be instructed to avoid contact with eyes. Pain relief takes anywhere from 2 to 4 weeks.

Moderate to severe pain, or failure to respond to Acetaminophen:

- NSAIDs (Naproxen 250–500 mg PO BID with meals, Etodolac 400 mg BID PO with meals, Ibuprofen 400–600 mg PO TID with meals, Celecoxib 100 mg BID or 200 mg daily with meals), *avoid in patients with renal dysfunction or h/o GI ulcers, caution in elderly as they are more susceptible to adverse effects.* To reduce adverse GI effects, prescribe misoprostol or proton pump inhibitor (PPI), e.g., omeprazole, pantoprazole. Caution should be taken with patients on anticoagulation, e.g., Coumadin, as it may potentiate anticoagulant effect.

Severe pain or refractory to above options:

- **Opioids (e.g., Tramadol, oxycodone)** may be beneficial for short-term use especially in patients with acute exacerbations of pain. *Adverse side effects, particularly sedation, confusion, and constipation should be explained to patients.* Be careful with drug–drug interactions. For example, Tramadol with SSRIs (selective serotonin reuptake inhibitors) may lead to increased risk for serotonin syndrome. These may also be considered for patients who are at high risk for adverse effects of both selective COX-2 inhibitors and nonselective NSAIDs.
- **Nutritional**: Glucosamine & Chondroitan sulfate supplementation still debated; fish oils (omega 3 fatty acids) may be beneficial. Both not studied with large trials.

Table 14.2 Viscosupplementation

Type and brand	Composition	Injections per cycle
Synvisc ® (Genzyme Corporation, Cambridge, MA, USA) (hylan GF-20)	Sodium hyaluronate, naturally derived, purified hyaluronic acid	1 (with Synvisc-One®) or series of 3
Orthovisc ® (Anika Therapeutics, Inc., Bedford, MA, USA) (high molecular weight hyaluronan)	Hylan polymers derived from hyaluronic acid and chemically modified to enhance viscosity	Series of 3 or 4
Euflexxa ® (Ferring Pharmaceuticals, Inc., Saint-Prex, Switzerland) (1% sodium hyaluronate)	Fermented, bacterial streptococcus Derived hyaluronic acid	Series of 3

From Stitik's injection procedures: osteoarthritis and other related conditions, Springer, New York: 2011, Table 3.2 [13]

- **Injections**

  ○ *Intraarticular steroid injections:* Triamcinolone or Depomedrol 40 mg for large joints (knee and shoulder), 20–30 mg for medium-sized joints (wrist, ankle, elbow), 10–20 mg for small-sized joints (PIP, MTP, tendon sheaths) [10, 12–14].

  ○ *Viscosupplementation:* for example, Hyaluronic acid. Indicated for patients with knee OA not responsive to trial of conservative therapy, weight loss, and conventional pain medications. May serve as an adjunct with pain medications [13, 14].

  ○ *Regenerative therapy:* 12.5–25% dextrose prolotherapy ("proliferation therapy") or autologous platelet-rich plasma (PRP); by injecting small volumes at areas of painful ligament and tendon insertions (entheses) and adjacent joint spaces. Premise is to promote new collagen deposition and remodeling in damaged tissue via healing process (inflammation, proliferation, and remodeling). Studies have shown benefit in pain control and function with safety, but thus far, have been uncontrolled with small sample sizes. Further study necessary to establish recommendations for use. Currently, advised for patients refractory to conservative management, medications, and established injections [15] (Table 14.2).

Rehabilitation Program: [6, 16–20] Knee OA

- Goals: decrease pain and inflammation, increase and preserve ROM, joint stability, increase aerobic capacity, improve body weight
- Education: joint protection via overuse avoidance, periods of rest while participating in therapy, e.g., decrease level of activities if pain persists >1–2 h(s) after therapy, proper sitting/standing postures
- Modalities: Therapeutic Heat/Cold, TENS, and/or cold laser
- ROM: AAROM/PROM to affected joint, muscle energy techniques (actively contracting one muscle, while relaxing its antagonist), joint protection as tolerated without pain
- Strengthening: Isotonic/Isokinetic closed chain exercises to hip flexors/extensors/abductors, quadriceps, and/or hamstrings, supine straight leg raises, side lying leg lifts
- Stretching: slow, gentle, and sustained stretching for 20–40 s to surrounding muscle group and joint mobilization (e.g., to affected joint capsule); for example, for hip and/or knee OA, focus stretching of quadriceps, hip flexors, and hamstring muscles groups
- Aerobic conditioning via pool, brisk walking, or ergometer
- Balance and propioceptive exercises, e.g., lower extremity side-stepping, tilt board balancing exercises, or tai-chi
- Functional gait training with appropriate orthotic (e.g., neoprene knee sleeve or medial/lateral offloading knee brace) and/or adaptive equipment, e.g., cane, walker, rollator
- Stair training

Rheumatoid Arthritis

Pathophysiology: Chronic systemic inflammatory disorder resulting in uncontrolled proliferation of synovial tissue, bony erosion, destruction of joint cartilage and extra-articular manifestations.

Diagnosis: previously based on American College of Rheumatology (ACR) 1987 classification of RA, fulfilling seven of the below criteria made the diagnosis of RA.

- Morning stiffness
- Arthritis of three or more areas
- Hand joint involvement
- Symmetric arthritis

Table 14.3 2010 American College of Rheumatology and European League against Rheumatism rheumatoid arthritis diagnosis criteria [21]

Joint involvement	Score
2–10 large joints	1
1–3 small joints (with or without involvement of large joints)	2
4–10 small joints (with or without involvement of large joints)	3
≥10 joints (at least one small joint)	5
Serology	
Low-positive RF or low positive ACPA	2
High-positive or high-positive ACPA	3
Acute-phase reactants	
Abnormal CRP or abnormal ESR	1
Duration of symptoms	
≥6 weeks	1

- Rheumatoid Nodules
- Serum rheumatoid factor positive
- Erosion on radiographic images

However, in 2010, the ACR and European League Against Rheumatism created a new criteria for diagnosis, where "definite RA is based on the confirmed presence of synovitis in at least one joint, absence of an alternative diagnosis that better explains the synovitis, and achievement of a total score of 6 or greater (of a possible ten) from the individual scores in 4 domains: number and site of involved joints (score range 0–5), serologic abnormality (score range 0–3), elevated acute-phase response (score range 0–1), and symptom duration (two levels; range 0–1)" [21] (Table 14.3).

Symptoms:

- Constitutional symptoms: malaise, low-grade fever without chills
- Morning fatigue and stiffness lasting at least 1 h or more
- Diffuse musculoskeletal pain
- Joint pain affecting MCP, PIP, MTP joints

Physical Exam: [1, 4, 21–23]

- Symmetric arthritis and joint swelling (most commonly, MCP, PIP, MTPs, followed by elbows, shoulders, knees, hip)
- Wrist and MCP ulnar deviation
- Rheumatoid Nodules (subcutaneous nodules over extensor surfaces, bony prominences)

- Swan-neck deformity (interosseous and hand flexor contractures causing MCP, DIP flexion, PIP hyperextension)
- Boutonniere's deformity (ruptured extensor hood with lateral bands migration causing DIP hyperflexion, PIP extension)
- Scleritis
- Entrapment neuropathies

Labs: [1, 22–25]

- CBC: to check for normocytic hypochromic anemia, Felty's syndrome (triad of RA, splenomegaly, leukopenia) [1]
- RF (rheumatoid factor): commonly found in patients with RA, but has poor specificity, as it may be positive and elevated in psoriatic arthritis, SLE, Sjoren's syndrome, cryoglobulinemia, cirrhosis, sarcoidosis, and other syndromes. May be found in 5–10% of healthy, normal individuals. Greatly elevated titers aid in serving as one criteria in confirming diagnosis, determining severity of disease, and generally indicate presence of systemic manifestations.
- ACPA: 95–98% specificity for RA
- ESR >20–30 mm/h, CRP >50 mg/L: acute-phase reactant markers, used to monitor severity and progression of clinical and radiological disease; CRP appears to correlate better than ESR [25].

Diagnostic studies: [1, 6, 25]

- C-spine films (open mouth, flexion/extension views) to assess for atlantoaxial instability, subluxation (greater than 3 mm from odontoid to C1 arch is abnormal) [25].

- Plain films of hands, wrist, feet show:
  - Uniform joint space narrowing
  - Ulnar deviation at MCP
  - Radial deviation of radiocarpal joint
  - Marginal erosions at MCP, PIP, ulnar styloid, and MTP joints
  - Periarticular osteopenia or in severe cases, juxta-articular osteoporosis
  - Subluxations (e.g., boutonniere or swan-neck deformities of the fingers, and palmar and ulnar subluxation of the proximal phalanges on the metacarpal heads)
  - Symmetric periarticular soft-tissue swelling

- Echocardiogram (to evaluate for cardiac valve abnormalities, pericarditis)

Treatment:
Nonpharmacologic: primarily used as adjuncts to pharmacologic therapy [22, 26]

- Weight loss
- Fish oils, omega 3-polyunsaturated fatty acid supplements
- Calcium and vitamin D supplementation for osteopenia, increased risk for patients who are exposed to glucorticoids, generally ≥7.5 mg/day of prednisone/prednisolone for ≥3 weeks (at least 1,200 mg of calcium and 800 units of vitamin D via combination of diet and supplements); for postmenopausal women, patients with history of osteoporosis, men ≥50 years old and/or fragility fractures, also begin biphosphonates (e.g., alendronate or risedronate).
- Orthotics: e.g., resting hand splints, Brunell ring splints for swan-neck deformities
- Acupuncture
- Tai-chi

Medications [22, 27]
- **Analgesics**: e.g., Tylenol please refer to medication section
- **NSAIDS**: all should be instructed to take with food to prevent GI upset, caution with renal pathology or in elderly. Effective daily anti-inflammatory doses include:

  ○ Ibuprofen 800 mg 1 PO TID
  ○ Naproxen 500 mg 1 PO BID
  ○ Celecoxib 100 mg BID or 200 mg daily

- **Opiates**: please refer to medication section
- **Intrarticular glucocorticoids**: 20–80 mg Depomedrol/Triamcinolone with 2–4 mL of local anesthetic depending on affected joint

1. **Mild disease** (meet basic diagnostic RA criteria, usually less than 6 inflamed joints, no extra-articular disease, and no evidence of erosions/synovitis/cartilage loss on plain film imaging) [27–29].

   - **Antimalarials**: **Hydroxychloroquine**: Initial: 400–600 mg/day taken PO with food or milk; increase dose gradually until optimum response level is reached; usually after 4–12 weeks dose should be reduced by $1/_2$ to a maintenance dose of 200–400 mg/day.

- **Sulfazalazine**: Oral (enteric coated tablet): Initial: 0.5–1 g/day; increase weekly to maintenance dose of 2 g/day in two divided doses; maximum: 3 g/day (if response to 2 g/day is inadequate after 12 weeks of treatment).
- **Minocycline**: 100 mg PO twice daily (unlabeled use)

2. **Moderate to Severe Disease** (meet basic diagnostic RA criteria with elevations in ESR, CRP; usually greater than 6–20 inflamed joints, presence of extra-articular disease, and/or evidence of ostepenia/erosions/synovitis/cartilage loss on plain film imaging) [26–29].

- **Glucorticoids**: consider oral prednisone as bridge to MTX or other DMARDs. Provide steroid-induced ulcer prophylaxis, e.g., PPI, monitor glucose and bone density (consider biphosphonate therapy as well).

- **Methotrexate (MTX)**:
    ◦ Oral (manufacturer labeling): 7.5 mg once weekly or 2.5 mg every 12 h for 3 doses/week dosage exceeding 20 mg/week may cause a higher incidence and severity of adverse events; recommend concomitant folic acid at a dose of least 5 mg/week (except the day of methotrexate) to reduce hematologic, gastrointestinal, and hepatic adverse events related to methotrexate.; alternatively, 10–15 mg once weekly, increased by 2.5–5 mg every 2–4 weeks to a maximum of 25 mg once weekly. Contraindicated in pregnancy.
    ◦ IM (intramuscular), subcutaneous (SubQ) (unlabeled route): 15 mg once weekly (dosage varies, similar to oral).

- **DMARDs**: alternative agents that may be used alone for patients with contraindications to and/or for patients who responded poorly to MTX.
    ◦ *Leflunomide*: Oral Loading dose: 100 mg/day for 3 days, followed by 20 mg/day; Note: The loading dose may be omitted in patients at increased risk of hepatic or hematologic toxicity (e.g., recent concomitant methotrexate). Dosage may be decreased to 10 mg/day in patients who have difficulty tolerating the 20 mg dose. Due to the long half-life of the active metabolite, serum concentrations may require a prolonged period to decline after dosage reduction.
    ◦ *Anakinra (Kineret)*: interleukin-1 receptor antagonist. Treatment of moderately to severely active RA in patients,

who have failed one or more DMARD, may be used in combination with DMARDS other than TNF blocking agents. 100 mg subcutaneously once daily.

- ∘ *TNF antagonists*: may be used alternatively to MTX or in combination (if no contraindications)
- ∘ *Etanercept (Enbrel)*: recombinant fusion (IgG-TNF receptor) protein that binds tumor necrosis factor (TNF) alpha and blocks its interaction with cell surface receptors. 50 mg subcutaneously once every week or 25 mg subcutaneously twice every week (72–96 h aparts).
- ∘ *Adalimumab (Humira)*: derived from fully human monoclonal antibody against TNF alpha. 20–40 mg subcutaneously every 2 weeks.
- ∘ *Infliximab (Remicade)*: chimeric (human/mouse) IgG1 monoclonal antibody directed against TNF alpha. 3 mg/kg IV every 6–8 weeks.

- **Statins**: may be considered in acute flare ups; some evidence in respect to decreasing and improving inflammation while providing some form of cardioprotective effect, but limited size and conflicting studies preclude any definite recommendations. However, this class of drugs should not be used as a substitute to above therapies.

Rehabilitation Program: [1, 6, 30–33]

- Goals: Pain control, control inflammation and disease progression, preserve and increase ROM, joint protection and conservation, improve endurance and reduce fatigue, emphasis on functional restoration (e.g., ability to carry out ADLs) over form (physical appearance)
- Education: joint protection via overuse avoidance, periods of rest while participating in therapy, e.g., decrease level of activities if pain persists >2 h after therapy, proper sitting/standing/bed postures (e.g., sitting upright with legs extended while in bed, not flexed to decrease hip flexion contractures)
- Modalities: Therapeutic cold for acute inflammation with effusion; deep heat for chronic inflammation and contractures; Paraffin, fluidotherapy for hands.
- ROM: AAROM/PROM to affected joints as tolerated
- Stretching: to affected joints, ideally after use of modality

- Strengthening: preferably closed chain exercises; gentle isometric strengthening to affected joints during acute flare-ups, light to moderate isotonic exercises may be slowly advanced to moderate-to high-intensity isokinetic exercises involving warm ups, dynamic weight-bearing exercises such as knee bending, step ups, with upper extremity and trunk strengthening [34].
- Aerobics: Low impact exercises such as swimming, bicycling tailored to patient's pain and symptoms
- Orthotic splinting as needed during ADL training, please refer to earlier section on nonpharmacologic management.

Gout

Pathophysiology: Monosodium urate crystal deposition in various articulating joints, cartilage, and soft tissues in the setting of hyperuricemia.

Risk factors:

- Trauma
- Surgery
- Starvation
- Fatty foods
- Dehydration
- Medications(allopurinol, uricosuric agents, thiazide, loop diruet-ics, low-dose aspirin).
- Alcohol
- Meat and seafood consumption.

Symptoms:

- Severe pain, swelling, erythema of joint:
  ○ Classically, 1st MTP (podagra)
  ○ Also found at knees, ankles, heels and elbows
    Patients with recurrent episodes are more likely to have involvement of the ankle or instep, wrist, finger, olecranon bursa, shoulders, hips, sternoclavicular joints, spine, and/or sacroiliac joints.

- *Symptoms of uric acid nephrolithiasis*: Flank pain with urinary hesitancy, dysuria.

Physical Exam: [1, 34]

- Pain, erythema and/or swelling of affected joint; may be associated with desquamation of overlying skin.
- Tophi (subcutaneous deposition of uric acid in joints, cartilage, and/or bone), stigmata of chronic gout

Diagnosis:

Largely based on history and physical exam. Uric acid tests may not be elevated in gout. Gold standard is diagnostic arthrocentesis of the affected joint, revealing *negatively bifringent* needle-shaped monosodium urate crystals under polarized light.

Differential diagnosis of acute gouty arthritis:

- Septic arthritis-fever, leukocytosis, elevated ESR
- Pseudogout (CPPD deposition disease)
- Trauma
- Osteoarthritis
- Rheumatoid arthritis

Labs/Procedures:

- Normal to low serum urate levels (<7 mg/dL) have been noted in cases of patients with acute gout. Conversely, pts may be hyperuricemic and be asymptomatic [35, 36].
- CBC (leukocytosis), Serum urate levels, CMP (assess renal function, electrolytes in setting of renal uric acid disease), ESR, and CRP (markers of inflammation).
- Joint aspiration and fluid analysis:

    ○ Xanthochromia inspection, clear vs. cloudy, total leukocyte count with differential, gram stain and culture, crystal analysis using polarizing microscopy. Aspiration of synovial fluid from the affected joint using polarized light microscopy revealing negatively bifringent crystals within neutrophils is diagnostic for gout.

Imaging: [6, 34, 35]

- X-ray of affected joint: Subcortical bone cysts with preserved joint space and no evidence of osteopenia.
- Ultrasound: synovial tophaceous deposits or linear density overlying cartilage. The finding hyperechoic cloudy areas (HCA), with

sensitivity and specificity for gout of 79% and 95%, respectively, and/or double contour sign (DCS), from hyperechoic enhancement overlying cartilage surface, with sensitivity and specificity of 44% and 99%, respectively, may be useful in clinical diagnosis. However, both of these findings may be found in asymptomatic patients [36].

- MRI: gouty erosions

Treatment: [37]

1. **NSAIDS/COX-2 inhibitors:** Initiate within 24 h, unless contraindicated.

   Naproxen: 500 mg twice daily or Indomethacin: 150 mg/day given in three divided doses.

   Reduce risks for GI complication: dose should be reduced by 1/2 as soon as improvement is noted, often *within 3 days*, and continue to decrease throughout course of treatment as most patients are on NSAIDs until resolution of symptoms, which may take 7–10 days.

   Avoid Aspirin: paradoxical effects of salicylates on serum urate, resulting from renal uric acid retention at low doses (<2–3 g/day) and uricosuria at higher doses.

2. **Colchichine**: FDA administration guideline:

   Acute Flare: 1.2 mg (two tablets) at the first dose followed 1 h later by 0.6 mg (one tablet), to give a total dose of 1.8 mg on the first day of colchicine treatment. Renal dosing: Creatinine clearance <30 mL/min: dosage reduction not required, but may be considered. Hemodialysis: 0.6 mg single dose. For renal impairment, repeat dosage should occur no earlier than 2 weeks.

   Prophylaxis: 0.6 mg qd-bid; maximum: 1.2 mg/day.

   Ensure no contraindications to use: concurrent use of interacting drugs or of end-stage renal disease/renal dialysis. Beware of P-gp and CYP3A4 interaction—may require dosing adjustment.

   Intravenous form—Life-threatening adverse effects, no longer used in USA.

3. **Glucocorticoids**

   a) **Intraarticular glucocorticoids**

      - Use in one or two actively inflamed joints
      - Triamcinolone or Depo-methylprednisolone: 40 mg for knee joints and lower doses for smaller joints.

b) **Systemic glucocorticoids**

- Patients who cannot take NSAIDs or colchicine, or depot glucocorticoid with polyarticular disease
- **Prednisone or Prednisolone**: 30–50 mg/day for 1–2 days, tapered over 7–10 days. Monitor for rebound attacks upon withdrawal.

c) **ACTH**: Patients that cannot take oral medications, intravenous glucocorticoids.

- 40–80 USP units, administered twice daily for 2 days and then once daily for several succeeding days as needed; or, 40 units as a single injection, with reinjection as needed; or, 25 units as a single injection when treating acute small joint monoarticular gout.

d) **Interleukin-1 inhibition (investigational)**

- Treatment of acute gout (or gout flare prophylaxis) with IL-1 inhibition remains off-label and cannot currently be recommended. Further studies are required.

Rehabilitation Program [6, 16]

- Goals: Minimize pain, prevent contracture formation, and preserve ROM
- Education: dietary and lifestyle changes to avoid hyperuricemic states, e.g., avoid alcohol, high purine diets, e.g., excessive red meat, seafood; avoidance of certain medications that may trigger attacks, e.g., thiazide diuretics
- Modalities: therapeutic cold for acute flare-ups, heat or ultrasound for chronic inflammation
- ROM: Gentle ROM exercises (at least once or twice a day even with affected, inflamed joint)
- Stretching: to affected joints, e.g., for knee, slow, sustained stretching of quads, hamstrings
- Strengthening: Isometric strengthening to muscles surrounding joint, e.g., quads, hamstrings, hip extensors for knee
- Orthotics: when appropriate, if 1st MTP, may use anterior offloading shoe

Fibromyalgia

Pathophysiology: Functional somatic syndrome of unknown etiology that affects muscles and soft tissues, causing widespread musculoskeletal pain with multiple tender points. Laboratory testing is often normal. It tends to occur more in females than in males.

Symptoms:

- Fatigue
- Diffuse musculoskeletal pain, tenderness
- Joint pain/stiffness
- Insomnia
- Headaches: Migraine or tension types
- Cognitive, mood disturbances
- Depression, anxiety
- Paresthesias
- Restless Leg syndrome
- Irritable bowel syndrome

Diagnosis: [38]
American College of Rheumatology Classification

- Pain involving both sides of the body
- Both above and below the waist
- Accompanied by axial skeletal pain
- Pain occurs when a pressure of 4 kg/cm^2, approximately the amount of pressure required to blanch the nail bed is applied.
- **At least 11 out of 18 defined tender points defined below** [38] (Fig. 14.1)

    ○ Occiput: suboccipital muscle insertions
    ○ Low cervical: anterior aspects of the intertransverse spaces at C5–C7
    ○ Trapezius: midpoint of the upper border
    ○ Supraspinatus: above the scapula spine near the medial border
    ○ Second rib: lateral to the second costochondral junction
    ○ Lateral epicondyle: 2 cm distal to the epicondyles
    ○ Gluteal: upper outer quadrants
    ○ Greater trochanter: posterior to the trochanteric prominence
    ○ Knee: medial fat pad proximal to the joint line

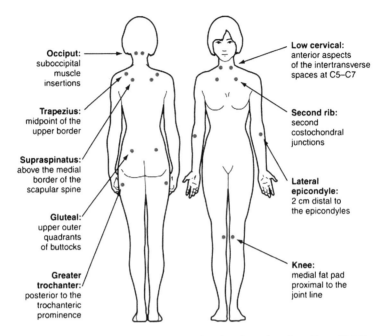

Fig. 14.1 Showing location of the nine pairs of tender points: from Freundlich B, Leventhal L. Diffuse pain syndromes. In: Klippel JH, editor. Primer on the rheumatic diseases. 11th ed. Atlanta: Arthritis Foundation; 1997. pp 123–127 [39]

Tests to Order (all must be ruled out to make a diagnosis of fibromyalgia)

- CBC, ESR, CRP, to ensure an inflammatory disorder is not present
- ANA, RF, if suspicion of systemic rheumatic disease
- Lyme ELISA/Western blot to rule out Lyme disease
- Thyroid function tests, if suspicion of thyroid disease
- CPK, if suspicion of inflammatory muscle disease
- Consider evaluations for restless leg syndrome, OSA, depression, anxiety
- Possible coexisting disorders: Inflammatory rheumatic conditions, OA, Inflammatory bowel syndrome

Treatment: [40, 41]

A. FDA-approved Medications for treatment of Fibromyalgia:

1. **Duloxetine**: inhibits both norepinephrine and serotonin reuptake

    Best tolerated in the morning. Start with 20–30 mg/day, and gradually increase to the recommended dose of 60 mg/day.
2. **Milnacipran**: also inhibits both norepinephrine and serotonin reuptake.

    Dose:100 mg/day or 200 mg/day
3. **Pregabalin**: binds to voltage-dependent calcium channels in the CNS

    Start with 25–30 mg at bedtime, then titrate as tolerated to the recommended dose of 300–450 mg/day. Some patients may respond to lower doses and may not require dose escalation to 300–450 mg/day.

B. Other commonly used medications:

1. **Amitriptyline**: inhibits reuptake of serotonin and noradrenaline.

    Start with 10 mg, titrate slowly up to 25 mg as a single bedtime dose, then increase by 5 mg at 2-week intervals. Final dose is patient dependent based on side effects, and efficacy. Monitor in patients with comorbid cardiac history (increases QT prolongation).
2. **Gabapentin**: binds to voltage-dependent calcium channels in the CNS

    Start with 100 mg at bedtime and titrate up to 900–3,600 mg/day in three divided doses.

    Some patients may respond to lower doses and may not require dose escalation to recommended levels.
3. **Tramadol** with acetaminophen: acts on GABAergic, noradrenergic, and serotonergic systems. Dose: 37.5 mg every 4–8 h, not to exceed 300 mg/day
4. **Bupropion**: Serotonin receptor agonist. Slow release 150–300 mg/day
5. **Cyclobenzaprine**: unknown mechanism of action, potentially increases norepinephrine release. Start at 10 mg at bedtime and increase as tolerated.

Other treatment options: [1, 6, 41, 42]

- Myofascial trigger point injections with local anesthetic: depending upon muscle region, 3–10 mL of 1% lidocaine with 25–27 gauge 1.5 in. needle.
- Acupuncture
- Cognitive behavioral therapy (CBT)
- Biofeedback
- Tai-chi

Rehabilitation Program: [6, 17, 34, 42–46]

- Goals: Patient and family education, pain control, improve endurance, preserve ROM, strengthening. Best responses occur with a multidisciplinary, individualized treatment program.
- Modalities: therapeutic heat/cold, preferably before beginning therapy
- ROM: AAROM/PROM exercises to spine, all four extremities, and trunk
- Stretching: gentle stretching to shoulder and hip girdle, quads, hamstrings
- Strengthening: graded isometric to isotonic resistive exercises to shoulder and hip girdle, quads, hamstrings as tolerated to pain level and fatigue
- Aerobic: low to moderate intensity aerobic activities such as walking, biking, swimming
- Balance and endurance training

Myositis

Polymyositis

Pathophysiology: Cause largely unknown, thought to be chronic inflammation of muscle tissue secondary to primarily autoimmune process, or less likely infection.

Symptoms:

- Systemic constitutional symptoms (fever, malaise)
- Symmetric proximal muscle weakness (not pain), affecting lower extremities and pelvic girdle greater than upper extremities
- Difficulty rising from chair, negotiating stairs, lifting objects
- Neck flexor weakness—difficulty keeping head up
- Typically does not involve ocular/facial muscles
- Dysphagia
- Dysphonia

Physical Exam:

- Proximal muscle weakness
- Deep tendon reflexes may be normal or diminished
- Muscle atrophy, in severe cases
- Interstitial lung involvement: velcro-like crackles
- CHF/arrhythmias
- Arthralgias
- Raynaud's phenomenon

Labs: [1, 6, 42, 47, 48]

- Elevated creatinine kinase(CK) levels, at least 10× ULN (upper limit of normal—references values vary, but ~1,500 U/L).
- Muscle-related markers also elevated: Aldolase, LDH, liver aminotransferases (AST, ALT)
- Consider Rheumatoid factor, ANA, anti-Jo-1 antibodies, to rule out presence of other rheumatologic conditions, e.g., lupus, scleroderma. However, both ANA and anti-Jo-1 antibodies may be positive in polymyositis.

Imaging/Special tests:

- MRI w T2-weighted images and STIR (short tau inversion recovery) sequence to evaluate soft tissue and muscle abnormalities. For example, may help to differentiate between active myositis vs. steroid-induced myopathies (edema, fascia enhancement found in myositis) [6, 48, 49].
- Consider screening CT imaging of chest/abdomen/pelvis as these patients may have associated malignancy (commonly include Non-Hodgkin's lymphoma, lung, and bladder cancers) [50].

EMG (*can refer to Electrodiagnostics chapter for more details*)

- Fibrillations, positive sharp waves, and increased insertional activity
- Spontaneous, high-frequency discharges
- Polyphasic motor unit potentials—low amplitude and short duration

Diagnosis:

Diagnosis of exclusion (rule out more common metabolic, toxic etiologies, e.g., hypothyroidism or alcohol first). **Gold standard is muscle biopsy**, showing T cell (CD8)-mediated autoimmune process with muscle fibers in different stages of necrosis, healing, and fibrosis.

Treatment:

- **Nonmedical**: Speech therapy for dysphagia/dysphonia

Medications: [48, 50]

1. **Glucocorticoids**
   Prednisone 1 mg/kg/day to maximum of 60–80 mg/day for 4–8 weeks, followed by monthly clinical reassessment and monitoring of CK levels. Be aware that steroid-induced myopathies tend to occur with normal CK levels.
2. **Immunosuppresants**: used when steroid therapy does not achieve results within 4–6 weeks' time or from intolerable side effects.

   - Methotrexate (MTX) 10–25 mg PO/week or 15 mg subcut/week or 50 mg IV weekly; use leucovorin 5 mg IV/IM/PO once per week 8–12 h post MTX administration until methotrexate level is <0.05 mmol/L or daily 1 mg daily folic acid when using more than 25 mg/week.
   - Azathioprine 2–3 mg/kg/day
     - No agreed-upon consensus for duration of immunosuppressive therapy, but assess monthly, with plan to taper and cease therapy by 6 months.

3. **IVIG** (intravenous immunoglobulin): based on Cherin et al. 2002 open label prospective study, patients given polyvalent human IVIG 1 mg/kg/day for two consecutive days per month for 4–6 months showed promise among patients in which standard therapy was unsuccessful [50]. In general, it is a temporary measure, with treatments often rendered every 4–8 weeks [48, 49].

Rehabilitation Program:

- Goals: improve muscle strength, preserve ROM to prevent contractures, increase endurance, and maximize mobility and ADLs; PROM programs initially preferred during periods of acute flare ups or exacerbations [6, 42, 47, 48, 51, 52].
- Modalities: Heat/cold/ultrasound as tolerated and appropriate (e.g., no heat or ultrasound to patients with concurrent active arthritis or swollen joints; no cold to patient's with Raynaud's); gentle muscle massage.
- ROM: PROM and AROM to shoulder/pelvic girdle musculature
- Stretching: Active assisted stretching to hip girdle, hamstrings
- Strengthening: Mild to moderate progressive isometric resistive and aerobic exercises to neck flexors/extensors, proximal muscles of shoulder, hip extensors/abductors, knee extensors, with at least 20 s rest periods.
- Balance exercises and trunk strengthening
- Ambulation with gait aids (rolling walker, bilateral canes, and/or standers)
- Stair training
- Breathing exercises
- Cardiovascular aerobic training (please refer to Cardiopulmonary chapter)

Dermatomyositis

Pathophysiology, diagnosis, workup similar to polymyositis, except also has classical skin findings on physical exam and patients have a higher risk for ovarian and stomach cancer [49].

Physical Exam: [1, 48]

- **Heliotrope rash**—violaceous discoloration of eyelids with periorbital edema
- **Shawl sign**—macular erythema of neck and posterior shoulders
- **V sign**—macular erythema of neck and upper chest
- **Gottron papules**—symmetric, violaceous raised lesions over dorsal aspect of IP and MCP joints.
- **Periungal telangiectasias** and **nailfold capillary changes**
- **Calcinosis cutis**—superficial calcium deposits, primarily found in juvenile dermatomyositis

Treatment: same guidelines as found for treatment of polymyositis except for cutaneous calcinosis—multiple agents used with inconsistent and variable success, though may try with diltiazem 5 mg/kg/day for up to 1 year [53, 54].

Rehabilitation Program: please refer to Polymyositis section

Polymyalgia Rheumatica

Pathophysiology: May occur alone or in same setting as giant cell arteritis, cause still unknown.

Symptoms:

• Systemic symptoms (fever, weight loss, malaise)
• Morning stiffness and aching >1 h involving cervical and proximal muscles (pelvic/shoulder girdle)

Physical Exam:

• May have decreased ROM, but otherwise neuromuscular exam is unremarkable.

Diagnosis:
Primarily clinical, elevated ESR (>40) is one criterion for diagnosis

Treatment:

Medications: [48, 55–58]

1. **Glucorticoids (First line)**

   ○ Prednisone 10–20 mg/d for 1–2 weeks, rapid response may be seen in few days
   ○ Maximum dosage of 30 mg/day if no response within first 1–2 weeks; if pt. does not improve with dose, consider other diagnoses besides polymyalgia rheumatica (PMR).
   ○ Once pt symptoms and lab abnormalities are resolved, may start to slowly taper by 3.5 mg decrements/week until 10 mg/day; at this point, may decrease by 1 mg/month.

2. **Glucocorticoid sparing drug**: **Methotextrate** 10–15 mg once/week for 48 weeks; long-term effect still controversial

Rehabilitation Program: [1, 6, 42, 58]

- Goals: improve muscle strengthening, increase endurance, and maximize mobility and ADLs
- Modalities: Therapeutic heat/cold/ultrasound as appropriate
- ROM: PROM and AROM to neck, shoulder, and hip girdle muscle groups
- Stretching: assisted stretching to neck, shoulder, and hip girdle muscle groups; focus may be on hip and knee flexors if iliopsoas or hamstring muscle tightness is present
- Strengthening: Progressive isometric resistive exercises to shoulder and hip girdle, trunk, quads, hip
- Extensors and abductors
- Balance exercises

Temporal Arteritis aka Giant Cell Arteritis

Pathophysiology: Affects large arteries (extracranial branches of carotid arteries) in primarily older individuals

Symptoms:

- Headaches
- Jaw claudication
- Temporal artery or scalp tenderness (for example, with combing/brushing hair)
- Visual loss/changes
- Constitutional symptoms (fever, weight loss, fatigue)
- Upper extremity intermittent claudication or paresthesias (suggests large artery involvement, e.g., subclavian, axillary branches).

Physical Exam: [1, 6, 48, 58–60]

- Tenderness of the scalp over the temporal region and in the muscles of mastication
- Visual field exam and fundoscopy (to assess for visual field deficits; abnormal optic disc size/shape; "Marcun Gunn pupil," aka afferent pupillary defect)
- May have diminished and unequal temporal artery, carotid, radial, pedal pulses
- Cardiac exam for bruits, signs of aortic regurgitation (may indicate aortic aneurysm involvement)

Diagnosis:
Predominantly clinical, fulfilling 3 out of the 5 following criteria: [57, 59, 60]

- Abnormal temporal artery (swollen, tender, thickened, or diminished pulse) on physical exam
- Positive temporal artery biopsy showing multinucleated giant cells
- Elevated ESR >50
- Age >50 years old
- New onset or different headaches compared to past

Treatment: [47, 48, 58–60]

- **Do not wait for temporal artery biopsy**
- For patients with active transient visual symptoms: patients should be admitted and initially given IV methylprednisolone 1 g/day for 3–5 days.
- If clinically suspected, prednisone 40–60 mg/daily for first 2 weeks, if no response, treat at maximum dose for at least 1 month and reassess.
- Optional to add low-dose 81 mg aspirin
- After 1 month, may taper depending upon clinical status and ESR/CRP levels. 10% decrease every week or every 2 weeks. Once 10 mg/day reached, may decrease by 1 mg every 2 weeks.
- Supplement with calcium 1,000–1,500 mg/day and vitamin D 800 IU/day, DEXA scan given that pt will be on oral steroids for months.

Rehabilitation Program: refer to polymyalgia rheumatica program. Overall, patients may benefit from a supervised program (with home exercise plan) involving general strengthening, endurance, ROM exercises while on steroid therapy to prevent/ameliorate steroid-induced myopathy or future flare-ups.

Sarcoidosis

Pathophysiology:
Autoimmune disease characterized by dysregulation of T-helper one immune response, leading to formation of noncaseating granulomas affecting various organ systems.

Symptoms:

- Multiorgan involvement, but more commonly pulmonary syndrome
- Constitutional symptoms (Fever, weight loss, fatigue)
- Uveitis
- Dry cough
- Dyspnea
- Polyarthritis, four to six joints (MCP, PIP, wrists, and/or knees).
- Generalized muscle weakness
- Sacroilitis
- Achilles tendonitis
- Cranial neuropathies (most common, Bell's palsy)
- Peripheral neuropathies
- Depression

Physical Exam:

- Usually fixed obstructive lung disease nonresponsive to bronchodilators
- Interstitial lung involvement: velcro-like crackles, but clubbing rare
- Erythema nodosum
- Arrythmias
- Lymphadenopathy
- Splenomegaly

Labs:

- Cell blood count (anemia, leukopenia)
- Comprehensive metabolic panel (hypercalcemia, renal insufficiency)
- Liver function tests (to screen for hepatic involvement)
- TB screening (rule out coexisiting caseating granulomatous disease)
- Urine: Hypercalciuria

Imaging/Special tests: [47, 48]

- Chest radiograph (abnormal in >90% of patients with sarcoidosis): revealing bilateral hilar adenopathy, interstitial infiltrates, and/or fibrocystic lung disease based on Scadding scale.
- Skeletal films may reveal "punched out" lesions with cystic changes
- MRI brain/spine (granulomatous basal meningitis/spinal cord lesions).

- EKG (screen for conduction abnormalities)
- Lumbar puncture-lymphocytic pleocytosis or elevated protein levels, providing support for inflammation.
- EMG/nerve conduction studies (axonal sensorimotor neuropathies).

Diagnosis: [1, 47, 48]

- Rule out malignancy (lymphoma, cancer) with biopsy and/or infection
- Primarily clinical with tissue biopsy (most common, pulmonary lymph node via bronchoscopy, though superficial tissues—nasal mucosa, peripheral lymph nodes may be used as well), showing noncaseating granulomas pattern.
- Lofgren's Syndrome: syndrome characterized by erythema nodosum, bilateral hilar adenopathy, polyarthritis

Treatment:
Medications: [47, 48, 61]

1. **Glucocorticoids**: mainly for pulmonary or systemic disease

   ◦ Controversy still exists as to optimal dosage and actual duration of therapy. However, prospective trials have shown that this group can provide prompt relief and prevent/reverse multiorgan pathology.
   ◦ Prednisone 20–40 mg/day for 2 weeks, then reassess. If patient responds, may decrease dose by 5 mg every 2 weeks until maintenance dose of 10–15 mg/day for 8–12 months. After routine clinical and laboratory follow up, may taper by 2.5 mg/day every 2–4 weeks.
   ◦ If patient has acute flare, retitrate toward original 20–40 mg/day dose.

2. **Antimalarials**: used to treat less serious skin, nasal mucosal, sinus sarcoidosis forms; reported to benefit those with bone, joint involvement or with hypercalcemia.

   ◦ Hydroxychloroquine 200 mg once or BID for up to 6 months
   ◦ Chloroquine 250 mg once a day or 500 mg every other day for 6 months followed by a 6-month drug holiday
   ◦ Hydroxychloquine preferred because of less risk for ocular toxicity; however, serial ophthalmologic examinations should be performed.

3. **Methotrexate** (MTX)

- Used as single agent or in conjunction with glucorticoid therapy in small doses.
- Effective in many patients, but benefits may take up to 6 months or longer to observe effects
- 10–20 mg/week plus folic acid 1 mg daily for 6 months or more

4. **Immunosuppressants**: alternatives used in patients where steroids no longer effective or side effects intolerable

- Azathioprine, preferred for patients who failed MTX; 100–200 mg/day with low-dose prednisone; duration not agreed upon, follow response on a monthly basis.

Rehabilitation Program: [6, 42, 62–64]
Goals: improve pulmonary function, muscle strength, increase endurance, maximize mobility and ADLs, maintain ROM of affected joints.

- Modalities (heat, ice, ultrasound) to affected joints, but not to affected limbs with neuropathy.
- ROM: AAROM/PROM to affected joints as tolerated
- Stretching: to affected joints as tolerated
- Strengthening: progressive resistive exercise to all four extremities and trunk
- Aerobic: treadmill, cycle ergometer, swimming
- Adaptive equipment, e.g., cane or orthotics, e.g., AFO in cases of lower extremity sensory peripheral neuropathy
- Please refer to cardiopulmonary rehabilitation chapter for pulmonary rehabilitation management

Amyloidosis (Primary Amyloid Light Chain Amyloidosis)

Pathophysiology: [48]
Deposition of insoluble extracellular protein (by plasma cells in bone marrow) in multiple tissue and organ sites. All have a basic B-pleated protein structure. Causes unexplained nephrotic syndrome, heart failure, hepatomegaly, and neuropathy.

Symptoms: primarily nonspecific and may mimic other rheumato-logic conditions (rheumatoid arthritis or giant cell arteritis)

- Constitutional symptoms (most common fatigue and unintentional weight loss)
- Symptoms consistent with:
  - Heart failure
  - Nephrotic syndrome
  - Idiopathic peripheral neuropathy: lower extremity paresthesias (pain and temperature lost before light touch, vibration, and proprioception).
  - Autonomic neuropathy: orthostatic hypotension, diarrhea, impotence, GU dysfunction (impotence, bladder control).
- Generalized muscle weakness and stiffness, but also depends upon areas of involvement.

Physical Exam: [1, 48, 65]

- Macroglossia
- Cardiomyopathy
- Arrhythmias
- Hepatomegaly
- Shoulder "fat pad" sign (glenohumeral soft tissue swelling).
- Muscle pseduohypertrophy
- Symmetric and bilateral Carpel tunnel syndrome
- Peripheral edema
- Charcot joint
- Flexion hand contractures (due to palmar fascia thickening).

Labs:

- Renal insufficiency
- Hypoalbuminemia
- Nephrotic range proteinuria (>3 g protein in 24 h urine)
- Serum and protein electrophoresis (monoclonal Ig light chain proteins)

Imaging/Special Tests:

- EKG
- CXR showing fluid overload
- Echocardiogram

- Plain skeletal films: osteoporosis, subchondral cysts, and erosions
- Immunohistochemical analysis (to identify light chain amyloid fibrils)
- Bone marrow biopsy (to detect monoclonal plasma cells)

Diagnosis: [47, 48]

Gold standard: **tissue biopsy demonstrating apple-green bifringence under polarized light with Congo red dye**; tissue may be obtained from subcutaneous abdominal fat. Identification of precursor protein helps to guide treatment and management.

Treatment: [48, 66, 67]
Medical therapy (usually given to patients who are not candidates for hematopoetic stem cell transplant)

- **First line**: **Melphalan** (0.22 mg/kg/day PO) **with dexamethasone** (40 mg/day PO) on days 1 through 4 every 28 days for 9 cycles. This regime is given with prophylactic omeprazole 20 mg/day, ciprofloxacin 250 mg PO BID, and itraconazole 100 mg/day for the first 10 days of each cycle.
- **Melphalan** (0.15 mg/kg/day orally for the same 7 days every 6 weeks) **and prednisone** (0.8 mg/kg/day orally for 7 days every 6 weeks)
- Supportive care for sequelae resulting from amyloid deposition (e.g., heart failure, renal failure)

- **Hematopoietic (bone marrow) cell transplantation**
  - ◦ Mayo Clinic eligibility criteria for transplantation based on a Dispenzieri et al. 2000 study [67]:

    - Biopsy-proven amyloid light chain (AL) amyloid
    - Symptomatic disease
    - Age <70 years
    - Serum troponin T<0.06 ng/mL
    - Left ventricular ejection fraction >55%
    - Creatinine clearance >30 ml/min (unless on chronic stable dialysis)
    - Performance status <2
    - New York Heart Association Class I or II
    - No more than two organs significantly involved
    - Serum direct bilirubin concentration <2.0 mg/dL

Rehabilitation Program: [1, 6, 42, 47, 48]

- Goals: optimize cardiopulmonary function, improve muscle strength, increase endurance, maximize mobility and ADLs, maintain ROM of affected joints and prevent contractures
- Patients should be first medically optimized in regards to cardiopulmonary disease.
- Strengthening to all four extremities
- PROM, AROM, and stretching to affected joints and extremities.
- Modalities to affected joints, but not to affected limbs with neuropathy
- Hand/wrist splints—refer to Rheumatoid arthritis chapter
- Rigid/solid plastic AFO to affected Charcot joints
- Ambulation with assisted device (straight cane, walker)
- Refer to cardiopulmonary chapter for management of CHF.

Systemic Lupus Erythematosis

Pathophysiology: production of autoantibodies that recognize various cellular antigens. The pathogenesis of systemic lupus erythematosis (SLE) is not yet well defined, and likely includes genetic and environmental factors (including infectious agents, medications, ultraviolet exposure, and stress). Because of its female predominance, sex hormones (which have immunomodulatory properties) may affect disease pathogenesis. Manifestations of SLE can range from mild to severe and life-threatening with chronic multi-organ system involvement [1, 48, 49, 68].

Symptoms:

- Constitutional symptoms: Fatigue (cardinal symptom), weight loss
- Multiple, symmetric joint pain in hands, wrists, and/or knees
- Photosensitivity—Malar rash
- Myalgias and weakness
- Raynaud's phenomenon
- Headaches, memory problems

Physical Exam and Diagnosis: [1, 6, 68, 69]

- Eleven criteria established by the ACR are used in the diagnosis of SLE. *Criteria for diagnosis of SLE: any 4 of the 11 criteria present.*
    1. Malar rash
    2. Discoid rash
    3. Photosensitivity
    4. Oral ulcers
    5. Arthritis: *Joint pain is frequently the presenting symptom of SLE.*
    6. Serositis
    7. Renal disorder
    8. Neurological disorder: seizures or psychosis (without other cause). Headaches and cognitive dysfunction are common neurologic manifestations in patients with SLE.
    9. Hematologic disorder: hemolytic anemia, or leukopenia, of lymphopenia, or thrombocytopenia.
    10. Immunological disorder:

        ○ Abnormal IgG or IgM anticardiolipin, or
        ○ Antibody to Smith, or
        ○ Positive test for antiphopholipid antibodies, including:

            – Abnormal IgG or IgM anticardiolipin
            – Lupus anticoagulant
            – False-positive serologic test for syphilis

    11. Positive antinuclear antibodies

        When >4 of these criteria are met, whether serially or simultaneously, the diagnosis of SLE can be established with 98% specificity and 97% sensitivity. Because these symptoms usually do not occur simultaneously, the diagnosis is usually not made at initial presentation. A high degree of clinical suspicion and reevaluation over time is needed before clinical criteria are met.

Other key points to remember regarding SLE symptoms include:

- **Joint involvement:** *usually the presenting symptom of SLE.* It generally is symmetric, migratory, involves multiple joints, both large and/or small joints, and is non-erosive.
- **Neurologic involvement:** may include seizures, encephalitis, stroke, transverse myelitis, psychosis, septic meningitis, or demyelinating

disease. Headaches and cognitive dysfunction are more common neurologic manifestations of SLE and do not correlate with disease activity.

Labs: [68, 69]

- ANA (Antinuclear antibodies): sensitive, but not specific for SLE, however best initial test, usually high titers >1:160
- Anti-Sm (Smith), Anti-Ds DNA (anti-double-stranded DNA) antibodies: both very specific for SLE and used to support diagnosis of SLE if ANA positive.
- Depressed complement: C3 and C4 levels

Imaging: [68–70]

- There is no universally accepted imaging criteria for the diagnosis of SLE.
- MRI brain: for evaluation of central nervous system lupus. Findings can include small white matter lesions, and cerebral atrophy
- MRI of the hip: avascular necrosis (AVN) of femoral hip
- Bone scan: can detect subclinical involvement of other sites

Treatment: [6, 47, 48, 71, 72]

Non-pharmacological:
- Lifestyle modifications such as weight loss, wearing sunscreen and reducing sun exposure, and smoking cessation.
- Neuropsychological evaluation if cognitive issues present.
- Treating comorbid conditions: Accelerated atherosclerosis, pulmonary hypertension, antiphospholipid antibodies, and osteopenia or osteoporosis.

Pharmacological: [71, 72]

- **NSAIDs**: Naproxen 500–1,000 mg/day in 2 divided doses; may increase to 1.5 g/day of naproxen base for limited time period.
- **Corticosteroids**: low dose used alone or in combination with immunosuppressive agents. High doses of prednisone 1–2 mg/kg/day with or without immunosuppressive agents is reserved with patients with significant organ involvement
- **Hydroxychloroquinolone**: significant organ involvement and/or patients who have had an inadequate response to glucocorticoids PO: 400 mg every day or twice daily for several weeks to months

depending on response; 200–400 mg/day for prolonged maintenance.

- **Methotraxate**: Oral (manufacturer labeling): 7.5 mg once weekly or 2.5 mg every 12 h for 3 doses/week (dosage exceeding 20 mg/week may cause a higher incidence and severity of adverse events); alternatively, 10–15 mg once weekly, increased by 2.5–5 mg every 2–4 weeks to a maximum of 20–30 mg once weekly has been recommended by some experts. IM, SubQ (unlabeled route): 15 mg once weekly (dosage varies, similar to oral). Contraindicated in pregnancy.
- **Cyclophosphamide**: (I.V.: 500 mg/m^2 every month; may increase up to a maximum dose of 1 g/m^2 every month), azathioprine: for lupus nephritis: Oral: Initial: 2 mg/kg/day; may reduce to 1.5 mg/kg/day after 1 month (if proteinuria <1 g/day and serum creatinine stable) or target dose: 2 mg/kg/day.

Rehabilitation Program: [1, 6, 42, 73]

- Goals: optimize cardiopulmonary function, improve muscle strength, increase endurance, maximize mobility and ADLs, maintain ROM of affected joints and prevent contractures. Rehab program similar to RA program. Patients should be first medically optimized in regards to cardiopulmonary disease.
- Education: joint protection and energy conservation techniques, e.g., 1–2 min rest periods between exercises
- Modalities: Therapeutic heat/cold/ultrasound/TENs unit as appropriate
- ROM: PROM, AROM, and stretching to affected joints and extremities as tolerated
- Stretching: gradual stretching to affected joints
- Strengthening: Low to moderate intensity isometric to Isotonic strengthening to all four extremities (if pain occurs post-exercise, switch to isometric exercises)
- Aerobic: bicycle, ergometer, treadmill, resistive aquatic exercises.
- Splinting/orthotic devices as necessary
- Balance and trunk exercises

Sickle Cell Disease (SCD)

Pathophysiology: Inherited homozygous disorder causing abnormal hemoglobin, hemoglobin S (HbS), to sickle. The sickling of the Hb causes decreased RBC deformability, hemolysis, and microvascular occlusion.

Symptoms:

- Fatigue
- Malaise
- Shortness of breath
- Joint pain
- Hand-foot pain
- Priapism

Physical Exam: [1, 6, 48, 74, 75]

- Stigmata of anemia: conjunctival pallor, generalized weakness.
- Splenomegaly
- Jaundice
- Musculoskeletal complications:

    ○ Painful crisis: abdomen, chest, and back and large joint pain
    ○ Dactylitis: painful non-pitting swelling of the digits (both fingers and toes)
    ○ Osteonecrosis, especially hips (femoral heads from avascular necrosis)
    ○ Osteomyelitis: most commonly caused by Salmonella
    ○ Cerebrovascular events: vaso-occulsion can cause CVA

Diagnosis:
Sickle-shaped RBCs and Howell-Jolly bodies found on peripheral smear, Hb electrophoresis (6)

Labs:

- CBC (assess for anemia, usually normocytic normochromic)
- Peripheral smear (to examine actually morphologic structure of red blood cells)
- Reticulocyte count, haptoglobin, LDH, LFTs (assess extent of erythrocyte destruction, hemolysis)
- Hemoglobin electrophoresis

Imaging: [74, 75]

- Plain radiography is excellent for identification of complications of bone infarction:

  - Bone infarctions commonly occur in proximal epiphysis of long bones (humerus, femur)
  - Dactylitis of extremities, e.g., hands, feet
  - **Fish mouth, Reynold's or "H-sign," and/or "fish-bone" appearance of vertebra** (depressions along upper and lower endplates of vertebra)

- Bone marrow expansion (e.g., in skull, widened trabeculae with decreased outer bone skull thickness and density secondary to bone marrow hyperplasia and immaturity, which is best appreciated on MRI).
- MRI is the preferred method for detecting osteomyeltis and early signs of osteonecrosis, followed by nuclear imaging.

Treatment: [76]

- **Hydroxyurea (ribonucleotide reductase inhibitor)**: PO: start at a dose of 15 mg/kg/day. Monitor blood counts for cytopenia, if none, may increase every 8 weeks to maximum tolerated dose of 30 mg/kg/day.
- **Blood transfusions**
- **Acute pain management**
- **Antibiotics** (if suspicious for osteomyelitis)

Rehabilitation Program: [1, 6, 16, 42]

- Goals: pain control, improve muscle strengthening, preserve ROM, increase endurance, maximize mobility and ADLs
- Modalities: Therapeutic cold to acutely inflamed painful, swollen joints
- ROM: AROM to affected joints, PROM as tolerated, careful with ROM at hip as patients have high risk for avascular necrosis
- Stretching: general stretching to
- Strengthening: gradual isometric to isotonic resistive strengthening to trunk, proximal shoulder, knee flexors/extensors, abductors; isometrics to hip girdle
- Refer to cardiopulmonary chapter for patients with cardiac and pulmonary symptoms.

References

1. Cuccurullo S. Physical medicine and rehabilitation board review. New York: Demos Medical Publishing; 2004.
2. Kalunian KC. Diagnosis and classification of osteoarthritis. In: Rose BD, editor. UptoDate. Waltham, MA: UpToDate; 2012.
3. Margaretten ME, Kohlwes J, Moore D, Bent S. Does this adult patient have septic arthritis? JAMA. 2007;297(13):1478–88.
4. Venables PJW, Maini RN. Diagnosis and differential diagnosis of rheumatoid arthritis. In: Rose BD, editor. UptoDate. Waltham, MA: UpToDate; 2012.
5. Klippel JH. Arthrocentesis and synovial fluid analysis (Chapter 3). In: Stone JH, Crofford LJ, White PH, editors. Pocket primer on the rheumatic diseases. 2nd ed. Atlanta, GA: Arthritis Foundation; 2010.
6. Joe GO, Hicks JE, Gerber LH. Rehabilitation of the patient with rheumatic diseases (Chapter 40). In: Frontera WR, editor. Delisa's physical medicine & rehabilitation: principles and practice. 5th ed. Philadelphia, PA: Lippincott Williams & Wilkins; 2010. p. 1–78.
7. Kalunian KC. Nonpharmacologic therapy of osteoarthritis. In: Rose BD, editor. UptoDate. Waltham, MA: UpToDate; 2012.
8. Vicnent HK, Heywood K, Connely J, Hurley RW. Obesity and weight loss in the treatment and prevention of osteoarthritis. PM R. 2012;4:S59–67.
9. De Luigi AJ. Complementary and alternative medicine in osteoarthritis. PM R. 2012;4:S122–33.
10. Kalunian KC. Pharmacologic therapy of osteoarthritis. In: Rose BD, editor. UptoDate. Waltham, MA: UpToDate; 2012.
11. Cheng DS, Visco CJ. Pharmaceutical therapy for osteoarthritis. PM R. 2012;4:S82–8.
12. Roberts Jr NW. Intraarticular and soft tissue injections: what agent(s) to inject and how frequently? In: Rose BD, editor. UptoDate. Waltham, MA: UpToDate; 2012.
13. Stitik TP. Injection procedures: osteoarthritis and other related conditions. New York: Springer; 2011.
14. Hameed F, Ihm J. Injectable medications for osteoarthritis. PM R. 2012;4:S75–81.
15. Vora A, Borg-Stein J, Nguyen RT. Regenerative injection therapy for osteoarthritis: fundamental concepts and evidence-based review. PM R. 2012;4:S104–9.
16. Kisner C, Colby LA. Therapeutic exercise: foundations and techniques. 5th ed. Philadelphia: F.A. Davis Company; 2007.
17. Semanik PA, Chang RW, Dunlop DD. Aerobic activity in prevention and symptom control of osteoarthritis. PM R. 2012;4:S37–44.
18. Brakke R, Singh J, Sullivan W. Physical therapy for osteoarthritis. PM R. 2012;4:S53–8.
19. Vincent KR, Vincent HK. Resistance exercise for knee osteoarthritis. PM R. 2012;4:S45–52.

20. Brander VA, Hinderer SR, Alpiner N, Oh TH. Rehabilitation in joint and connective tissue diseases. 3. Limb disorders. Arch Phys Med Rehabil. 1995;76:S47–56.

21. Aletaha D, Neogi T, Silman AJ, et al. 2010 rheumatoid arthritis classification criteria: an American College of Rheumatology/European league against rheumatism collaborative initiative. Ann Rheum Dis. 2010;69(9):1580–8.

22. Temprano K, Smith H. Rheumatoid Arhritis. Diamond DS, et al., editor. eMedicine. 23 April 2012. http://emedicine.medscape.com/article/331715-overview. Accessed 7 May 2012

23. Schur PH, Matteson EL, Turesson C. Overview of the systemic and nonarticular manifestations of rheumatoid arthritis. In: Rose BD, editor. UptoDate. Waltham, MA: UpToDate; 2012.

24. Kushner I. Acute phase reactants. In: Rose BD, editor. UptoDate. Waltham, MA: UpToDate; 2012.

25. Venables PJW, Maini RN. Clinical features of rheumatoid arthritis. In: Rose BD, editor. UptoDate. Waltham, MA: UpToDate; 2012.

26. Schur PH, Maini BA, Gibofsky A. Nonpharmacologic and preventive therapies of rheumatoid arthritis. In: Rose BD, editor. UptoDate. Waltham, MA: UpToDate; 2012.

27. Schur PH, Moreland LW. General principles of management of rheumatoid arthritis. In: Rose BD, editor. UptoDate. Waltham, MA: UpToDate; 2012.

28. Schur PH, Cohen S. Treatment of early, moderately active rheumatoid arthritis in adults. In: Rose BD, editor. UptoDate. Waltham, MA: UpToDate; 2012.

29. Schur PH, Cohen S. Treatment of persistently active rheumatoid arthritis in adults. In: Rose BD, editor. UptoDate. Waltham, MA: UpToDate; 2012.

30. Leonard JB. Joint protection for inflammatory disorders. In: Lichtman DM, Alexander AH, editors. The wrist and its disorders. 2nd ed. Philadelphia: WB Saunders; 1997. p. 1377.

31. Van den Ende CH, Breedveld FC, le Cessie S, et al. Effect of intensive exercise on patients with active rheumatoid arthritis: a randomised clinical trial. Ann Rheum Dis. 2000;59(8):615.

32. Bilberg A, Ahlmen M, Mannerkorpi K. Moderately intensive exercise in a temperate pool for patients with rheumatoid arthritis: a randomized controlled study. Rheumatology. 2005;44(4):502–8.

33. Pan JC, Bressler DN. Fatigue in rheumatologic diseases. Phys Med Rehabil Clin N Am. 2009;20:373–87.

34. Becker MA. Clinical manifestations and diagnosis of Gout. In: Rose BD, editor. UptoDate. Waltham, MA: UpToDate; 2012.

35. Becker MA. Asymptomatic hyperuricemia. In: Rose BD, editor. UptoDate. Waltham, MA: UpToDate; 2012.

36. De Miguel E, Puig JG, Castillo C, Peiteado D, Torres RJ, Martín-Mola E. Diagnosis of gout in patients with asymptomatic hyperuricemia: a pilot ultrasound study. Ann Rheum Dis. 2012;71(1):157–8.

37. Becker MA. Treatment of acute gout. In: Rose BD, editor. UptoDate. Waltham, MA: UpToDate; 2012.

38. Goldenberg DL, Schur PH. Clinical manifestations and diagnosis of fibromyalgia. In: Rose BD, editor. UptoDate. Waltham, MA: UpToDate; 2012.

39. Freundlich B, Leventhal L. Diffuse pain syndromes. In: Klippel JH, editor. Primer on the rheumatic diseases. 11th ed. Atlanta: Arthritis Foundation; 1997. p. 123–7.

40. Goldenberg DL, Schur PH. Treatment of Fibromyalgia in Adults. In: O'Dell JR, editor. UptoDate. Waltham, MA: UpToDate; 2012.

41. Braddom RL. Physical medicine and rehabilitation. 4th ed. Philadelphia: W.B. Saunders; 2010.

42. Gilliand RP. Rehabilitation and Fibromyalgia. Childers MK, Talavera F, Foye PM, editor. eMedicine. 28 June 2011. http://emedicine.medscape.com/article/31277-overview#aw2aab6b5. Medscape. 7 May 2012.

43. Kingsley JD, Panton LB, Toole T, Sirithienthad P, Mathis R, McMillan V. The effects of a 12-week strength-training program on strength and functionality in women with fibromyalgia. Arch Phys Med Rehabil. 2005;86:1713–21.

44. Sañudo B, Galiano D, Carrasco L, Blagojevic M, de Hoyo M, Saxton J. Aerobic exercise versus combined exercise therapy in women with fibromyalgia syndrome: a randomized controlled trial. Arch Phys Med Rehabil. 2010;91:1838–43.

45. Kingsley JD, McMillan V, Figueroa A. The effects of 12 weeks of resistance exercise training on disease severity and autonomic modulation at rest and after acute leg resistance exercise in women with fibromyalgia. Arch Phys Med Rehabil. 2010;91:1551–7.

46. Busch AJ, Barber KA, Overend TJ, Peloso PMJ, Schachter CL. Exercise for treating fibromyalgia syndrome. Cochrane Database Syst Rev. 2007;(4):CD003786. doi:10.1002/14651858.CD003786.pub2.

47. Firestein GS, Kelley WN. Kelley's textbook of rheumatology. 8th ed. Philadelphia: Saunders; 2009.

48. Imboden JB, Stone JH, Hellmann DB. Current rheumatology diagnosis and treatment. 2nd ed. New York: McGraw-Hill Co.; 2007.

49. Hill CL, et al. Frequency of specific cancer types in dermatomyositis and polymyositis: a population-based study. Lancet. 2001;357(9250):96.

50. Cherin P, Pelletier S, Teixeira A, et al. Results and long-term follow-up of intravenous immunoglobulin infusions in chronic, refractory polymyositis: an open study with thirty-five adult patients. Arthritis Rheum. 2002;46:467.

51. Hicks JE, Miller F, Plotz P, et al. Isometric exercise increases strength and does not produce sustained creatinine phosphokinase increases in a patient with polymyositis. J Rheumatol. 1993;20:1399–401.

52. Wiesenger GF, et al. Benefit of 6 months long-term physical training in polymyositis/dermatomyositis patients. Br J Rheumatol. 1998;37(12):1338–42.

53. Ichiki Y, Akiyama T, Shimozawa N, Suzuki Y, Kondo N, Kitajima Y. An extremely severe case of cutaneous calcinosis with juvenile dermatomyositis, and successful treatment with diltiazem. Br J Dermatol. 2001;144(4):894–7.

54. Stringer E, Feldman BM. Advances in the treatment of juvenile dermatomyositis. Curr Opin Rheumatol. 2006;18(5):503–6.

55. Frearson R, Cassidy T, Newton J. Polymyalgia rheumatica and temporal arteritis: evidence and guidelines for diagnosis and management in older people. Age Ageing. 2003;32(4):370–4.

56. Michet CJ, Matteson EL. Polymyalgia rheumatica. BMJ. 2008; 336(7647):765.

57. Saad Ehab R., et al. Polymyalgia rheumatica. Kristine M. Lohr, et al., editor. eMedicine. 26 Nov 2007. http://emedicine.medscape.com/article/330815-overview. Medscape. 31 Dec 2011.

58. Oh TH, Lim PA, Brander VA, Kaelin DL. Rehabilitation of orthopedic and rheumatologic disorders. 2. Connective tissue diseases. Arch Phys Med Rehabil. 2000;81(3 Suppl 1):S60–6. quiz S78–86. Review.

59. Hunder G. Clinical manifestations of giant cell (temporal) arteritis. In: Rose BD, editor. UptoDate. Waltham, MA: UpToDate; 2012.

60. Weyland CM, Goronzy JJ. Giant-cell arteritis and polymyalgia rheumatica. Ann Intern Med. 2003;139(6):505–15.

61. King TE. Treatment of pulmonary sarcoidosis with alternatives to glucocorticoids. In: Rose BD, editor. UptoDate. Waltham, MA: UpToDate; 2012.

62. Spruit MA, Wouters WFM, Goselink R. Rehabilitation programmes in sarcoidosis: a multidisciplinary approach. Sarcoidosis. 2010;1:316–26.

63. Stubblefield M, O'Dell M. Cancer rehabilitation: principles and practice. New York: Demos Medical Publishing; 2004.

64. Carter GT. Rehabilitation management of peripheral neuropathy. Semin Neurol. 2005;25(2):229–37.

65. Gorevic PD. Musculoskeletal manifestations of amyloidosis. In: Rose BD, editor. UptoDate. Waltham, MA: UpToDate; 2012.

66. Rajkumar V. Prognosis and treatment of immunoglobulin light chain (AL) amyloidosis and light and heavy chain deposition diseases. In: Rose BD, editor. UptoDate. Waltham, MA: UpToDate; 2012.

67. Dispenzieri A, et al. Eligibility for hematopoietic stem-cell transplantation for primary systemic amyloidosis is a favorable prognostic factor for survival. J Clin Oncol. 2001;19(14):3350.

68. Schur PH, Wallace DJ. Diagnosis and differential diagnosis of systemic lupus erythematosus in adults. In: Rose BD, editor. UptoDate. Waltham, MA: UpToDate; 2012.

69. Petri M. Clinical research in systemic lupus erythematosus: immediate relevance to clinical practice. Int J Rheum Dis. 2011;14:1–5.

70. Lalani TA, Kanne JP, Hatfield GA, Chen P. Imaging Findings in Systemic Lupus Erythematosus. Radiographics. 2004;24:1069–86.

71. Schur PH, Wallace DJ. Overview of the therapy and prognosis of systemic lupus erythematosus in adults. In: Rose BD, editor. UptoDate. Waltham, MA: UpToDate; 2012.

72. Falk RJ, Schur PH, Appel GB. Clinical features and therapy of membranous lupus nephritis. In: Rose BD, editor. UptoDate. Waltham, MA: UpToDate; 2012.

73. Alpiner N, Oh TH, Hinderer SR, Brander VA. Rehabilitation in joint and connective tissues. 1. Systemic diseases. Arch Phys Med Rehabil. 1995;76:S32–40.

74. Vichinsky EP. Clinical manifestations of sickle cell disease. In: Rose BD, editor. UptoDate. Waltham, MA: UpToDate; 2012.

75. Ivan Ramirez I. Sickle cell anemia: skeletal imaging. Choi, MJH, et al., editor. eMedicine. 15 July 2011. http://emedicine.medscape.com/article/413542-overview. Medscape. 5 May 2012.

76. Rodger GP. Specific therapies for sickle cell disease. In: Rose BD, editor. UptoDate. Waltham, MA: UpToDate; 2012.

Chapter 15
Prosthetics

Gregory Burkard Jr., John-Ross Rizzo, Jeffrey Heckman, and Jeffrey Cohen

1. Introduction

In this growing field, the physiatrist's role has evolved to be the team leader prior to the amputation and continued throughout the patient's life. It is most important to convey the patient's needs and functional level in creating the prosthesis to ensure a highly functioning amputee. In addition, it is necessary to manage the patient's comorbidities to enhance the patient's quality of life and preserve the residual limb (Fig. 15.1).

2. ISO Classification

In 1989, the International Standards Organization (ISO) defined terms intended for descriptive use in prosthetics, orthotics, and related allied health professionals. Previously accepted American practices used the terms "above," "below," or "through" the joint to describe levels of limb amputation in acquired amputees [1]. The ISO nomenclature system replaced this terminology with three adjectives: trans, disarticulation, and partial (Table 15.1).

G. Burkard Jr., D.O. • J. Rizzo, M.D. • J. Heckman, D.O. (✉) • J. Cohen, M.D.
Department of Rehabilitation Medicine, New York University,
Langone Medical Center, New York, NY, USA
e-mail: gregburkard@gmail.com; Jeffrey.Heckman@nyumc.org;
cohenj01@nyumc.org

K.A. Sackheim (ed.), *Rehab Clinical Pocket Guide:*
Rehabilitation Medicine, DOI 10.1007/978-1-4614-5419-9_15,
© Springer Science+Business Media, LLC 2013

3. K Levels
- Define expectations of an amputee's capacity for mobility after rehabilitation. The Durable Medical Equipment Regional Carrier (DMERC) K codes or Medicare's Functional Classification Level (MFCL) index provides a means to describe an amputee's potential ability to ambulate with a prosthesis.
- Assign K-levels based on several factors, including the patient's past history (including prior prosthetic use, if applicable), the patient's current condition (including the status of the residual limb), co-morbid medical problems and the patient's desire to ambulate [2].
- Categorization by K-levels provides physicians with a consistent method for evaluating and reporting patients' expected functional outcome, and then matching the patients with prosthetics that are appropriate for their potential ability. K-levels have been found to be a valid measure of function as it pertains to an amputee's ability to ambulate [2] (Table 15.2).

4. Epidemiology
In 2005, 1 in 190 Americans, were estimated to be living in the United States with the loss of a limb and this number is expected to almost double by the year 2050 [3]. This increase is related to the aging population and the associated increase in the number of people living with diabetes and other dysvascular conditions [4]. These numbers draw attention to the need for effective programs and policies that will address the necessity of appropriate healthcare and prosthetic services to ensure the well-being of persons with limb loss [3].

5. Etiology
Major etiologies for lower limb deficiency are *vascular* disease (pertaining to the blood vessels), *trauma*, *malignancy* and *congenital absence* [5]. Each year the majority of new lower limb amputations occur due to complications of the vascular system.

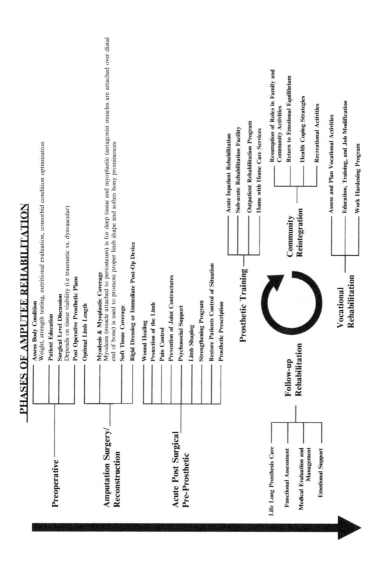

PHASES OF AMPUTEE REHABILITATION

Preoperative
- Assess Body Condition
  Weight, strength testing, nutritional evaluation, comorbid condition optimization
- Patient Education
- Surgical Level Discussion
  Depends on tissue viability (i.e traumatic vs. dysvascular)
- Post Operative Prosthetic Plans
- Optimal Limb Length

Amputation Surgery/ Reconstruction
- Myodesis & Myoplastic Coverage
  Myodesis (muscle attached to periosteum) is for deep tissue and myoplastic (antagonist muscles are attached over distal end of bone) is used to promote proper limb shape and soften bony prominences
- Soft Tissue Coverage
- Rigid Dressing or Immediate Post-Op Device

Acute Post Surgical Pre-Prosthetic
- Wound Healing
- Protection of the Limb
- Pain Control
- Prevention of Joint Contractures
- Psychosocial Support
- Limb Shaping
- Strengthening Program
- Restore Patients Control of Situation
- Prosthetic Prescription

Prosthetic Training
- Acute Inpatient Rehabilitation
- Sub-acute Rehabilitation Facility
- Outpatient Rehabilitation Program
- Home with Home Care Services

Community Reintegration
- Resumption of Roles in Family and Community Activities
- Return to Emotional Equilibrium
- Health Coping Strategies
- Recreational Activities

Follow-up Rehabilitation
- Life Long Prosthesis Care
- Functional Assessment
- Medical Evaluation and Management
- Emotional Support

Vocational Rehabilitation
- Assess and Plan Vocational Activities
- Education, Training, and Job Modification
- Work Hardening Program

Fig. 15.1 Phases of amputee rehabilitation: a visual overview

Table 15.1 ISO classification: application to prosthetics

Descriptive	Definition	Example
Trans	The amputation is across the axis of a long bone. **Note**: When there are two contiguous bones (i.e.: tibia/fibula), only the primary or large bone is identified during description.	Transtibial amputation
Disarticulation	The amputation is between long bones (through the center of a joint).	Knee disarticulation
Partial	Describes amputations of the foot (or hand) distal to the ankle (or wrist) joint	Partial foot amputation

From: Schuch, C.M. & Pritham, C.H. (1994). International Forum—International Standards Organization Terminology: Application to Prosthetics and Orthotics. *J Prosthet Orthot,* 6, 29. Reprinted by permission of the publisher

Table 15.2 K-level categorization

K-levels	Potential ability
Level 0	**No ability or potential to ambulate or transfer safely**
	The patient does not have the ability or potential to ambulate or transfer safely with or without assistance and a prosthesis does not enhance his/her quality of life or mobility.
Level 1	**Household ambulator**
	The patient has the ability or potential to use a prosthesis for transfers or ambulation on level surfaces at fixed cadence. Typical of the limited and unlimited household ambulator.
Level 2	**Limited community ambulator**
	The patient has the ability or potential for ambulation with the ability to traverse low-level environmental barriers such as curbs, stairs, or uneven surfaces. Typical of the limited community ambulator.
Level 3	**Community ambulator**
	The patient has the ability or potential for ambulation with variable cadence. Typical of the community ambulator who has the ability to traverse most environmental barriers and may have vocational, therapeutic, or exercise activity that demands prosthetic utilization beyond simple locomotion.
Level 4	**Child, active adult, or athlete**
	The patient has the ability or potential for prosthetic ambulation that exceeds basic ambulation skills, exhibiting high impact, stress, or energy levels. Typical of the prosthetic demands of the child, active adult, or athlete.

HCFA Common Procedure Coding System

A. **Dysvascular**

Lower limb loss is most commonly due to vascular disease (~82%) [5]. An estimated 65,000 lower-limb amputations are performed each year in the United States for adults with vascular disease. Vascular disease can present as an episode of acute arterial insufficiency or a progressive small vessel occlusion, both resulting in pressure ulcers, infection of the skin (cellulitis) and bone (osteomyelitis). Lower limb amputations secondary to vascular disease are most commonly due to complications from diabetes mellitus [6]. Ultimately, limb amputation may be necessary if medical management is unable to control soft tissue or bone infection or unrelenting pain due to muscle ischemia.

B. **Trauma**

18% of lower extremity amputations, are related to trauma [5]. Motor vehicle accidents, falls or industrial accidents comprise the majority of such traumatic events. They most commonly occur among young males. Trauma to the limb may result in a direct limb transection or an open fracture that may be associated with nerve injury, soft tissue loss, and ischemia. If feasible, limb salvage techniques may be attempted. However, often multiple surgical procedures are required at the expense of time and money. Ultimately, this may result in a painful, nonfunctional limb that will require amputation surgery.

C. **Malignancy**

Lower limb amputation due to malignancy comprises only 0.9% of persons undergoing such amputations [5]. Osteosarcoma is a common cancer that may lead to limb loss.

D. **Congenital**

Congenital limb deficiencies comprise 0.8% of cases of lower limb deficiency. Congenital limb deficiency occurs as a result of the failure of the formation of part or all of a limb bud during the first trimester. The etiology is often unclear, but teratogenic agents, e.g., thalidomide and radiation exposure, and maternal diabetes are major risk factors.

6. **Medical Complications of Prosthetic Management**

There are multiple complications associated with prosthetic management. Common complications include incisional pain, phantom pain, contractures, bone problems, and dermatologic complications. It is important to ensure a proper fitting prosthetic to minimize many of these complications. It is also necessary to educate the patient on proper skin management and prosthetic care to prevent any problems and maximize patient comfort.

A. Pain

Pain in an amputee can be categorized into incisional and neurologic in origin. Incisional pain can be secondary to the healing process in the acute phase. A chronic cause of pain is secondary to adhesions and scar tissue. Adhesions are decreased and prevented by gentle massage to free the healing skin from the subcutaneous tissue during wound healing. Shear forces extended through the prosthetic into the stump puts a great deal of tension on the stump. A fixed skin can put traction on the pain fibers directly stimulating pain and discomfort.

B. Phantom Pain

Phantom pain is a common cause of limb pain that is not fully understood. Studies have shown that about two-thirds of amputees have phantom pain within the first half year following amputation [7]. Although many patients experience phantom pain following amputation, it appears that this pain diminishes with time. It has not been associated with the amputee's age or sex, the level of amputation or the reason for the amputation [8]. Despite many proposed mechanism for the origin of phantom pain, we are still unsure the cause; but studies lead to a multifactorial cause due to peripheral nervous system and central nervous system input, and preamputation pain [8]. Amputees with phantom pain gain some type of relief from a multimodal approach to the remaining limb: prosthetic adjustment, sensory modulation (TENS), exercise, medications like antidepressants, anticonvulsants, opioids, tramadol, anesthetics, surgery and psychosocial support [9].

C. Contractures

Contractures occurs secondary to a limb being flexed into a position for a prolonged period of time (4–7 days) resulting in a shortening of the muscle and collagen fibers. Contractures can results in a decreased ROM, pain and crepitus. It is important to prevent contractures to give amputees the best potential function for the existing limb. Contractures can be prevented and treated with proper bracing, passive and active ROM exercises, stretching and medications.

D. Bone Pain

Bone pain is typically secondary to spurs and heterotrophic ossification. Bone spurs result from periosteum stripping secondary to trauma or during the surgical procedure. Treatment is through prosthetic adjustment and last resort, surgical excision. Heterotrophic ossification is excessive bone growth in soft tissue which occurs commonly in traumatic amputation. Heterotrophic ossification is treated with radiation therapy, medications like bisphosphonates and surgical excision.

E. Skin Complications

Skin complications are common in amputees due to the direct skin contact between the residual limb and the prosthetic device. Hyperhydrosis of the residual limb secondary to functional use, friction and the prosthetic material creates the perfect environment for bacterial and fungal skin infections to occur. It is important to monitor for signs of infection and to treat the patient immediately with the proper antibiotics and antifungal medications. Hyperhydrosis alone or in combination with infections can lead to skin breakdown so it is necessary to maximize the prosthetic fit, practice and educate good limb and prosthetic hygiene and use antiperspirants when necessary. Poor socket fit can disrupt the venous outflow resulting in choked stump syndrome (brawny edema, induration and discolored limb bud) and verrucous hyperplasia.

7. Prosthetic Management Complexity

K-level assignments may change with time. New prosthetic technology such as microprocessor-controlled knees enable greater knee control compared with passive mechanical prosthetic knees. These knees may increase safety and mobility; therefore promoting transition to the next K-level [10]. For example, K-2 level amputee, using an active microprocessor control knee, may potentially improve in function, acquiring the ability to ambulate at various speeds and to traverse most environmental barriers, thus advancing to a K-3 level. These advances are highly beneficial to the patient who improves in safety, functionality and flexibility.

LOWER EXTREMITY

1. *Hemipelvectomy/Hip Disarticulation:*

Hip disarticulations encompass any amputation proximal to the greater trochanter. Contemporary prosthetics are based on the Canadian design which allows for stability in the stance phase and hip and knee flexion during the swing phase. It consists of a molded plastic socket which encompasses the ischial tuberosity for weight bearing, extends over the iliac crest providing suspension and wraps around the contralateral pelvis to provide trunk stability. An extension hip strap prevents unwanted hip flexion during stance and swing phase in combination with a posterior hip bumper to resist hyperextension. Generally any knee, shank and ankle-foot device can be used, but an endoskeleton is beneficial secondary to the decrease in weight. Amputees do however benefit from a hydraulic knee or locking mechanism for stance support, and an extension aid of the knee unit secondary to the decreased cadence in hip disarticulations.

2. *AKA (Above Knee Amputation):*
   The transfemoral prosthesis includes five major components from the ground up: foot-ankle prosthetic, shank, knee unit, socket and suspension. The foot-ankle prosthetic and shank are the same components used in the BKA however many patients prefer more stability so a single axis foot-ankle prosthesis with a light shank (endoskeleton) are more commonly prescribed.

   A. AKA: Knee Unit
   The knee unit has to provide support during the early to mid stance phase and provide flexion during the swing phase and when the amputee sits. The knee unit accomplishes this through different combinations of some or all of the features:
   a. Axis: Connection between residual limb and shank
      There are two types of connections, the single-axis and polycentric-axis knee unit. The single-axis allows for knee flexion and extension around a transverse bolt. This design is easy to maintain and makes little noise. The polycentric-axis contains two or more pairs of bars that pivot shifting the center of rotation of the knee. This maintains the knee behind the center of gravity allowing a more natural motion. The polycentric-axis knee unit is heavier and more stable, but is expensive and requires additional maintenance. The polycentric design is used in amputees with short transfemoral residual limbs, knee disarticulations, or weak hip extensors.
   b. Friction mechanism: Controls shank/ankle-foot prosthetic through the swing phase
      The friction mechanism prevents both, excessive and acute flexion of the knee unit during early swing phase

(high heel rise), and excessive and acute extension of the knee unit during late swing phase (terminal impact). This friction mechanism is accomplished through a constant friction mechanism or a variable friction knee unit. The constant friction unit applies uniform resistance throughout the swing phase by a pair of clamps on the knee bolt. This is the most common friction mechanism used based on simple design, low cost and ability to adjust and maintain. The variable friction unit is generally applies more friction during early swing phase and late swing phase preventing high heel rise and terminal impact, but allows for smooth swing during the midswing phase. This is accomplished through a sliding friction unit or a fluid filled friction mechanism, either air (pneumatic) or oil (hydraulic). Pneumatic units provide modest resistance and are best for moderately active amputees. They are bulky units and aren't suitable in high altitudes due to gases compressibility. The hydraulic unit provides greater resistance and is best used in very active individuals (K-3, K-4).

c. Extension aid: Aids shank extension during terminal swing phase

The extension aid provides amputees with extra assistance during the late swing phase which allows the patient to heel strike with a fully extended knee. This is achieved through internal or external extension aid. The internal extension aid uses elastic webbing or springs, and the external uses an elastic strap on the extensor surface spanning the knee unit. The internal can be noisy and difficult to adjust. Most fluid-resistance knees incorporate internal extension aid springs. It is also recommended that all fixed cadence ambulators (K-1 and K-2) use one of the extension aid devices since the knee momentum during a slower cadence sometimes does not generate enough force to fully extend the knee during the terminal swing phase.

d. Stabilizer: Mechanism that maintains a fixed knee through resisting flexion during stance phase

Some knee units include a mechanical stabilizer that resists knee flexion during early and midstance phase resulting in increased knee stability. This is obtained through a manual locking mechanism or a weight-activated friction brake.

- **Manual lock** is a spring-loaded pin that locks in complete extension when the amputee stands. This maintains full extension through the entire stance phase so it is sometimes necessary to shorten the prosthesis by 1 cm to allow for proper ground clearance. This is reserved for amputees who are household amulators (K-1) who require standing for prolonged period of time. They are also used for amputees who lack proper musculature to support the knee during stance phase.
- **Weight-activated friction brake** uses a wedge that is lodged into a groove when the amputee transfers full weight to the prosthesis during early stance phase (knee flexion angle must be less than 25°). This unit is heavy and requires routine maintenance every 3–6 months. However, many K1 and K2 ambulators benefit from the friction brake.

   e. <u>Extension mechanism</u>: A motor that extends the knee during stance phase

Note: The prosthetic prescription is guided by the patient's functional level. Medicare will cover certain prosthetic knee components as seen in the chart below (Table 15.3):

B. AKA Socket

The transfemoral socket is usually made of flexible thermoplastic inside a rigid plastic frame (ISNY design). Compared to the original rigid socket, the flexible socket is more comfortable (especially when sitting), has better heat dissipation, and is modifiable as the thermoplastic can be reshaped with heat. However, the thermosplastic is more expensive and not as

Table 15.3 K-levels and medicare coverage

K-level	Function	Medicare Coverage
K-0	Nonambulator	No prosthesis
K-1 and K-2	Fixed cadence ambulator	Constant-friction knee unit
K2 and K3	Fixed to variable cadence, moderately active amputee	Pneumatic-friction knee unit
K-3 and K-4	Variable cadence ambulatory, very active amputee	Fluid-friction knee unit, microprocessor knee

durable which may tear under marked stress. Most transfemoral amputees have a total contact configuration with two socket shapes: **quadrilateral** (ischial-gluteal bearing) or a **narrow mediolateral (ischial containment)** sockets.

a. The original design is the quadrilateral socket. It has four distinct sides with four distinct convexities to promote tendon relief (medial to lateral: adductor, rectus femoris, gluteus maximus and hamstring) with an anterior concavity to protect the sensitive femoral triangle. The majority of weight bearing is accomplished through a posterior horizontal shelf that allows for ischiogluteal support. The anterior and lateral brims are about 3 in. higher dispersing the weight posteriorly sparing the femoral triangle and residual limb. Many amputees have skin irritation over the ischium and pubis, discomfort while sitting, and poor cosmesis.

b. The narrow mediolateral socket is narrower than the anteroposterior side with the ischial tuberoisty contained inside the socket. Most of the weight bearing is directed through the medial aspect of the ischium and inferior pubis ramus. A study by Lee comparing the ischial containment verses quadrilateral socket design showed that the ischial containment socket distributed pressure more evenly, especially on the anterior and posterior socket walls [11]. Amputees prefer the added support and comfort of the narrow mediolateral socket.

C. **AKA Suspension**
   a. Suction Suspension
      - **Total Suction Suspension**: the suction suspension system is the most popular suspension system used. It is ideal for amputees with a mid to long residual femur. This system has a one-way escape valve that forms a snug fit with the residual limb during the stance phase. This system requires a tight fitting socket and a well formed and solid residual limb to maintain a proper fit. This system is recommended for active amputees with good lower extremity muscle strength and good hand dexterity and contraindicated in patients with cardiac conditions or poor balance. This system allows the amputee to ambulate without the need of a cumbersome belt or torso strap.

- **Partial Suction Suspension**: an alternative to the total suction system. The partial suction suspension systems are available for patients with varying limb sizes and who have difficulty donning the prosthesis. This system uses a hyperbaric sock to assist in donning the prosthesis. Since the sock is a potential site for air leakage, the patient requires an additional suspension system (Silesian belt).

b. Belt suspension

Patients may also use a belt suspension to support the socket.

- **Soft Belt Suspension:**
    - The Silesian belt and total elastic suspension are two soft belt suspension system. The Silesian belt rests on the opposite iliac crest. It is easy to don, comfortable, inexpensive and easy to maintain. It is often used when the total elastic suspension doesn't provide enough rotational control. It is not recommend in patients with hip instability and weak abductors, in addition to any skin condition where the belt would rest (scars, grafts, etc.). The total elastic suspension (TES) belt is a neoprene sleeve that encompasses the proximal 8 in. of the prosthesis and then wraps around the waist being connected via Velcro. This suspension system is very comfortable and provides good prosthetic control, however, the neoprene material retains heat and has poor durability. It also tends to slide and rotate with activity.

- **Rigid Belt Suspension:**
    - A rigid belt system is the pelvic band and belt suspension is a single-axis joint that is made of metal or plastic with a leather or fabric strap. This system prevents prosthetic rotation and provides mediolateral pelvic support. This suspension system also allows for the amputee to have a looser socket and tends to be easier to don. It is however heavy and bulky and can interfere with sitting. It is recommended in obese patients, amputees with weak abductors, or short or poorly formed residual limbs.

3. *Knee Disarticulation:*

Amputations through the tibiofemoral joint or through the cortical bone of the distal femur.

Advantages: a long lever arm with intact hip extensors and flexors, a distal weight bearing residual limb and a surgical benefit.

Disadvantages: result of a bulbous socket secondary to the prominent femoral condyles.

Design considerations: The socket design traditionally is made of leather with an anterior buckle or lace to assist in donning the prosthesis. More modern sockets are molded polyester with a window to make the donning process easier. The socket is usually molded to be quadrilateral shaped to minimize rotation. There are multiple interfaces that could be used to maximize patient comfort like gel liners with suction, hyperbaric socks, pneumatic bladders and silicone. Usually a suspension system is not necessary if the socket is snug. The socket does not need to extend to the ischial tuberocity if the residual limb is able to fully weight bear. Patients gain the best functional outcome using a fluid-friction knee unit with a four bar polycentric-axis to ensure knee stability and improve cosmesis during sitting. This polycentric knee-unit also proves to be more functional as it pushes the knee center of gravity more proximally and allows for greater toe clearance during swing phase. It is also better to use a single walled socket to minimize socket width ultimately improving cosmesis.

4. *BKA (Below Knee Amputation):*

   An important concept to ensure comfort and functional improvement in transtibial amputations is to maximize the residual limb contact with the socket to distribute the pressure even, over a larger surface area. In addition, it is important to keep the functional prosthetic unit aligned by having the limb in balance with the socket. This is a achieved using a proper suspension system and having the socket and foot-ankle prosthetic working as a unit. The transtibial prosthesis requires a four part construction: **suspension, socket, shank, and foot-ankle prosthesis**.

   A. BKA Suspension:

   The transtibial suspension system maintains the prosthesis in proper alignment during the swing phase of walking. There are multiple styles of suspension systems that can be tailored to the patients' needs.

   a. Supracondylar Cuff Suspension: the most basic suspension system is a supracondylar cuff. It is an adjustable leather or fabric strap that attaches to the medial and lateral aspect of the socket and secures proximally to the posterior aspect around the femoral condyles and anteriorly it is rests superior to the patella. A supracondylar cuff with fork strap and waist-belt suspension is intended for the more active amputees who need additional support when the leg is not supported by the ground as in mountain climbers or people who climb ladders. The fork strap and waist-belt suspension is easily removable when the extra support is not needed.

b. Brim Suspension System: is a elongation of the socket to extend above the femoral epicondyles. This design is considered in patients with prominent epicondyles who want a prosthetic that is easy to don. One such design is the supracondylar brim suspension that extends medially and laterally to form a firm fit with the femoral epicondyles sparing the patella. A similar design is the suprcondylar/suprapatellar brim suspension which includes an anterior socket margin that encompasses the patella. This type of suspension system is used primarily with short residual limbs for the extra suspension and improved mediolateral knee control.

c. Sleeve Suspension: is used with patients with a well-formed and slender thigh with good hand dexterity. It is constructed of neoprene, latex and other elastic material and used as a primary suspension system or in combination with another suspension system for additional support. It is not used in patients with short residual limbs, poor mediolateral support, and patients who need control with hyperextension.

d. Suction Suspension: uses negative pressure to maintain a snug fit between the residual limb and socket. A silicone lining with an air-leak valve creates a suction seal with the limb when the socket is donned. Suction suspension can be mechanical or electric. The electric design utilizes a miniature electric pump in the distal socket that creates the vacuum seal. It is primarily used in patients with increased prosthetic demands, who have short residual limbs, and whose skin is unable to withstand shear forces. A study by Ferraro found that patients with the vacuum suspension have a lower incidence of predicted future falls, less skin problems and increased activity in comparison to pin suspension [12]. Caution is used in patients with knee stability issues and poor bimanual dexterity.

e. Thigh Corset Suspension: consists of a leather corset that attaches to metal rails on the medial and lateral side of the socket connected by single-axis hinges. This design provides maximal mediolateral support while decreasing the force on the residual limb through transferring weight to the thigh. Some disadvantages of this suspension are that overtime, the thigh muscles atrophy secondary to disuse, it is cumbersome, and is difficult to don.

B. **BKA Socket:**

There are primarily two socket designs used, a patellar tendon-bearing and a total surface-bearing socket.

a. **Patellar Tendon-Bearing Socket (PTB)**: the oldest and most commonly used socket design. A hand molded plaster socket is used to distribute the socket pressures through interior convex bulges over pressure-tolerant areas (patellar tendon, gastrocnemius belly, etc.) of the residual limb sparing the pressure-sensitive areas (fibular head and common peroneal nerve, tibial condyles, and distal ends of the remaining fibula and tibia). A more modern approach is to use computer-aided manufacturing to construct plastic sockets.

b. **Total Surface-Bearing Socket (TSB)**: It is similar to the PTB socket except more pressure is evenly distributed throughout the residual limb by decreasing the anterior convexity that support the patellar tendon. This design decreases skin irritation over the anterior knee. Hachisuka found that patients subjectively preferred the TSB over the PTB socket secondary to its greater comfort, less skin irritation, increased ability to flex the knee, and greater durability. Although this is a much better design, it is less commonly used due to the difficulty attaining a proper fit due to the limbs changing shape. A new addition to the TSB has been a vacuum assisted socket system which has shown to be promising but lacks scientific evidence.

C. **BKA Shank:**

The socket is connected to the ankle-foot prosthetic through a rigid shank that restores leg length and transmits weight from the socket to foot. There are two types of shanks: endoskeletal and exoskeletal design.

a. **Endoskeletal shanks** are metal shafts, usually titanium, called **pylons**. It has adjustable screws to alter the shaft in the frontal and coronal plane to improve the biomechanics of walking. They are usually covered with rubber or other material to resemble skin.

b. **Exoskeletal shanks** are custom made from rigid material (wood or plastic) that are shaped and designed to replicate the preserved skin. Exoskeletal shanks are more durable and cheaper to make, but are unable to be adjusted. More advanced shank systems include shock absorbers and rotators. Shock absorbers may assist people in walking at faster paces [13]. Rotators are commonly used in the avid golfer with the desire to continue golfing.

D. **Foot/Ankle Component:**
   The foot/ankle component is the ground support for the prosthesis. It serves to restore foot shape and provides the necessary functionality for walking. There are two styles of foot-ankle assembly: non-articulated and the articulated prosthetic foot.

a. **Non-Articulated**: the non-articulated or SACH (solid ankle cushion heel) design is the most popular prosthetic foot. It is a simple design which lacks both an ankle joint and moveable parts making it durable, inexpensive and lightweight. The SACH functions best on flat surfaces and does consume energy.

b. **Articulating**: the articulating foot improves foot range of motion but also increases moving parts, which are at risk for breakdown. There is the *single-axis* prosthetic foot and the *multi-axis* prosthetic foot. Single-axis results in improved ankle dorsiflexion and plantarflexion and the multiple-axis provide slight passive motion in all planes (plantarflexion/dorsiflexion, inversion/eversion, and rotation). The single-axis is generally used in active transtibial amputees who ambulate up and down multiple steps/ramps and is also used with transfemoral amputations. The multiple-axis articulating prosthetic foot is preferred in active amputees who are traversing varying surfaces. The multiple-axis tends to be heavier and more expensive.

    c. **Energy-Storing Foot**: the energy-storing foot is used for the K3 and K4 amputees who run, jump and participate in multiple sports. This foot/ankle component stores energy during midstance of the gait cycle and release it during push-off. It has the advantage of conserving overall energy expenditure and allowing the amputee to participate in activities for a longer period of time. There has been numerous studies comparing the energy-storing foot to the SACH, however, the studies are inconclusive regarding clinical effectiveness but many patients prefer the dynamic prosthesis. Unfortunately, the foot/ankle component is expensive and can be difficult to align.

5. *TMA/Partial Foot/Toes:*
Partial-foot prosthetics are used to restore both, functionality and forefoot contour while dispersing weight evenly decreasing focal pressure points. Toe amputations require toe fillers constructed of cork or plastic foam. Depending on the digit amputated, different insoles with arch support are used. For example, small-toe amputations do not drastically affect gait so only toe fillers are necessary and big-toe amputations require the most support since the big-toe is used for push off in the gait cycle.

    A. **Transmetatarsal** amputations (TMA) require a molded socket to prevent pes equinas. The socket attaches to a rigid plantar sole plate which extends distal to the normal toe length. Toe fillers and padding are used to create a leverage to improve toe-off. Alternative design of a thin carbon-fiber plate beneath a custom-molded insole with toe fillers significantly improved gait dynamics by increasing power through toe-off [14].

    B. **Lisfranc** disarticulation is an amputation at the tarsometatarsal joint. This amputation results in loss of the extrinsic toe extensors and the foot is primarily plantar flexed. Patients are best fitted with a custom socket and attached toe filler. In addition, a longitudinal arch support is helpful. Shoes are generally designed with a rocker bar to aid in dorsiflexion and prevent contractures.

    C. **Syme** amputations are transmalleolar amputations where the calcaneal heal pads are attached to the anterior skin to aid in cushioning the residual limb. The patient is left with a limb length discrepancy and they benefit the most from a custom prosthetic. Depending on the patients need, physicians and patients can use a calf socket or a patellar tendon-bearing socket which allows for more weight bearing. Calf sockets have two designs: an elastic socket or a side opening socket. The elastic socket is a streamlined socket that is used for well-shaped distal limbs, and side opening sockets are generally used for bulbous residual limbs due to the ease of donning the prosthetic. There are primarily four syme prosthetic devices used with the sockets described:

a. **Original Syme Prosthesis**: a leather socket, steel side bars and a single-axis prosthetic foot. Not used in clinical practice due to patient discomfort and loss of energy transfer.

b. **Canadian Syme Prosthesis**: plastic socket attached to a modified solid-ankle cushioned heel (SACH). The socket is a two-piece design with a removable posterior panel to allow donning of bulbous residual limbs.

c. **Removable-window design**: similar to the Canadian Syme Prosthesis but the window is on the medial aspect of the prosthetic which allow for increase prosthetic strength in plantar and dorsiflexion.

d. **Flexible posterior build-up Syme Prosthesis**: a non-fenestrated plastic socket that is shaped to fit a streamline distal residual limb. The socket is padded with soft and flexible build-ups to add extra protection. This one-piece design allows for a stronger prosthetic.

UPPER EXTREMITY

1. *Forequarter/Shoulder Disarticulation (F/S D):*
   There are three categories of upper limb prosthetics: ***body-powered***, ***myoelectric***, and ***hybrid*** systems. It is important to consider the prosthetic attachment, socket construction and the materials to ultimately help the patient gain the most function.

   A. F/S D Socket:
   a. **Open frame** design **or closed encapsulated** sockets are used to attach the prosthesis directly to the thorax. The open frame design is made of aluminum, carbon fiber or carbon-reinforced plastic. The frame design serves to stabilize the shoulder and allows for heat dissipation while minimizing weight [15]. The socket design must take into the consideration the

overall motion and use of the prosthetic. The glenohumeral
socket can be shaped using traditional shaping practices.
Although, more modern techniques are employed using laser
surface scanning techniques to maximize socket fit. In addition, adjustments are made through a dynamic trial fitting
procedure [16].

B. F/S D Suspension:
    a. The prosthetic is suspended via a **chest strap** that attaches
       to the *anterior* and *posterior* portion of the socket with a
       waist band.

C. F/S D Control:
    a. **Body-powered** or cable operated systems needs to maxi-
       mize shoulder range of motion to maintain prosthetic
       function. Biscapular abduction controls elbow flexion and
       the terminal device, and shoulder elevation is used for
       elbow locking and unlocking.
    b. A **myoelectric** controlled system is best fitted for a patient
       on a stable platform. This allows for electromyograms to
       maintain proper contact with the residual muscle contrac-
       tions and promote maximal limb control.
    c. The **hybrid** system is combination of both. The patient
       has myoelectric control of the shoulder while using a
       cable-lock mechanism to direct elbow motion. It must
       provide a platform for EMG placement while maintaining
       shoulder range of motion to maximize overall effect.

2. *Transhumeral/Elbow Disarticulation (TH/E D):*
A transhumeral or elbow disarticulation provides a long lever arm
and allows for humeral rotation which accounts for maximum
terminal device control.
  A. **TH/E D Socket**: for transhumeral amputations, a double wall
     construction is utilized. The lateral socket wall extends to the
     acromium, and the medial socket wall flattens out just below
     the axilla. The medial wall flattening prevents inadvertent
     socket rotation. Elbow disarticulation socket construction are
     flat and broad to accommodate for the medial and lateral epi-
     doyldes. A more modern anatomic contoured socket that takes
     the persons residual bone structure into account has proven to
     increase rotational control, decrease need for harnessing,
     increase limb range of motion, and improve overall patient

comfort [17]. For example, compression of the anterior and posterior wall from the mid-humerus to the distal limb improved both, rotational control and flexion/extension [17].

B. **TH/E D Suspension**: the suspension system used in a transhumeral and elbow disarticulation is a figure-of-eight harness or shoulder saddle with chest strap.

C. **TH/E D Elbow Unit**: the elbow unit consists of a hinge and cable system to allow for flexion and extension. An external flexion-locking elbow is used with elbow disarticulations because of space limitations. An internal flexion-locking elbow is used for transhumeral and more proximal prosthetics.

D. **TH/E D Control**: patients are able to control the elbow and terminal device through cables, myoelectrics or a microswitch. The cable activated elbow unit utilizes a two cable system that is controlled through shoulder and scapular motion. If the elbow is locked, activation of the dual cable system controls the terminal device. Myoelectric examples are the Utah Arm and Utah Elbow which controls elbow flexion via biceps activation and elbow extension via triceps. The microswitch-controlled elbows control elbow motion via a push-button or pull switch. Two examples are the Boston Elbow and NY-Hosmer Electric Elbow.

3. *Transradial/Wrist Disarticulation (TR/W D):*
   All patients with upper-limb prostheses with amputation at the wrist or above will use a terminal device. A terminal device can be a passive or active terminal device. Passive devices do not have a functional component and serve primarily for cosmetic purposes. Active terminal devices are intended to replace the prehensile function of the hand. The active terminal devices are shaped into hooks and hands which are voluntary-opening (more common in practice) and voluntary-closing mechanism. Hooks are lighter, more durable, cheaper and far superior for gripping small objects based on the fine control and unobscured visual field.

   A. **Wrist units** are metal devices that attach terminal devices to the prosthetic. Wrist units come in three designs:
       a. **Wrist friction units** fix the terminal device in pronation or supination by friction resistance.
       b. **Wrist flexion units** are generally used with bilateral amputations and are preferred to be on the side of longer residual

limb. They are used for activities midline to the body like brushing one's teach and dressing oneself. A study by Bertels showed that 40° of flexion has proven to be the most comfortable in daily activities. It also has been shown to decrease compensatory movement in the forearm, shoulder and trunk which supports that this is an optimal setup with energy conservation being maximized [18].

c. **Locking wrist units** allow for quick interchange of terminal devices. This is of great use in patients who require multiple terminal devices.

B. **TR/W D Socket**: the socket design of a transradial and wrist disarticulation depends on the residual limb length and suspension system desired. All sockets are a double walled design with the inner wall in direct contact forming a snug fit with the residual limb, and the outer wall is contoured to mimic the length and shape of the contralateral forearm. The socket extends proximally on the posterior aspect to the olecranon and anteriorly to the antecubital fossa. A study by John Miguelez found that patients with wrist disarticulation benefit the most from a contoured flexible thermoplastic suction socket with a micro expulsion valve [19]. The contoured shape in this study provided compression of the interosseous soft tissue capturing supination and pronation and maintaining firm contact with the residual limb through all ranges of motion [19]. They found that patients had better prosthetic function and subjective comfort.

C. **TR/W D Suspension:**
The sockets in transradial and wrist disarticulations are suspended through three different suspension systems: harness-suspended socket design, self-suspended socket design, and a split socket design.

a. The **harness-suspended** socket design is a three-part system that includes the shoulder harness (commonly a figure-of-nine harness) that connects to the upper arm via half-cuff or triceps pad which in turn connects to the socket. The half-cuff pad is generally used in transradial amputations, and the triceps pad is used with amputations distal to and including a long transradial amputations.

• Harness suspension systems are used for both socket support, and to transmit scapular and shoulder motion via a cable system in order to operate the terminal device. There are three common systems used: figure-of-eight, figure-of-nine, and cross-chest strap harness with shoulder straddle. Harness systems are unnecessary with myoelectric controlled or static terminal devices.

- **Figure-of-eight** is the most common harness in upper extremity prosthesis.
- **Cross-chess strap** harness with shoulder straddle is used when the amputee is unable to handle an axillary load or when heavy lifting is required.
- **Figure-of-nine** is used in self-suspending transradial prosthetics that only need to be controlled via cables. This configuration is lighter, more comfortable and provides greater limb range of motion since there lacks a shoulder strap, arm cuff or triceps pad.

  b. A **self-suspended** socket design is a popular design because it is less cumbersome and doesn't restrict shoulder range of motion. Different material like a silicone bladder, latex rubber, elastic sleeve or neoprene attach to different anatomical sites (i.e. suprastyloid, sleeve and supracondylar) to provide a snug fit depending on the length of amputation and if power or range of motion is desired.

  c. A **split** socket design is specifically used in short residual limbs in transradial amputations. They are constructed to be used with a step-up elbow hinge or locking elbow hinge. The residual limb is in total contact with the socket that is connected by hinges to a separate forearm socket that serves to attach to the wrist unit and terminal device (Table 15.4).

Note: Elbow hinges are primarily used in the harness-suspended socket system. A different hinge system is utilized depending on the residual limb length and function.

4. *Partial Hand/Digits:*

Partial hand and digit amputations make up the vast majority of upper extremity amputations. Partial hand and digit prosthetic fitting are used for primarily three reasons: to restore prehensile grip, cosmetic appeal and to protect sensitive areas or fragile areas (neuromas, skin grafts). A cosmetic finger may also provide opposition to an intact first digit. These partial prosthetics used to

Table 15.4 Transradial and wrist disarticulation elbow hinge recommendations

Amputation	Elbow hinge	Function
Wrist disarti- culation—long transradial	Flexible elbow hinge	Preserves voluntary pronation/ supination
Short transradial	Single-axis rigid elbow hinge	Provides stability
Very short transradial —limited ROM	Polycentric rigid elbow hinge or split socket with step-up elbow hinge and locking elbow hinge	Provides increased range of motion

restore grasping function of the hand use static and dynamic configurations. Chris Lake described that physicians and prosthetists should take into consideration four major goals when fitting a patient for a partial hand or digit prosthetic. These are: (1) protection of the residual limb, (2) maintain bimanual mobility, (3) restore prehensile function, and (4) provide a cosmetically appealing hand while maintaining durability [20].

The static partial hand and digit prosthesis are made of a variety of composite rubbers; however polyvinylchloride (PVC) is most common. It can also be made of more rugged material like stainless steel, plastic formed over balsa wood, or lightweight aluminum rods covered with polyurethane foam. The electric controlled prosthetics use a stiff interface that is durable and made of material like prepreg carbon and fiber glass. Silicone is used for its protective role.

PROSTHETICS IN PRACTICE:

In the pages that follow are two prescription templates are two prescriptions templates that physicians may use to communicate effectively and efficiently with their prosthetics team.

UPPER EXTREMITY PROSTHETIC PRESCRIPTION

NAME: _____ DOB: _____ PRACTITIONER: _____

REFERRING M.D./D.O.: _____ PRESCRIBING M.D./D.O.: _____

DIAGNOSIS: _____ AMPUTATION TYPE: _____

PROGNOSIS: _____

FUNCTIONAL: _____

CONSTRUCTION/TYPE OF PROSTHESIS: _____ Endoskeletal _____ Exoskeletal _____

Shoulder Disarticulation: _____ Above Elbow: _____ Below Elbow: _____ Wrist Disartic: _____ Partial Hand: _____

ABOVE ELBOW/SHOULDER DISARTICULATION

BELOW ELBOW

SOCKET:
Test Socket: _____
Shoulder Cap: _____
Double Wall: _____
Flexible Socket: _____
Rigid Frame: _____
Suction: _____

SOCKET:
Test Socket: _____
Double Wall: _____
Triple Wall: _____
Supracondylar: _____
Flexible Socket: _____
Rigid Frame: _____
Split: _____
Suction: _____

ELBOW DISARTICULATION
SOCKET:
Self Suspending: _____

ELBOW HINGE:
Flexible: _____
Single Axis: _____
Polycentric: _____
Step Up: _____
Other: _____

SHOULDER JOINT:
Universal (Flexion/Abduction): _____
Fixed: _____

ELBOW UNIT:
Passive Friction: _____
Internal Lock: _____
External Lock: _____
Manual Lock: _____
Nudge Control: _____
Flexion Spring Assist: _____
External Power: _____
        Utah: _____
        Boston: _____

CUFF:
Triceps Cuff: _____
Triceps Pad: _____

Other: _____

HARNESS:
Figure Eight: _____
Figure Nine: _____
Chest Strap: _____
Fixed Cross: _____
O Ring: _____
Waist Belt: _____
Shoulder Saddle: _____

CONTROLS:
Body Powered: _____
        Single: _____
        Dual: _____
        Excursion Amplifier: _____
Externally Powered: _____
        Pull Switch: _____
        Myoelectric: _____
                Single Site: _____
                Dual Site: _____
        Button Switch: _____
        Proportional Control: _____
Other: _____

WRIST UNIT:
Friction: _____
        Internal: _____
        External: _____
Quick Disconnect: _____
Flexion Unit: _____
Electric Wrist Rotator: _____

TERMINAL DEVICE:
Passive Mitt: _____
Cosmetic Hand: _____
Hook: _____
Voluntary Opening: _____
Voluntary Closing: _____
Greifer: _____
Sleeper: _____
Protective Glove: _____
Other: _____

MISCELLANEOUS:
Stump Socks: _____
Sheaths: _____

LINERS:
Soft Foam: _____
Silicone: _____
        Cushion: _____
        Pre-Fab: _____

Special Features/Instructions: _____

The above prescribed devices are a medical necessity to increase the patient's safety and functional status.

Duration of Necessity: _____

Date: _____ Physician Signature: _____

LOWER EXTREMITY PROSTHETIC PRESCRIPTION

NAME: _____ DOB: _____ PRACTITIONER: _____

REFERRING M.D./D.O.: _____ PRESCRIBING M.D./D.O.: _____

DIAGNOSIS: _____ AMPUTATION TYPE: _____

PROGNOSIS: _____

FUNCTIONAL: _____

CONSTRUCTION: Temporary _____ Permanent _____ Exoskeletal _____ Endoskeletal _____ Adjustable _____

ABOVE KNEE

SOCKET:
Ischial Containment Total Contact: _____
Hip, Knee Disartic: _____
Quad Total Contact: _____
Test Socket: _____
Socket Replacement Only: _____
Flexible Socket & Rigid Frame: _____
Other: _____

MATERIAL:
Thermoplastic: _____
Laminated: _____
Other: _____

SUSPENSION:
Total Suction: _____
Silicone Gel Suction: _____
Semi Suction: _____
TES Belt: _____
Silesian Band: _____
Other: _____

COMPONENTS:
Titanium: _____
Stainless Steel: _____
Carbon Graphite: _____
Other: _____

KNEE JOINTS:
Manual Knee Lock: _____
Polycentric, 4-Bar: _____
Safety, Stance Control: _____
Hydraulic Swing Phase: _____
Pneumatic Swing Phase: _____
Hydraulic SNS: _____
Micro-Processor Control: _____

Ankle-Foot: _____
Light Weight SACH: _____
Single Axis: _____
Bock Dynamic: _____
Greisinger: _____
Multi Flex: _____
College Park: _____
Seattle: _____
Flex Foot: _____
Other: _____

MISCELLANEOUS:
Wool Stump Socket: _____
One Ply Socks: _____
Nylon Sheaths: _____
Stump Shrinker: _____
Other: _____

BELOW KNEE

SOCKET:
PTB, Total Contact: _____
Liner Material: _____
Test Socket: _____
Socket Replacement Only: _____
Other: _____

MATERIAL:
Thermoplastic: _____
Laminated: _____
Other: _____

SUSPENSION:
Cuff: _____
Supracondylar Wedge: _____
Supracondylar/Suprapatellar: _____
Silicone Suction (3S): _____
Custom: _____
Pre-Fab: _____
Elastic Sleeve: _____
Other: _____

THIGH CORSET:
Laced: _____
Velcro: _____
Knee Joint: _____
Other: _____

SYMES/PARTIAL FOOT:
Specify: _____

SHOES:
Orthopedic/Blucher: _____
Sneaker Style: _____
Surgical: _____
High Top: _____
Extra Depth: _____
High Toe Box: _____
Bunion Lasts: _____
Deer Skin: _____
Heel/Sole Lift: _____
Type of Sole: _____
Other: _____

CLOSURE TYPE:
Laces: _____
Velcro Patch: _____
Velcro D-Ring: _____

CUSTOM FOOT ORTHOTICS:
Left: _____
Right: _____
Accommodative: _____
Corrective: _____

MATERIAL:
Plastazote: _____
PPT: _____
Neoprene: _____
Polypropylene: _____
Thermocork: _____
Other: _____

The above prescribed devices are a medical necessity to increase the patient's safety and functional status.

Duration of Necessity: _____

Special Features/Instructions: _____

Date: _____ Physician Signature: _____

References

1. Schuch CM, Pritham CH. International forum—international standards organization terminology: application to prosthetics and orthotics. J Prosthet Orthot. 1994;6:29–33.

2. Gailey RS, Roach KE, Applegate EB, Cho B, Cunniffe B, Licht S, Maguire M, Nash MS. The amputee mobility predictor: an instrument to assess determinants of the lower-limb amputee's ability to ambulate. Arch Phys Med Rehabil. 2002;83(5):613–22.

3. Ziegler GK, Mackenzie EJ, Ephraim PL, Travison TG, Brookmeyer R. Estimating the prevalence of limb loss in the United States: 2005 to 2050. Arch Phys Med Rehabil. 2008;89:422–29.

4. Wild S, Roglic G, Green A, Sicree R, King H. Global prevalence of diabetes. Diabetes Care. 2004;27:1047–53.

5. Dillingham TR, Pezzin LE, MacKenzie EJ. Limb amputation and limb deficiency: Epidemiology and recent trends in the United States. South Med J. 2002;95:875–83.

6. Boulton AJ, Kirsner RS, Vileikyte L. Clinical practice. Neuropathic diabetic foot ulcers. N Engl J Med. 2004;351:48–55.

7. Jensen T, Krebs B, Nielsen J, Rasmussen P. Phantom limb, phantom pain and stump pain in amputees during the first 6 months following limb amputation. Pain. 1983;17:243–56.

8. Jensen T, Krebs B, Nielsen J, Rasmussen P. Immediate and long-term phantom limb pain in amputees: Incidence, clinical characteristics and relationship to pre-amputation limb pain. Pain. 1985;21:267–78.

9. Tan J. Practical manual of physical medicine and rehabilitation. China: Elsevier Inc., 2006. p. 660.

10. Hafner BJ, Smith DF. Differences in function and safely between medical Functional Classification Level 2 and 3 transfemoral amputees and the influence of prosthetic knee joint control. J Rehabil Res Dev. 2009;46(3): 417–33.

11. Lee VS, Solomonidis S, Spence WD. Stump-socket interface pressure as an aid to socket design in prosthesis for trans-femoral amputees—a preliminary study. Proc Inst Mech Eng H. 1997;211:167–80.

12. Ferraro C. Outcomes study of transtibial amputees using elevated vacuum suspension in comparision with pin suspension. J Rehabil Res Dev. 2011;23:78–81.

13. Gard SA, Konz RJ. The effect of a shock-absorbing pylon on the gait of persons with unilateral transtibial amputation. J Rehabil Res Dev. 2003;40:109–24.

14. Tang S, Chen C, Chen M, Chen WP, Leong CP, Chu NK. Transmetatarsal amputation prosthesis with carbon-fiber plate: enhanced gait function. Am J Phys Med Rehabil. 2004;83:124–30.

15. Farnsworth T, Uellendahl J, Mikosz M, Miller L, Petersen B. Shoulder region socket considerations. J Prosthet Orthot. 2008;20:93–106.

16. Farnsworth T. Trial fittings of upper-extremity prostheses. in-Motion. 2001;11:33–5.

17. Andrew J. Transhumeral and elbow disarticulation anatomically contoured socket considerations. J Prosthet Orthot. 2008;20:107–17.
18. Bertels T, Dipl-Ing, Schmalz T, Ludwigs E. Objectifying the functional advantages of prosthetic wrist flexion. J Prosthet Orthot 2009;21:74–9.
19. Miguelez J, Conyers D, Lang M, Dodson R, Gulick K. Transradial and wrist disarticulation socket considerations: case studies. J Prosthet Orthot. 2008;20:118–25.
20. Lake C. Experience with electric prostheses for the partial hand presentation: an eight-year retrospective. Prosthet Orthot. 2009;21:125–30.

Part IV
Additional Diagnostics
and Therapeutics

Chapter 16
Electrodiagnostic Studies

Emerald Lin, Jason W. Siefferman, and Joyce Ho

Tests that are an extension of the physical exam, allowing for objective evaluation of the central and peripheral nervous systems, neuromuscular junctions, and muscles.

Nerve Conduction Studies

Definitions:

Latency—Time between stimulation and recorded response

For Motor, it is the time to waveform onset (change in baseline >2SD of mean)

For Sensory, *peak latency*, or time to maximal negative depolarization, is used

E. Lin, M.D. (✉) • J.W. Siefferman, M.D.
Department of Anesthesiology, The Mount Sinai School
of Medicine, 1 Gustave Levy Place, Box 1010, New York, NY 10029, USA
e-mails: lin.emerald@gmail.com; jsiefferman@gmail.com

J. Ho, M.D.
Department of Anesthesiology and Perioperative Care,
University of California Irvine, 1 Medical Plaza Drive,
Irvine, CA 92697, USA
e-mail: joyceh3@uci.edu

K.A. Sackheim (ed.), *Rehab Clinical Pocket Guide:*
Rehabilitation Medicine, DOI 10.1007/978-1-4614-5419-9_16,
© Springer Science+Business Media, LLC 2013

Amplitude—Voltage recorded over muscle (mV) or nerve (μV). Measured from onset to peak for muscle and either *onset to peak* or *peak to peak* for nerve.

Normal values reported include the mean and two standard deviations (SD).

1. MOTOR NERVE CONDUCTION STUDIES (MNCS)

- **R1** (Black, Active) placed over motor point of muscle
- **R2** (Red, Reference) placed over the distal osseous attachment
- Stimulus is applied with cathode (-) distal and repeated with ↑ current until waveform amplitude is maximized and latency minimized
- The stimulator is then moved to a defined proximal landmark over the same nerve, and stimulation is repeated with R_1 and R_2 unchanged.
  - The distance between the two stimulation points is measured, allowing for calculation of conduction velocity (CV).
- For late responses (i.e., F-wave), the distal stimulus is repeated, but with the cathode and anode reversed (Table 16.1).

2. SENSORY NERVE CONDUCTION STUDIES (SCNS)

- R_1 and R_2 placed **4 cm apart** (to optimize amplitude) along the course of a sensory nerve, R_1 is proximal
- Stimulus is applied with the cathode distal, 10–20 cm proximal to R_1 (varies by nerve)
- Ground is placed between R_1 and the site of stimulus
- Current is slowly ↑ to maximize SNAP without motor artifact if possible
  - Pulse width (duration of stimulation) may be ↑ from 0.1 ms to 0.2 or 0.5 ms to preferentially activate sensory fibers (Tables 16.2, 16.3, 16.4, 16.5).

Pitfalls of NCS & Troubleshooting Tips

- Anomalous innervation or anastomosis may yield false (+) or (-) findings.
- Skin temperature: Goal 30° (lower limbs), 32°C (upper limbs) for reference values
  - ↓Temperature: ↓CV (2.4 ms/s per 1°C), ↑ amplitude, ↑ latency

Table 16.1 Motor nerve landmarks [1, 2]

Nerve	R$_1$ (active)	R$_2$ (reference)	ground	Distal stim	Proximal stim
Median	APB	1st MCP	Dorsum of hand	**8 cm** prox. to R$_1$, between FCR and PL tendons	Medial to biceps tendon
Ulnar	ADM	5th MCP	Dorsum of hand	Ulnar wrist, **8 cm** prox. to R$_1$	*Below elbow:* **4 cm** prox. to med. epicondyle *Above elbow:* **10 cm** prox. to the *below elbow* site
Radial	EIP	5th digit	Dorsum of hand	**6 cm** prox. to lat. epicondyle in groove between brachialis and BR	
Axillary	Deltoid	Acromion	Scapula	Erb's point– just above clavicle lat. to clavicular head of SCM	–
Musculocutaneous	Biceps just distal to midportion	Proximal to antecubital fossa	Postero-lateral shoulder	Erb's point	
Fibular (peroneal)	EDB	5th MTP	Dorsum of foot	Ant. ankle, **8 cm** prox. to R1 slightly lateral to AT tendon	Slightly posterior and inferior to fibular head
Tibial	AH, 1 cm post. & inf. to navicular	1st MTP	Dorsum of foot	Post. to med. mall., **8 cm** prox. to R$_1$	Mid-popliteal fossa

Table 16.2 Sensory nerve landmarks (antidromic) [1]

Nerve	R₁	Stimulus site
Median	Digit 3, proximal phalanx	**14 cm** (**7 cm** for mid-palm)
Ulnar	Digit 5, proximal phalanx	**14 cm**
Dorsal ulnar cutaneous (DUC)	Last web space	**10 cm**
Radial	1st web space	**10 cm**
Medial antebrachial cutaneous (MAC)	**10 cm** distal to stimulus in a line to ulnar styloid	Bisection of biceps tendon and med. epicondyle
Lateral antebrachial cutaneous (LAC)	**10 cm** distal to stimulus in a line to radial styloid	Bisection of biceps tendon and lat. epicondyle
Lateral femoral cutaneous N. (LFCN) [1]	**20 cm** below ASIS	**1 cm** medial to ASIS, above inguinal ligament
Superficial fibular N. (SFN)	1/3 from lat. malleolus to med. malleolus	**14 cm** (ant. aspect of fibula)
Saphenous	Medial edge of tibial, 4 cm above med. malleolus	**14 cm** (med. edge of tibia)
Sural	Posterior to lateral malleolus	**14 cm** (mid calf/just lateral to mid calf)

Table 16.3 Normal values (NCS) for motor nerve landmarks [2]

Motor nerve	Distal latency (ms)	Amplitude (mV)	Conduction velocity (m/s)
Median	≤4.4	≥4.0	≥49
Ulnar	≤3.3	≥6.0	≥49
Ulnar segmental (across elbow) [2]		≤20% drop	≤10 m/s difference
Fibular	≤6.5	≥2.0	≥44
Tibial	≤6.3	≥3.0	≥41

Table 16.4 Normal values (SNCS) for sensory nerve landmarks [1, 2]

Sensory nerve	Peak latency (ms)	Amplitude (μV)
Median	≤3.5	≥20
Ulnar	≤3.1	≥17
Dorsal ulnar cutaneous	≤2.5	≥8
Radial	≤2.9	≥5
MAC	≤3.2	≥5
LAC	≤3.0	≥10
LFCN [1]	≤3.6	≥9.0*
Superficial fibular	≤4.4	≥6
Saphenous	≤4.4	≥4
Sural	≤4.4	≥6

*Measured *peak to peak*

Table 16.5 Late responses [1–3]

	Technique	Normal values	Significance
H-reflex (Tibial)	R$_1$ at bisection between popliteal crease and posterior calcaneus where R$_2$ is placed, cathode at mid popliteal crease	Most subjects: ≤35.1 ms Side–side latency ≤1.5 ms Side–side amp <50% Must normalize for height	S1 nerve roots Electrical correlate of stretch reflex
H-reflex (FCR)	R$_1$ over belly of FCR, usually 1/3 distance from med epicondyle to radial styloid, R$_2$ over BR	Most subjects: ≤18.9 ms Side–side latency ≤1.0 ms	C6,7 nerve roots Electrical correlate of stretch reflex
F-wave	Same setup as MNCS of APB or ADM in UE, or EDB or AH in LE, but **reverse cathode/anode**	≤31 ms median ≤32 ms ulnar ≤56 ms fibular and tibial	Electrical volley to/from anterior horn cells (motor neuron cell bodies)

- Skin impedance: Clean skin, no lotion/cream, may debride skin with alcohol, electrode prep, or sandpaper
- Electrical interference (60 Hz)—Ensure wires are uncrossed, or evenly twisted together, turn off equipment not in use, use dedicated line if possible, may use 60 Hz notch filter.
- Waveform with initial (+) deflection:
  ◦ R_1 may be off motor point
  ◦ Collateral innervation (i.e., Martin-Gruber) if proximal stimulation only
  ◦ Volume conduction to another nerve innervating a muscle near R_1
- Stimulus artifact obscuring CMAP or SNAP onset:
  ◦ Rotate stimulator around fixed cathode
  ◦ ↓ stimulus intensity
- Unable to obtain waveform:
  ◦ Ensure everything is plugged into the correct channel(s)
  ◦ Test stimulator
  ◦ Confirm electrode(s) placement and stimulation site
  ◦ ↑ Current/pulse width (to compensate for thick tissue/edema)
  ◦ ↓ Gain if small waveform
  ◦ Motor—Attempt proximal stimulus, if obtainable, consider anastomosis or anomalous innervation
  ◦ Sensory—Check skin impedance, attempt another nerve
- Timing of injury may also yield false (+) or (−) findings
  ◦ See nerve injury classifications discussed in next section for details.

Electromyography

- Intramuscular needle exam—records electrical activity of muscle fibers
  ◦ Characterizes pathology (muscle vs. nerve)
  ◦ Determine chronicity, severity, recovery
- On the screen: Negative is Up, Positive is Down
- Normal waveform begins with a positive deflection followed by upward deflection followed by a return to baseline, sometimes crossing baseline and peaking above (negative peak) before returning to baseline.

There are four components to the electromyography (EMG) test

1. INSERTIONAL ACTIVITY (Muscle at rest)

- Muscle's response to needle penetration
- **Normal**: discharge lasts **<300 ms**, followed by electrical silence unless in end-plate
- **Increased**: 300–500 ms [4] represents membrane instability and may be abnormal
  - ° Tapping the muscle without moving the needle in an affected muscle will also often produce ↑ discharges compared to an unaffected muscle.
- **Decreased**: <300 ms [4] may occur in fatty, fibrotic, or edematous muscle, or with electrolyte abnormalities
  - ° May also indicate needle not correctly placed in muscle (i.e., connective tissue)

2. SPONTANEOUS ACTIVITY (Muscle must be at rest)

- **Normal**:
  - ° No activity (silent)
  - ° End-plate potentials—seen at NMJ, these regions can be painful
    - ▪ End-plate noise (seashell sounds)
    - ▪ End-plate spikes (similar to fibrillations in that they are narrow complexes but end-plate spikes have initial **Negative** deflection.)
- **Abnormal**:
  - ° **Fibrillation potentials (Fibs)**—initial Positive deflection, "rain on the roof," suggestive of denervation
  - ° **Positive Sharp Waves (PSWs)**—initial positive phase with prolonged negative phase, "dull pop," suggestive of denervation
  - ° **Complex Repetitive Discharges (CRDs)**—"machine gun-like," indicative of chronic denervation
  - ° **Myotonic discharges**—waxing and waning in amplitude and frequency, "dive-bomber," associated with various myotonias
  - ° **Fasiculations**—large irregular MUAP-like units, "pop-corn" [2], axon-mediated, appear like motor units, very slow firing, may be normal or not depending on other findings
  - ° **Myokymic discharges**—rhythmic, clustered, spontaneous repetitive "marching" discharges (grouped fasiculations) [2], classically associated with radiation plexopathy

- ° **Neuromyotonic discharges**—high frequency, decreasing, repetitive discharges, "pinging;" seen in Isaac's syndrome, associated with Myasthenia Gravis, malignancy, inflammatory demyelinating polyneuropathy, familial neuromyotonia [2].
- ° **Cramp discharges**—high frequency repetitive discharges of normal MUAP's, slight irregularity, may be benign (nocturnal cramps, post-exercise) or associated with different neurologic, endocrine or metabolic conditions [2].
- Artifact potentials may also be seen from a pacemaker or external electrical source.
  - ° Very consistent, regularly spaced, nonphysiologic spikes

3. MOTOR UNIT ANALYSIS

- Goal: Assess individual type I motor unit action potentials (MUAP's)
- MUAPs best analyzed with *slight* activation of the muscle.
  - ° If ↑ Activation → recruitment of additional type I units and eventual recruitment of type II units.
  - ° Individual type I MUAPs cannot be analyzed in presence of type II or summated type I MUAPs.
- Sample 4 regions of muscle, and advance needle slowly
  - ° From a distance, MUAP appear broad and have a dull sound, but as you approach, they become more narrow and crisp.
  - ° Normal MU may also look like PSWs or polyphasics from a distance.
  - ° Advance slowly, may tilt needle different directions to localize MU
  - ° Rise time should be <500 μs [4]
- Often difficult for patients to sustain low-level contractions for a long period of time.
  - ° Allow brief periods of rest (Table 16.6)

4. INTERFERENCE PATTERN (IP)

- Maximum voluntary contraction
- **Normal**: full overlap of multiple MUAP with obliteration of baseline

Table 16.6 MUAP analysis normal values [2]

Characteristic	Normal	Long duration, large amplitude (neuropathic)	Short duration, small amplitude (myopathic)
Amplitude	100 µV–2 mV	>4–5 mV	<2 mV
Duration	5–15 ms	Normal or ↑, >15 ms	↓, <5 ms
Phase Count	2–4 or 12–35% polyphasia [3]	Normal/↑ polyphasia	↑ polyphasia
Firing rate	5–20 Hz	Normal/increased	Normal
Recruitment	At 5–10 Hz	Late/reduced	Early

- **Incomplete**: "Picket fence"—Associated with decreased recruitment
    - ° Typically due to neuropathic process
    - ° Normal muscle may appear incomplete due to ↓ activation—either voluntary or involuntary (i.e., pain, stroke).

PITFALLS OF EMG [1]

- Cannot be interpreted in isolation, i.e., Positive findings can help to establish a diagnosis but negative findings do not exclude a diagnosis.
- **Sampling error**
    - ° Area of muscle may be more heavily innervated by one root than another
    - ° Anomalous muscle innervation (prefix/postfix spine)
    - ° Needle may not be in intended muscle
    - ° Too few MUAPs evaluated (goal 20 per muscle)
- **Technical error**
    - ° Type II or summated type I fibers may be mistaken for giant MUAPs
    - ° Distant MUAPs may be mistaken for polyphasia or PSWs
    - ° Background noise/voluntary activity may obscure/appear like spontaneous activity
    - ° Scar tissue may be associated with spontaneous activity
- **Chronology**
    - ° Acute findings may not appear for up to 21 days after nerve injury
    - ° Chronic findings may take up to 3–6 months to appear (Table 16.7)

Table 16.7 Classification of nerve injury (Seddon Classification) [4]

	Neurapraxia	Axonotmesis	Neurotmesis
Etiology	Compression injury	Crush injury	Transection injury
Description	Axon is intact	Axonal interruption	Axonal interruption
	Focal myelin injury	Connective tissue intact	Connective tissue disruption
NCS	Conduction block ↓Amp/↓CV	Conduction failure	Conduction failure
Across lesion	NL	↓Amp/↓CV	↓Amp/↓CV
		↓Amp/↓CV (after >4 days)	↓Amp/↓CV (after >4 days)
Distal to lesion	Recovery with compression release	May see recovery after 5 weeks	No recovery
EMG proximal to lesion	No Fibs, PSW	<2 weeks: NL	<2 weeks: NL
	NL/↓recruit	2–3 weeks: fibs, PSW, ↓recruit	2–3 weeks: fibs, PSW, ↓recruit
EMG distal to lesion	No Fibs, PSW	>4 days: fibs, PSW, ↓recruit	>4 days: fibs, PSW, ↓recruit
	NL/↓recruit	>5 weeks: may see reinnervation	Never reinnervated

Basic Approach to NCS/EMG for UE

NCS

Sensory: Median and ulnar nerve, include radial over superficial radial nerve if suspect radial nerve lesion or C6 lesion
Motor: Median and ulnar nerve (proximal and distal)

EMG

– Evaluate insertional activity, spontaneous activity, voluntary activity with minimal contraction, and interference pattern at maximal contraction, look at recruitment pattern.

Muscles: APB (median, T1 > C8) ADM (ulnar, C8 > T1), radiculopathy screen—usually test deltoid (C5/6, axillary), biceps (C5/6, musculocutaneous), triceps (C6,7,8, radial), FCR (C7 > C6, lateral cord, median), FDI (C8/T1, most distal ulnar), paracervicals (mostly looking for spontaneous activity and giant MUAPs (3–4 mV))

Pearls:
• If APB/FDI (both C8/T1) positive can also test EIP to rule in/out *C8* nerve root.
• *Most common cervical radiculopathy is at the level of C7*: pattern should mostly fit positive findings in triceps and FCR, but not in deltoid, biceps, FDI, or APB.
• *C6*: pattern should mostly fit positive findings in deltoid and biceps, but not the rhomboids or the other muscles mentioned above
• To help isolate a *C5* lesion (if positive findings in deltoid and biceps muscles), test the rhomboids (pure C5).

Basic Approach to NCS/EMG for LE

NCS
Sensory: superficial fibular and sural nerve, may test saphenous for medial leg sensory complaint.
Motor: tibial and fibular nerve (proximal and distal), may test fibular nerve above and below knee for lesion across fibula head, may also test femoral for proximal weakness.

Late responses:

H-reflexes: submaximal stimulus detects and can be first sign of S1 radiculopathy, once abnormal, always abnormal

F-responses: supramaximal stimulus, limited utility except for diffuse/uniform demyelinating disease such as CMT or GBS

EMG

Muscles for radiculopathy screen—tibialis anterior (L4/L5, deep fibular), medial gastrocnemius (*S1*, S2, tibial), VMO (L2-4, femoral), TFL/gluteus medius (L4, *L5*, S1, superior gluteal nerve), gluteus maximus (L5, *S1*, S2, inferior gluteal nerve), lumbar paraspinals (mostly looking for spontaneous activity and giant MUAPs (3–4 mV))

Pearls:

- *Foot drop* has a broad differential (stroke, L5 radic, sciatic injury, fibular nerve injury…)
- *L4 radiculopathy*: pattern should mostly fit positive findings in tibiablis anterior, VMO, TFL/gluteus medius, but not the other muscles in the screen above.
- *L5 radiculopathy*: pattern should mostly fit positive findings in tibialis anterior, TFL/gluteus medius, gluteus maximus, but not the other muscles in the screen above.
- If suspect diffuse **peripheral neuropathy**, must test 3 limbs. May see a pattern of prolonged latencies and slowed conduction velocities in the NCS in addition to decreased amplitude.

Specific Diagnostic NCS/EMG Approach

Radiculopathy

Injury to a spinal nerve root

CC: Dermatomal pain or paresthesias generally radiating from spine to extremity ± myotomal weakness or sensory loss

Pathophysiology:

- Most commonly injury at the neuroforamen due to disc herniation, osseus/ligamentous/synovial hypertrophy, mass, or spondylolisthesis.

Anatomy: Sensory root cell bodies reside within dorsal root ganglion (DRG), just outside neuroforamen; Distal to DRG, roots join to form spinal nerve

PE: Myotomal weakness/atrophy, dermatomal sensory impairment, dermatomal hypo/ hyperalgesia, ↓/absent reflexes, (+) neural tension/ provocative tests such as SLR, Slump test, cross-SLR, Spurling, Shoulder abduction (Bakody)

Study Components:

CERVICAL RADICULOPATHY [5]

NCS:

- Minimum of 1 MNCS (Motor Nerve Conduction Study) and 1 SNCS (Sensory Nerve Conduction Study) in symptomatic limb to determine if other concomitant neuropathy exists.
- MNCS/SNCS—median or ulnar nerve (only one needed to rule out gross peripheral neuropathy)
- May also include:
  - MNCS/SNCS—Both median & ulnar
  - NCS of other nerves such as tibial or fibular nerve if one or more 1+ NCS abnormal or suspect peripheral neuropathy (PN).
  - FCR H-reflex—corroborate pathology of C6 and C7 nerve roots (if suspect C7 radiculopathy)
  - Cervical nerve root stimulation—aid in identifying radiculopathy
  - F-wave—Median and/or ulnar studies in suspected C8 or T1 radiculopathy
- Compare with contralateral side if necessary

EMG:

- Test ≥5 muscles in symptomatic limb covering all myotomes + paraspinals at 1+ levels [6]
- 1–2 muscles innervated by a suspected root and different peripheral nerves.
- If any muscle abnormal, may test 1+ contralateral muscles (Table 16.8)

LUMBAR RADICULOPATHY [8]

NCS:

- Minimum of 1 MNCS and 1 SNCS in symptomatic limb to determine if other concomitant neuropathy exists.
- May include both tibial/fibular MNCS, sural SNCS
- NCS of other nerves if 1+ NCS abnormal or suspect peripheral neuropathy (PN)
- H-reflex (tibial) (↓/absent H-reflex may be early sign of an S1 radiculopathy)

Table 16.8 Cervical muscles by peripheral nerve and spinal root [2, 7]

Muscle	Nerve	C5	C6	C7	C8	T1
Rhomboids	Dorsal scapular	++				
Deltoid	Axillary	++	++			
Biceps	Musculocutaneous	++	++			
Brachioradialis	Radial	++	+++			
Pronator teres	Median		++	++		
FCR	Median		++	+++		
Triceps	Radial		++	+++	+	
EIP	PIN			+	++	
FCU	Ulnar			+	+++	+
FDI	Ulnar			+	++	++
Pronator quadratus	AIN				++	+
APB	Median				++	+++

Table 16.9 Lumbar muscles by peripheral nerve and spinal root [2, 7]

Muscle	Nerve	L4	L5	S1	S2
Vastus M/L	Femoral	++	+		
Fibularis long	Superficial fibular	++	++	+	
Tib. ant.	Deep fibular	++	+		
EHL	Deep fibular	+	++	+	
Biceps fem. L	Sciatic (tibial)		+	++	+
Biceps fem. S	Sciatic (fibular)		+	++	+
Med. gastroc.	Tibial		+	++	+
Lat. gastroc.	Tibial		+	++	+
TFL	Superior gluteal	+	++	+	
Glut. med.	Superior gluteal	+	++	+	
Glut. max.	Inferior gluteal		+	++	++
Piriformis	N. to piriformis			++	++

EMG:

- Test ≥5 muscles in symptomatic limb covering all myotomes + paraspinals at 1+ levels [9]
- 1–2 muscles innervated by a suspected root and different peripheral nerves

Not recommended:

- F-waves of fibular/tibial (low sensitivity)
- Dermatomal/segmental SEP of L5 or S1 dermatomes
- Paraspinal mapping in sacral radiculopathy (Table 16.9)

Diagnostic Criteria:
1. Normal SNCS
2. MNCS may be normal or ↓amplitude
3. EMG findings in 2+ muscles innervated by same nerve root but different peripheral nerves [5]
4. Demonstration of normal muscles above and below the involved root

Other Notes:
- Difficult to diagnose with concomitant peripheral neuropathy
- May be difficult to distinguish from plexopathy in lumbar spine if SNCS technically difficult and (+) posterior rami irritation.
- H-reflexes really only helpful for S1 and C7

Treatment: Please see Musculoskeletal chapter

Lumbar Spinal Stenosis

Multilevel, bilateral radiculopathies

CC: Neurogenic claudication—Burning pain in lower extremities associated with lumbar extension (but may also be with flexion) relieved with flexion (or extension). In vascular claudication, pain does not abate with position change.

Pathophysiology:
- Generally spondylosis resulting in neuroforaminal or central impingement at multiple levels
  - With facet/ligamentum flavum hypertrophy, extension exacerbates
  - With disc herniation, flexion exacerbates
- Vascular supply of nerve roots is compromised
- May also occur with a single central disc herniation catching multiple nerve roots

PE: Loss of lordosis and extension ROM, forward-flexed posture.
± Bilateral weakness and sensory deficits, ↓/absent reflexes, neural tension tests often negative

Study Components: Bilateral radiculopathy study, please see previous section.

Diagnostic Criteria: Multilevel (usually sequential), bilateral radiculopathies

Other Notes: [2]
- May be few/no EMG abnormalities in lumbosacral Spinal Stenosis (SS) since symptoms may be intermittent→ insufficient compression for denervation
- In elderly may be difficult to differentiate mild chronic distal polyneuropathy from mild chronic bilateral L5–S1 radiculopathies (due to age-related changes in NCV and SNAP)
- DDx: peripheral neuropathy, chronic arachnoiditis, vascular claudication, amyotrophic lateral sclerosis (ALS)

Treatment:
- PT: manual therapy, walking, core strengthening [10]
- Surgery: case-dependent
- Medication: limited evidence for any drug

MONONEUROPATHIES

NOTE: Mononeuropathies are not limited to those listed below. If a lesion does not fit any of the descriptions below, consider other possibilities.

Median Nerve Pathology

Carpal Tunnel Syndrome

Focal compression of the median nerve at the wrist within the carpal tunnel

CC: Paresthesias and dysesthesias in median hand distribution with pain which may radiate proximally, often worse at night, associated with manual labor, thumb weakness

Pathophysiology: May be due to repetitive stress injury. Compensatory hypertrophy of lumbricals (attach to flexor tendons → encroach into tunnel) and tendons within carpal tunnel. Other associations include DM, hypothyroidism, RA, and pregnancy.

Anatomy:
- Course: from anterior wrist, median n. courses beneath palmaris longus (PL) and FCR tendons
- *Ten structures in the carpal tunnel*: Tendons (4 FDS, 4 FDP, FPL) & median n.
- Sensory: only the digital sensory branch travels through tunnel
  - Palmar nerve: thumb to middle finger and radial half of ring finger
  - Palmar cutaneous branch (palm sensation) arises BEFORE entering carpal tunnel
- Motor: 2**LOAF**—Lumbricals 1&2 (2), **O**PB, **A**PB, and **F**lex pol. brev. (superficial half only)

PE: Sensory deficits as in CC, weakness in APB (thumb abduction in plane perpendicular to palm), (+)Tinel's over carpal tunnel, (+) Phalen's; no signs of radiculopathy

Study Components:
NCS:
- Median SNCS on symptomatic side, if abnormal:
- Ipsilateral ulnar or radial SNCS, AND one of the following:
  - Median/Ulnar cross-wrist SNCS (7 cm) comparison
  - Ringdiff (SNCS to ring finger for median/ulnar comparison, 14 cm)
  - Thumbdiff (SNCS to thumb for radial/median comparison, 10 cm)
  - Median mid-palmar SNCS at 7 cm with median wrist SNCS at 14 cm
- Median MNCS, and if abnormal: ipsilateral ulnar MNCS

EMG (optional):
- May consider APB or OPB to differentiate neurapraxia from axon loss, evaluate for ongoing axon loss (spontaneous activity), and recovery
- May also consider radiculopathy screen if concerned about a second pathology (*double crush*), or if SNCS was normal

Diagnostic Criteria: (see Tables 16.10, 16.11)
- Abnormal median MNCS or SNCS across the carpal tunnel, including comparison studies [11]
- Abnormal EMG of APB or OPB (optional)

Table 16.10 Carpal tunnel syndrome diagnostic criteria [11]

Median/ulnar MNCS dL	>1.2 ms
Thumbdiff	>0.5 ms
Ringdiff	>0.4 ms
Mid-palmar: wrist stimulation	<1:2 ratio
Median/ulnar cross-wrist	>0.4 ms

Table 16.11 Grading of carpal tunnel syndrome [11]

Grade	Motor	Sensory	EMG
Mild	Normal	Prolonged (>4 ms)	Normal
Moderate	Prolonged (>4.5 ms)	Prolonged	Normal
Severe*	Low amplitude (<5 mV) or Absent	Low amplitude (<10 μV) or absent	Axon loss

*Findings only required in one category to be designated *severe*

Notes:

- Martin-Gruber anastomosis (MGA, motor fibers only) may cause false (+) in ↓ CMAP/impression of axonal loss
  - ○ ↓ CMAP at the APB from the wrist but not the elbow
  - ○ (+)deflection from elbow stimulation, due to activation of ulnar fibers
  - ○ Falsely ↑ conduction velocity
- C6 or C7 radiculopathy may clinically mimic sensory symptoms of carpal tunnel syndrome (CTS)
- Similar findings may occur after wrist injury/distal forearm fracture, and should be differentiated from CTS.

Treatment: [12]

- Evaluation and medical management of underlying medical condition if present
- NSAIDS, topical or oral
- Neutral wrist splint limiting MCP extension (to induce lumbrical atrophy)
- Corticosteroid injection
- Surgical release by hand surgeon (most effective long term) [8]
- Conservative treatment of choice in pregnancy (symptoms expected to resolve after delivery)

Anterior Interosseus Nerve (AIN)

Motor branch of the median n. (with deep sensory, not cutaneous innervation)

CC: Weakness in hand, may complaint of "achy" wrist

Pathophysiology: Trauma or compression syndrome

Anatomy:
- Course: Branches off from median n. distal to pronator teres (spared)
- Sensory: no cutaneous
- Motor: Radial ½ of FDP, FPL, and PQ

PE: Focal weakness in flexion of DIP of thumb and index finger, wrist pronation, (+) OK sign, no sensory deficits, must rule out compartment syndrome

Study Components: [2]

NCS
- Median MNCS/SNCS similar to study components for CTS
- Median MNCS with needle pickup at PQ

EMG
- 1+ of following: PQ, FPL, FDP
- Upper extremity screen to include distal median muscles and muscles innervated by same cervical root (C8) to exclude median neuropathy and/or C8 radiculopathy

Diagnostic Criteria:
Focal EMG findings in anterior interosseus nerve (AIN) muscles in setting of normal routine median NCS

Note: MGA with AIN may also have hand findings

Treatment: [13–15]
- Relative rest (avoidance of pain-producing activities: elbow flexion, wrist pronation, and grasp)
- Medications (NSAIDs)
- Immobilization for 7–10 days
- Progressive stretching and strengthening of elbow flexors, wrist flexors and pronators, and grip exercises
- If no interval improvement seen in 6–8 weeks, consider surgical decompression. However, may recover spontaneously up to 12 months after onset of symptoms.
- Tendon transfer indications vary with level of injury, quality of motor return, functional needs, surgeon preference.

Radial Nerve

CC: Weak grasp, sensory change to posterior arm/forearm/dorsal radial hand including thumb, index, middle, and radial half of ring fingers

Pathophysiology: injection, compression (crutches, honeymooner's, arcade of *Frohse*, wristwatch/handcuff), RA, Monteggia fracture, lead poisoning

Anatomy: [2]

- Innervation: all 3 trunks of brachial plexus from C5–T1 → posterior cord becomes the radial nerve after the axillary nerve branches off
- Course: posterior cord in high arm → posterior cutaneous and lower lateral cutaneous n. of arm, posterior cutaneous n. of forearm → triceps and anconeous→ spiral groove → BR, long head of ECR, supinator at arcade of Frohse →distal to lateral epicondyle → bifurcates into superficial radial n (thru extensor retinaculum) and posterior interosseus (PIN) (see below)
- Sensory: posterior arm and forearm, dorsal hand to thumb and digits 2, 3, radial half of 4th not including fingertips
- Motor: three heads of triceps and anconeous, BR, long head of ECR, supinator

PE:

- *Crutch compression*—weakness in all radial n. innervated muscles, weak grip due to loss of tenodesis, sensation changes over posterior arm/forearm/dorsal hand as above
- *Spiral groove compression*—sparing of triceps and anconeous (EE), weak elbow flexion in neutral position, wrist drop, weak WE/FE, weak grip due to loss of tenodesis, sensation changes over posterior arm/forearm/dorsal hand as above
- *Superficial radial compression*—pure sensory abnormalities in dorsal hand only as above

Study Components:

  NCS

- Radial SNCS on symptomatic side, if abnormal:
  - Contralateral radial SNCS
  - Thumbdiff (thumb for radial/median SNCS at 10 cm)
  - Radial MNCS to EIP and/or triceps

EMG
- Screen including EIP/BR/triceps and other muscles innervated by same nerve roots (especially C7 but different peripheral nerves, i.e., median innervated FCR)

Diagnostic Criteria: [2]

Spiral groove: ↓/absent radial SNAP, ↓amp distal radial CMAP to EIP, normal MNCS to triceps, EMG findings in all radially innervated muscles except for triceps/anconeus

Axilla: ↓superficial radial SNAP, ↓amp distal and proximal radial CMAP to EIP/triceps, EMG findings in all radially innervated muscles including triceps/anconeus

Other Notes: many lesions produce wrist drop: PIN, radial neuropathy at spiral groove, axilla; posterior cord brachial plexus lesion, C7 radiculopathy, CNS lesion [2]

Treatment: [16]
- Occupational therapy
- Cock-up wrist splinting for tenodesis to ↑hand function
- Surgical release of compression
- Tendon transfer

Posterior Interosseus Nerve (PIN)

Motor branch of the radial n. (deep sensory only)

CC: Wrist and finger weakness with sparing of elbow extension, some people complain of elbow pain

Pathophysiology:
- Trauma, compression
- May be seen with lateral epicondylitis–entrapment at Arcade of Frohse

Anatomy:
- Course: Bifurcation proximal to supinator, courses under Arcade of Frohse
- Sensory: no cutaneous
- Motor: ECRB, supinator, EDC, EDM, ECU, APL, EPL/B, EIP

PE:
- Focal weakness, typically of wrist extension ulnar more than radial direction due to **ECRL sparing**

- Normal EE, normal EF in wrist neutral position
- No cutanenous sensory deficits

Study Components:
   NCS
   - Radial MNCS to EIP, if abnormal, contralateral MNCS to EIP
   - Radial SNCS

   EMG
   - Minimum of 2 of PIN muscles as listed above
   - Upper extremity screen to include BR/triceps and other nonradial muscles for radial neuropathy and/or possible C7 or C8 radiculopathy

Diagnostic Criteria: Abnormal radial MNCS to EIP, focal EMG findings in PIN muscles only, normal radial SNCS
Treatment:
- Partial denervation: low lesion—buddy splint
- Surgical release of entrapped nerve at Arcade of Frohse [15]

Ulnar Nerve

CC: *Cubital tunnel*: numbness along ulnar hand, weak grasp
Guyon's canal: weak grasp and tingling in pinky and ring finger
Pathophysiology: trauma, compression (cycling), RA, tardy ulnar palsy
Anatomy:
- Course: from C8, T1 → lower trunk → medial cord→ ulnar n.→ Arcade of Struthers→ retrocondylar groove between medial epicondyle and olecranon → cubital tunnel → DUC branches off → Guyon's canal
- Sensory: recurrent branch comes off before Guyon's canal and innervates the hypothenar area, superficial branch continues within Guyon's canal to supply finger sensation (5th digit, ulnar ½ 4th digit)
- Motor:
   ○ Forearm (FCU, ½ FDP); branch to FCU may arise prox. or distal to cubital tunnel

○ Hypothenar branch passes through Guyon's canal to supply hypothenar muscles, deep motor branch also passes through Guyon's canal to supply almost all hand muscles other than LOAF (median), with FDI being the last muscle supplied.

PE: Weak hand, interosseus wasting, radially deviated wrist flexion, ulnar claw hand, (+) Froment's sign, (+)Wartenberg's sign, (+)Tinel's at cubital tunnel or at ulnar wrist (Guyon's canal)

Study Components: [17]

NCS
- Ulnar SNCS at 14 cm
- Ulnar MNCS ulnar to ADM at wrist, below and above elbow
  ○ Elbow flexed 70–90°
  ○ Approximately 10 cm between stimulation sites across elbow
  ○ Consider inching to localize lesion
- If ulnar SNCS/MNCS abnormal, perform NCS of other nerves to exclude a diffuse process
- If ulnar MNCS inconclusive, repeat MNCS with pickup at FDI

EMG
- FDI and 1+ additional ulnar innervated muscles distal to suspected lesion
- Non-ulnar C8/medial cord/lower truck muscles to exclude brachial plexopathy
- Cervical paraspinals to exclude C8/T1 radiculopathies

Diagnostic Criteria:
- **Cubital tunnel**: Abnormal ulnar MNCS/SNCS including DUC SNCS, 10 m/s ↓in CV across elbow, 20% ↓ in amplitude or CV, or CV < 50 m/s; EMG findings in ulnar innervated muscles below and above wrist
- **Guyon's canal study**: Abnormal ulnar MNCS/SNCS but normal DUC SNCS, normal EMG findings in ulnar innervated muscles below but not above wrist

Other Notes: Normal DUC does not completely rule out proximal ulnar neuropathy

Treatment: [18, 19]

Conservative:
- If mild–moderate neuropathy with intermittent/persistent sensory loss and weakness without wasting; mod–severe but stable neuropathy <6 month duration; (for reference moderate is conduction block on NCS); or older/less healthy patient

- Biomechanical modification of daily activities
- Guyon's canal: neutral position wrist brace
- Cubital tunnel: Soft foam/towel wraps to keep elbow straight at night

Surgery:
- If persistent weakness and numbness >6 month, refractory to conservative therapy, moderate–severe findings on EMG/NCS, or mod–severe progressive signs and symptoms, younger/ healthy patient
- Ulnar nerve decompression or transposition

Lateral Femoral Cutaneous Nerve/Meralgia Paresthestica

CC: Numbness, tingling, or burning in lateral thigh(s)
Pathophysiology: compression by repeated low-grade trauma, belt, pannus, pregnancy, tight clothing; may be associated with obesity, DM, tumor, infection.
Anatomy:
- Course: Direct nerve from L2, L3 roots, passes over iliacus towards anterior iliac spine and through inguinal ligament
- Sensory: Lateral thigh
- Motor: none

PE: Causes of nerve compression, sensory deficit in the lateral thigh, no motor abnormalities
Study Components:
  NCS
  - SNCS of lateral femoral cutaneous nerve (LFCN) bilaterally (may perform above or below inguinal ligament)
  - May consider other SNCSs and/or MNCSs if LFCN SNCS abnormal to exclude other processes (plexopathy, peripheral neuropathy)

  EMG (optional)
  - L2/3 innervated muscles to r/o radiculopathy [4]
    - (Iliacus, Gracilis, Adductor longus, Vastus medialis, TA)
    - Paraspinals

Diagnostic Criteria: Abnormal LFCN SNCS
Other notes:
- Difficult to obtain a response on a normal individual
- Normal EMG findings help to rule out more serious etiologies (i.e., lumbar radiculopathy, plexopathy, diabetic amyotrophy)

Treatment: [20]
- Most resolve spontaneously
- Looser clothing and/or weight loss
- Gabapentin (or other neuropathic agents), NSAIDs for pain
- Nerve blockade, corticosteroid injection
- Surgical release

Sciatic Nerve [21]

CC: Leg weakness, numbness/tingling, pain in buttock radiating down leg, foot drop
Pathophysiology: Compression, trauma, iatrogenic (hip replacement), piriformis entrapment, pregnancy; compression at pelvic outlet preferentially affects fibular component
Anatomy: [4]
- Course: L4, L5, S1, S2 S3 nerve roots→ lumbosacral plexus→ exit pelvis through greater sciatic foramen as sciatic n. proper (tibial and fibular divisions) → bifurcates into tibial and common fibular nn.
- Motor (thigh):
  - Tibial division: hamstrings (long head of biceps femoris (LHBF), semitendinosis, semimembranosis, half Adductor magnus)
  - Fibular division: short head of biceps femoris (SHBF)
- Sensory: Lateral calf (superficial fibular n.), dorsal (deep fibular n.) and plantar foot
PE: Weakness/sensory loss in sciatic distribution, preserved quad strength, and patellar reflex. Piriformis synd. aggravated by FADIR
Study Components:
  NCS
  - MNCS ipsilateral tibial & fibular, may compared with contralateral
  - SNCS ipsilateral sural & SFN, may compared with contralateral
  - Bilateral tibial H-reflexes

EMG
- Tibial and fibular innervated muscles below and above knee (i.e., Short Head of the Biceps Femoris (SHBF) is innervated by Common Fibular nerve above the knee; Fibularis Longus is innervated by Superficial Fibular nerve below the knee, Medial Gastrocnemius is innervated by tibial nerve below the knee).
- 1+ muscle innervated by L5/S1 nerve roots outside sciatic distribution (i.e., for L5: gluteus medius and TFL; S1: gluteus maximus) to exclude plexopathy and radiculopathy
- L5/S1 paraspinals to exclude radiculopathy

Diagnostic Criteria:
- Abnormal fibular and/or tibial MNCS (especially fibular)
- Abnormal Sural/SFN SNCS (especially SFN) with normal saphenous SNCS
- Prolonged H-reflex compared to contralateral side
- Abnormal EMG of tibial and fibular innervated muscles below and above knee
- Normal EMG of low lumbar paraspinals and non-sciatic muscles innervated by L5/S1 nerve roots

Other notes:
- Need to differentiate from radiculopathy, plexopathy
- May only see evidence for fibular n. injury, even though it occurs in the sciatic n. (more susceptible to injury than tibial portion)
  - SHBF is helpful in confirming sciatic injury and ruling out radiculopathy (since it is a branch of the sciatic as the common fibular nerve) in these cases

Treatment:
- Rehabilitation concentrating on lower legs including hamstrings and piriformis
- Surgery to release entrapment

Fibular Nerve/Foot Drop

CC: foot drop with changed sensation over lateral calf and dorsum of foot

Pathophysiology: Usually occurs at fibular neck, associated with trauma, stretch, compression, surgical positioning, and crossing legs

Table 16.12 Clinical localization of injury in footdrop [2]

			DFN	CFN	Sciatic	LS plexus	L5
Weakness	Ankle	Dorsiflexion	+	+	+	+	+
		Eversion		+	+	+	+
		Inversion			+	+	+
	Knee flexion				+	+	+
	Hip abd/ext					+	+
Sensory	1st web space		+	+	+	+	+
loss	Dorsum of foot			+	+	+	+
	Lateral calf			+	+	+	+
	Lateral knee				+	+	+
	Sole of foot				+	+	+
	Post. thigh					+	+
Tinel's	Fibular neck		+	+	+		

Anatomy:[2]
- Course: L4-S1 nerve roots→ lumbosacral plexus→ sciatic n. (FIBULAR division) → Common Fibular N. (CFN) to posterior of fibular head → bifurcates into Deep and Superficial Fibular NN. (DFN, SFN) → DFN dives deep and bifurcates into medial and intermediate dorsal cutaneous nn. of foot
  - 15–20% have accessory fibular n. which runs posterior to lateral malleolus
- Motor: DFN: fibularis tertius, TA, EDL, EHL, EDB
  SFN: fibularis longus and brevis
- Sensory: DFN: webspace between 1st and 2nd toes
  SFN: mid- and lower lateral calf, dorsum of foot except 1st webspace

PE: Tenderness and (+)Tinel's over fibular neck, weak DF/eversion, decrease/absent sensation as described above, compensatory gait (hip hike or circumduction). **See Table 16.12**.

Study Components: [2]

  NCS
- MNCS DFN with pickup over EDB or AT stimulating behind fibular head and lateral popliteal fossa
- SNCS SFN (orthodromic and/or antidromic)
- 1+ additional MNCS & SNCS to demonstrate lack of other abnormalities

EMG
- SHBF, 1+ DFN, and 1+ SFN muscles
- 1+ non-fibular sciatic muscle (**also see Table 16.9**)

Diagnostic Criteria: [22]
- Abnormal NCS limited to CFN, DFN, or SFN
- Abnormal EMG in 2+ muscles innervated by CFN, DFN, or SFN
- Normal findings in non-fibular muscles of the same spinal roots

Other Notes
- Abnormal SHBF will rule out a lumbar radiculopathy
- Most common mononeuropathy of LE
- CFN injury occasionally found in popliteal fossa, most commonly by Baker's cysts [23]
- Consider other causes of foot drop: brain injury, SCI, L4/5 radiculopathy, LS plexopathy, diffuse diabetic polyneuropathy, nerve infarctions due to mononeuropathy multiplex [23] (see chart below).

Treatment: Surgical release (if indicated) [4, 23] and rehabilitation

Tibial Nerve/Tarsal Tunnel Syndrome (TTS)

CC: Pain and numbness in foot/big toe, perimalleolar, burning, worse with weight-bearing or at night

Pathophysiology: Tibial n. entrapment underneath flexor retinaculum of medial ankle (tarsal tunnel). Usually trauma, degenerative bone, or connective tissue disorder.

Anatomy: [4]
- Course: Tibial n (L4–S2) → posterior tibial n. (at soleus) → post. to medial malleolus → below flexor retinaculum through tarsal tunnel (with FHL, FDL, TP, a, v) → distal tibial n. → splits into calcaneal sensory n. and plantar n.
- Sensory: Calcaneal sensory n.: sole
  - Medial plantar n.: medial 3 ½ toes
  - Lateral plantar n.: 1/2 4th and 5th toes
- Motor: Medial plantar n.: AH, FHB, FDB
  - Lateral plantar n.: abductor digiti minimi pedis (ADMP)

PE: Decreased sensation on sole, normal ankle tendon reflex and sensation over sural and SFN distribution, possible intrinsic foot muscle atrophy, (+)Tinels over tarsal tunnel.

Study Components: [2, 24]
  NCS
  - MNCS bilateral tibial with pickup over AH and ADMP
  - SNCS bilateral Medial/lateral plantar mixed

  EMG (limited usefulness, optional) [24]
  - AH or ADMP
  - Distal tibial-innervated muscles proximal to tarsal tunnel

Diagnostic Criteria: [24]
- Prolonged DL in tibial MNCS
- Prolonged PL/slow CV in medial/lateral plantar mixed NCS
- Slow CV across TT and/or ↓/absent SNAP in medial/lateral plantar SNCS

Specific Pitfalls:
- Significant technical difficulties: may need needle pickup for SNCS
- Intrinsic foot EMG may be (+) in normal or related to aging
- Difficult to diagnose in setting of other neuropathies

Treatment: [23]
- Footwear: reduce compression, use orthotics
- NSAIDs, topical or oral
- Corticosteroid injection
- Surgical tarsal tunnel release

Polyneuropathy

- Large spectrum of systemic neuropathy with multiple presentations and etiologies
- Important to determine the primary process, therefore detailed H&P is important

Pathophysiology:
- Axon, myelin, or vascular supply of peripheral nerves may be affected
- May be due to inflammatory, autoimmune, paraneoplastic, metabolic, endocrine, or other systemic process

PE: Document pattern of weakness and sensory loss, reflexes, absence of UMN signs, and use thorough ROS to guide exam. Presentations variable (see Table 16.13)

Table 16.13 Clinical patterns of polyneuropathies [2, 7]

Symmetric*	Weakness	Sensory loss	Considerations	Examples
Yes	Diffuse	Yes	Inflammatory demyelinating neuropathy	Acute/chronic inflammatory demyelinating polyradiculoneuropathy (AIDP/CIDP)
Yes	Distal	Yes	Hereditary motor and sensory neuropathy (HMSN), metabolic disorders, toxic	Charcot-Marie-tooth disease (CMT), DM, uremia
No	Distal	Yes	Mononeuropathy multiplex: vasculitis, sarcoidosis, infection, multifocal acquired demyelinating motor, and sensory neuropathy (MADSAM), hereditary neuropathy with liability to pressure palsies (HNPP)	HIV, DM, herpes zoster, lyme, leprosy
No	Distal	No	Motor neuron disease, multifocal motor neuropathy (MMN)	ALS
No	Diffuse	Yes	Polyradiculopathy or plexopathy related to DM, tumor infiltration, idiopathic	DM
Yes	None	Distal loss	Metabolic, toxic, infection, anti-MAG associated neuropathies, idiopathic	DM, HIV
Variable	Variable	Sensory ataxia	Paraneoplastic, Sjogren's syndrome, toxic, idiopathic sensory	Anti-Hu, sulfa, vitamin B6 toxicity, cisplatin, etoposide, antinucliosides
Significant autonomic involvement			DM, amyloidosis, GBS, porphyria, idiopathic autonomic neuropathy	

*Symmetry may not be exact

Study Components: [2, 25]

Goal: Determine the pattern of involvement of functional fiber types (motor, sensory, autonomic) to narrow the differential (see Tables 16.13, 16.14)

NCS (for most PN)
- SNCS: bilateral sural and unilateral ulnar; optional bilateral SFN
- MNCS: bilateral fibular, bilateral tibial, unilateral ulnar, possibly unilateral median
- F-waves: bilateral fibular, unilateral ulnar
- Consider autonomic responses [26]

EMG
- 1+ distal and 1+ proximal muscles in bilateral LE and unilateral UE
- Paraspinals ↑ increase sensitivity

Diagnostic Criteria: (see Tables 16.13, 16.14)

Classify based on:
- Diffuse vs. Focal
- Proximal vs. Distal
- Generalized vs. Segmental
- Sensory vs. Motor vs. Sensorimotor
- Axonal vs. Demyelinating
- Presence of autonomic involvement
- Symmetric vs. asymmetric (Symmetric not necessarily perfectly symmetrical).

Definitions:
- Demyelination: NCV < 70% lower limit, varying degrees of conduction blocks, may see PSWs, fibrillation potentials if secondary axonal loss present on EMG
- Axonal: ↓ in CMAPs/SNAPs, signs of denervation on EMG

Other Notes:
- Small sensory and autonomic fibers not well tested by NCS
- Skin punch biopsy may be helpful for diagnosis [27]
- Additional reference on diabetic polyneuropathy [25]

Treatment:
- Treat underlying condition
- Skin care to prevent complications
- Dysesthesias:

Table 16.14 Electrodiagnostic patterns of polyneuropathies [7]

Symmetric demyelinating sensorimotor

Uniform demyelination	*Segmental demyelination*
HMSN 1,3,4, metachromatic leukodystrophy, Krabbe's globoid leukodystrophy, adrenomyeloneuopathy, Tangier's disease, cerebrotendinous xanthomatosis, Cockayne's syndrome, Refsum's disease	HNPP, AIDP, CIDP, MMN, MADSAM, leprosy, diphtheria, HIV, Lyme, Lymphoma, Castelman's disease, Osteosclerotic myeloma, Waldenstrom's macroglobulinemia, monoclonal gammopathy of undetermined significance (MGUS), acromegaly, hypotheyroidism, post-portocaval anastomosis

Symmetric axonal

Sensory>motor	*Mixed sensorimotor*	*Motor>sensory*
Hereditary sensory & autonomic neuropathies (HSAN I-V), Friedrich's ataxia, spinocerebellar degeneration, vit E deficiency, abetalipoproteinemia, ataxia telangiectasia, AIDP Fischer variant, remote effects of cancer- anti-Hu syndrome, Sjogren's syndrome, idiopathic, other complications of systemic disease	Hereditary: HMSN 2, spinocerebellar ataxia	HMSN 2, porphyria, AIDP (acute motor axonal neuropathy (AMAN)), vasculitis, Toxic: hexa carbon inhalation, amiodarone, chloroquine
	Vasculitic: polyarteritis nodosa (PAN), Churg-Strauss, SLE	
	Endocrine: acromegaly, hypotheyroidism	
	Nutritional deficiencies: B1, B12, folate	
	Infectious: HIV, Lyme	
	Other systemic: amyloidosis, paraprotein-related neuropathies, sarcoidosis, COPD	
Toxic: anti-nucelosides, vincristine	Toxic: ETOH, pharmaceuticals-phenytoin, nitrofurantoin, amitriptyline, chemotherapeutics, industrial agents, metals	
	AIDP (acute motor-sensory axonal neuropathy (AMSAN))	
	Chronic idiopathic	

Symmetric mixed demyelinating and axonal sensorimotor	
DM, Uremia, CIDP, paraproteinemic polyneuropathies	
Asymmetric sensorimotor	
Demyelinating	Axonal
AIDP, CIDP, MMN, HIV	PAN, SLE, atherosclerotic vascular disease
Compression neuropathy	Drug-induced
DM, Neoplastic/Granulomatous infiltration	HIV, CMV, Lyme, Herpes zoster, Hep B/C

- ○ Gabapentin 300 mg po qhs, progress to tid and titrate as tolerated for effect (max 3,600 mg/day)
- ○ Duloxetine 30 mg po daily, may increase to 60 mg after 2 weeks
- ○ Memantine 5 mg po qhs, increase to 10 mg after 2 weeks
- PT for weakness, balance, gait training as indicated

Plexopathy

CC: weakness, sensory complaints, dysesthesias (see Table 16.15)
Pathophysiology: Trauma, inflammatory, compression
Anatomy: C5–T1 nerve roots → 3 trunks (Upper, middle, lower) → 6 divisions (3 anterior, 3 posterior) → 3 cords (lateral, posterior, medial) → 5 major terminal nerves
(Musculocutaneous, axillary, radial, medial, ulnar)
PE: See following diagnosis-specific subsections and Table 16.15.
Study Components: (depends largely on where the suspected lesion is)
Brachial Plexus:

NCS
- Upper trunk: axillary MNCS, Musculocutaneous MNCS, radial MNCS/SNCS, median SNCS to thumb, LAC SNCS on both affected and unaffected sides as well as ulnar SNCS and either median or ulnar MNCS on affected side
- Middle trunk: radial MNCS/SNCS, median SNCS, H-reflex on both affected and unaffected sides as well as median MNCS and/or ulnar MNCS/SNCS on affected side
- Lower trunk: median, ulnar MNCS/SNCS/F-waves, MAC SNCS on both affected and unaffected sides
- Lateral cord: musculocutaneous MNCS, median/LAC SNCS, median H-reflex on both affected and unaffected sides as well as ulnar SNCS and either median or ulnar MNCS on affected side
- Medial cord: median/ulnar MNCS/SNCS/F-waves, MAC SNCS
- Posterior cord: axillary MNCS, radial MNCS/SNCS

EMG
- Upper trunk: 3+ muscles innervated by C5/6 nerve roots and different peripheral nerves including serratus anterior/rhomboids, latter expected to be **normal** (long thoracic n. and dorsal

Table 16.15 Brachial plexopathies [2, 28]

Lesion	Major contributions	Muscle involvement	Common SNCS abnormalities	Notes
Panplexus	All	All (SA & rhomboids spared)	All	Sparing of SA & rhomboids indicates plexus >> root [2]
Upper trunk (UT)	C5/C6	Supraspinatus, infraspinatus, teres minor, deltoid, BR, biceps, brachialis, triceps, PT, FCR, ECR (Erb's palsy, Stinger (transient), Rucksack palsy)	Median/radial (thumb), LAC (lateral forearm)	Sparing of SA & rhomboids separates plexus vs. root pathology [2] Rehabilitation, intermittent splinting, activity restriction [4]
Middle trunk (MT)	C7	PT, FCR, triceps, anconeus, ECR, EDC, EIP	Median/radial (index and middle fingers)	Sparing of serratus anterior separates plexus vs. root pathology [2]
Lower trunk (LT)	C8/T1 → ulnar n.	APB, FPL, PQ, EIP, EPB, ECU, FDI, ADM, ADP, FDP (ulnar), FCU (Klumpke's palsy)	Ulnar (little finger), MAC (medial forearm)	Rehabilitation with incomplete lesions or surgical exploration with avulsion [4]
Lateral cord	MCN, C6/7 part of median n.	Biceps, brachialis, PT	Median (thumb, index and middle fingers), LAC (lateral forearm)	
Posterior cord	All roots → radial, axillary, TD n.	Ld, deltoid, teres major and minor, triceps, anconeus, BR, ECR, EDC, EPB, ECU, EIP	Radial (all)	Must differentiate from complete radial palsies
Medial cord	Extension of anterior division of LT from C8/T1	APB, OP, FPL, FDI, ADP, ADM, FCU, FDP (ulnar)	Ulnar (little finger), MAC (medial forearm)	Very similar to LT pathology with exception of intact radial C8 fibers

SA serratus anterior, MCN musculocutaneous, TD thoracodorsal

scapular n. come directly off roots), additional muscles similar to a cervical radiculopathy screen to exclude other diagnoses

- Middle trunk: Same as a C7 radiculopathy screen including serratus anterior, which is expected to be **normal** (long thoracic n. come directly off roots)
- Lower trunk: Same as a C8/T1 radiculopathy screen
- Lateral cord: 3+ muscles innervated by C5/6 nerve roots and different peripheral nerves including supraspinatus or infraspinatus, latter expected to be **normal** (suprascapular n. exits before formation of lateral cord at trunk level), additional muscles similar to a cervical radiculopathy screen to exclude other diagnoses
- Medial cord: Same as a C8/T1 radiculopathy screen including ≥1 muscle innervated by C8/radial such as EIP, which is expected to be **normal**
- Posterior cord: Same as a cervical radiculopathy screen including ≥2 muscles innervated by radial and axillary nn and ≥1 muscle not innervated by posterior cord
- For all: Paraspinals at level, and one level below/above

Lumbosacral Plexus: [2]

NCS

- Lumbar plexus: (roots L1–L4), MNCS and SNCS of obturator and femoral nn., SNCS LFCN./saphenous n.
- Lumbosacral plexus: (roots L4–S2 (S3)), MNCS and SNCS of sciatic n-tibial and peroneal, SNCS of sural and superficial peroneal nn

EMG

- Lumbar plexus: L1-L4 (radic screen for upper roots, i.e., ≥5 muscles for each limb)
- Lumbosacral plexus: L4-S2 (S3) (radic screen for lower roots)
- Paraspinal muscles (L2–S1).

Diagnostic criteria:

- Abnormal NCS corresponding to site of injury
- Abnormal EMG in same muscles as abnormal NCS
- Normal paraspinal EMG helpful, but not required

Treatments: see Table 16.15 and following sections

Parsonage Turnor/Brachial Plexitis

Also called neuralgic or brachial amyotrophy
CC: Sudden onset of shoulder pain with significant weakness, followed by muscle atrophy [2]
Pathophysiology: Unknown, often occurs after activation of immune system or surgery, often onetime event/self-limited; if recurrent, may be hereditary [28]
Anatomy: Varied involvement of brachial plexus, usually unilateral; predisposition to pathology in: **Long thoracic, Suprascapular, Axillary, AIN** [2, 29]
PE: Shoulder girdle weakness, sensory loss, scapular winging, dysmorphic features
Diagnostic criteria: Spontaneous activity in long thoracic, AIN, axillary, and/or spinal accessory n., along with other findings of brachial plexopathy [4]
Treatment: [4, 28]
• May resolve spontaneously
• PT for ROM and positioning to prevent contracture

Radiation Plexopathy

CC: Progressive, usually PAINLESS weakness with parasthesias in arms. May occur during, a few weeks after, or many years after radiation therapy. Usually slowly progressive [28, 30].
Pathophysiology: Unclear, likely microvascular ischemia and soft tissue fibrosis. Most commonly associated with treatment for breast cancer [29, 30].
Anatomy: Predilection for upper trunk [4] and lateral cord [28].
PE: Muscle fasciculations, deltoid & biceps weakness, sensory loss, edema
Other notes:
• **Myokymic discharges** and fasciculations common
• Must rule out direct invasion from recurrent tumor

Treatment:
• Transient type: Short course of corticosteroids [30], usually self-limited

- Delayed type: No established treatment, some evidence for anticoagulants [30–32]
- TENS or dorsal column stimulator [30, 33]

Thoracic Outlet Syndrome (TOS)

CC: Arterial: limb ischemia/necrosis, vague pain/fatigue, cold
Venous: bluish, swollen, and achy
Neurogenic: pain and numbness along ulnar forearm and hand, intrinsic wasting.
Pathophysiology:
- Neurogenic type: Entrapment of brachial plexus during exit from shoulder and axilla into arm
- Vascular type: compression of subclavian and axillary vessels
- Fibrous band from cervical rib to first thoracic rib entrap lower trunk (esp. **T1**)

Anatomy: Outlet borders: 1st rib, 1st thoracic vertebra, clavicle, sternum and space between anterior & middle scalenes [34]
PE:
- **Weak APB** > hand intrinsics, C8/T1 sensory impairment
- Cervical rib, first rib, muscle hypertrophy (scalene), fibrous bands
- (+)Adson's, (+)Wright's hyperabduction, (+)Roos, (+)Costcoclavicular tests

Study Components:
- MNCS & SNCS Ipsilateral Median/ulnar
- SNCS Bilateral MAC
- EMG to include APB

Diagnostic Criteria: [2]
- Abnormal ulnar and MAC SNAPs, relative sparing of median SNAP
- Abnormal median CMAP, relative sparing of ulnar CMAP
- Abnormal EMG in C8/T1 innervated muscles, worse in the median distribution
- Normal EMG in lower cervical paraspinals

Specific Pitfalls: May be confused with ulnar neuropathy at or above elbow, plexopathy involving medial cord, or C8/T1 radiculopathy
Treatment:
- Rehabilitation focusing on ROM, stretching, strengthening of scapular stabilizers, postural mechanics to open up area of compression [4, 35, 36]
- Resection of cervical rib, release of fibrous bands [4] (but risk of iatrogenic plexopathy) [35]

Diabetic Amyotrophy

Also known as proximal diabetic neuropathy/plexopathy, or femoral neuropathy [37]
CC:
- Initial severe pain deep in pelvis/proximal thigh, worse with movement
- Pain later resolves leaving only weakness, primarily in hips/quads (LE>>UE/thoracic involvement)
- Weight loss, difficulty climbing stairs, usually bilateral [37, 38]
Pathophysiology: debatable: one theory—abnormality of vaso-nevorum; more common with DM2, unrelated to duration of insulin insensitivity
Anatomy: Affects combination of upper lumbar roots and peripheral nerves (femoral, obturator, fibular) [38], therefore often called a radiculoplexopathy [2]
PE: Weakness/atrophy of anterior and medial thigh muscles, ↓/absent knee jerk, minimal sensory loss in L2-L4 distribution
Study Components:
- MNCS of b/l LE: consider femoral and fibular or tibial n.
- SNCS of b/l LE: saphenous, fibular, sural
- EMG similar to LE radiculopathy screen

Diagnostic Criteria: Variable findings in NCS, EMG [28]
- Axonal loss >> segmental demyelination [39]
- NCS: markedly ↓CMAP (tibial and fibular n) and SNAP (sural n), with CV mild slowing [40]
- EMG: denervation initially in proximal muscles and paraspinals.
- Distal and bilateral involvement likely to develop a few months after disease onset

Specific Pitfalls:
- May coexist with other neuropathies, such as diabetic polyneuropathy, making diagnosis difficult. May be difficult to differentiate from: [38]
- A mild, primarily axonal, length-dependent sensorimotor polyneuropathy
- Mononeuropathies at typical sites of compression (i.e., CTS)
- Thoracic/high lumbar radiculopathy: increased fibs and PSW in corresponding paraspinals

Other Notes:
- Onset in distal leg is not uncommon
- In nearly all cases, progresses to involve contralateral and distal LE's [38]
- Spontaneous partial improvement common

Treatment: Nothing proven [38]
- Glucose control
- Neuropathic pain treatment

Neuromuscular Junction Disorders

CC: Weakness and easy fatigability of proximal, bulbar, and/or extraocular muscles without mental fatigue, motor control deficits, or sensory complaints

Pathophysiology:
- Myasthenia Gravis (MG): Anti-ACh receptor antibody binds postsynaptically
- Lambert Eaton Myasthenic Syndrome (LEMS): Antibody binds to presynaptic voltage-gated Ca^{2+} channel (VGCC), preventing ACh release
  - Paraneoplastic usually Small Cell Lung CA; immunoglobulin cross-reactivity
- Botulism: Toxin cleaves SNAP-25/Synaptobrevin/Syntaxin protein preventing presynaptic vesicles from fusing with terminal button and releasing ACh
- Congenital: Defective synthesis/packaging of ACh, or deficiency of ACh receptors

Table 16.16 Neuromuscular junction disorders—clinical [4, 28, 41]

	Myasthenia gravis (MG)	LEMS	Botulism
Location	Post-synaptic	Pre-synaptic	Pre-synaptic
PE	Easy fatigability	Predilection for LE's	Respiratory (vital capacity), bulbar weakness (dysphagia), generalized paralysis, low resting heart rate, and decreased HR variation
	Usually symmetric, proximal: eyes droop with prolonged upward gaze	Worse with rest, improves with exercise: viselike grip	
	Bulbar: nasal speech, oromotor weakness, dysphagia		

Anatomy: Calcium influx → migration and fusion of vesicles in nerve terminals, releasing ACh into synaptic cleft. Post-synaptic ACh receptors allow influx of Na^+ and muscle contraction.

PE:
- Proximal >distal fatigability and weakness (see Table 16.16).
- MG: "Ice bag" test for ptosis—apply ice over frontalis for 4–5 min → may improve dramatically [2].

Study Components: [42, 43] (**see Table 16.17**)
- MNCS of nerves on which Repetitive Nerve Stimulation (RNS) will be performed, if abnormal additional MNCS to evaluate for other processes
- SNCS of nerves on which RNS will be performed if available, otherwise, SNCS in adjacent nerves

RNS for MG (based on presentation):
- Limb-axial: Trapezius, ADM, and/or other affected muscles
- Bulbar: Anconeus and Nasalis
- Orbicularis oculi more controversial

RNS to be performed under the following settings:
- Anticholinesterase medications withheld 12 h prior to testing, if can be done safely
- Immobilization of limb when possible
- Frequency of stimulation between 2 and 5 Hz

- Baseline and immediate post-exercise or post-tetanic 2–5 Hz nerve stimulation followed by stimulation at regular intervals of 30–60 s, and continuing to 5 min.
- Maintain skin temperature over recording site as close to 35°C as possible

Single Fiber (SFEMG):
- If normal RNS, SFEMG of 1+ symptomatic muscle should be performed
- If 1st SFEMG normal but high clinical suspicion → study 2nd muscle.

SFEMG under the following conditions:
- Acceptable muscle fiber potentials: amplitude >200 mV, rise time <300 μs
- Abnormal if >10% of fiber potential pairs exceed normal jitter, have impulse blockade, and/or mean jitter exceeds normal limits

Other Notes: RNS of ADM easiest but least sensitive, facial muscle most sensitive but technically difficult [43]
Diagnostic Criteria and Treatment: Please see Table 16.17

Motor Neuron Disease

Amyotrophic Lateral Sclerosis [2]

Degenerative, progressive, usually sporadic, occasionally hereditary, affects both upper and lower motor neurons (UMN, LMN), characteristically in the same myotome, many variants
CC: Insidious weakness in distal extremity, some with sensory complaints
Pathophysiology: unknown, UMN and LMN affected.
PE: Weakness, spasticity and/or flaccidity, UMN and LMN signs (hyper- or hyporeflexia), normal sensation
Study Components: [2]
Role of NCS/EMG is to help establish the LMN component and exclude other diagnoses [45]
  NCS:
  - MNCS/F-waves of unilateral median, ulnar, tibial, and fibular (more symptomatic side)
  - SNCS of unilateral median, ulnar, and sural

Table 16.17 Neuromuscular junction disorders—electrodiagnostic [4, 44]

Test	Parameter	Myasthenia gravis (MG)	LEMS	Botulism
MNCS	Distal latency	NL	NL	NL
	Amplitude	NL	↓/borderline	↓/absent
	Conduction velocity	NL	NL	NL
SNCS	Peak Latency	NL	NL	NL, ↓ sympathetic skin responses [41]
	Amplitude	NL	NL	NL
RNS (1)	2–5 Hz	Reproducible >10% decrement in CMAP when comparing 1st to 4th or 5th response in 1+ muscle	Reproducible >10% decrement in CMAP when comparing 1st to 4th or 5th response in 1+ muscle	Reproducible >10% decrement in CMAP when comparing 1st to 4th or 5th response in 1+ muscle
RNS (2)	2–5 Hz post-exercise or post-tetanic stim for 10 s (facilitation)	Repair of decrement to, or close to, baseline	Reproducible ↑ Amp ≥100% of baseline	May or may not have repair of decrement
RNS (3)	2–5 Hz post-exercise or post-tetanic stim for 60 s	>>10% decrement in CMAP	>>10% decrement in CMAP	>>10% decrement in CMAP
EMG	Spont. Activity	NL	NL	Fibs, PSW
	MUAP	NL/unstable MUAP's	NL/unstable MUAP's	Acute: NL/unstable MUAP's
				Chronic: ↑D↑A MUAP's
	Interference Pattern	NL/↓IP, early recruitment	NL/↓IP, early recruitment	Acute: NL/↓IP, early recruitment
				Chronic: ↓recruitment, ↑firing

(continued)

Table 16.17 (continued)

Test	Parameter	Myasthenia gravis (MG)	LEMS	Botulism
SFEMG		↑fiber density, ↑jitter, blocking	↑fiber density, ↑jitter, blocking	↑fiber density, ↑jitter, blocking
Diagnostic Criteria		Reproducible >10% decrement in CMAP when comparing 1st to 4th or 5th response in 1+ muscle in RNS(1) Repair of decrement to, or close to, baseline in RNS(2)	Reproducible ↑ Amp [3]**100%** of baseline in RNS(2)	Reproducible >10% decrement in CMAP when comparing 1st to 4th or 5th response in 1+ muscle in RNS(1) with denervation on EMG
Treatment		Thymectomy, anticholinesterase drugs (edrophonium), corticosteroids, immuosuppressive agents, plasmapheresis, rehabilitation	Treat malignancy, corticosteroids, immusuppressive agents, plasmapheresis, guanidine	Supportive Botulism antitoxin (types A, B, E) blocks toxin in circulation only

- Bilateral tibial H-reflexes
- Consider contralateral MNCS

EMG:
- 3+ limb muscles, including distal and proximal, with different nerve and root innervations
- 3+ mid-thoracic paraspinals (to avoid cervical or lumbar roots)
- Bulbar muscles: 1–2 of tongue, masseter, SCM, or facial

Diagnostic Criteria: Signs of denervation and reinnervation. Please see neuromuscular chapter for further details.
Specific Pitfalls:
- DDx: cervical or lumbar stenosis, PN, NMJ d/o
- Craniobulbar findings eliminate spinal etiology

Treatment: see neuromuscular chapter
- Riluzole—glutamate inhibitor; only medication to enhance survival [46]
- Symptomatic management of respiratory, dysarthria, nutritional, musculoskeletal, pain, pseudobulbar, and fatigue; psychosocial counseling [47]

Post-poliomyelitis Syndrome [4]

CC: Muscle and joint pain, fatigue, weakness especially in previously affected muscle groups, 25–30 years after acute polio
Pathophysiology: Unknown, likely due to combination of normal aging process with perpetually denervated muscles
PE: Diffuse asymmetric weakness with LMN findings (atrophy, fasciculations) [48]
Study Components: Varies upon other differentials, consider macro/surface EMG
Diagnostic Criteria:
- NCS/EMG primarily used to rule out other pathologies since cannot differentiate between history of polio and post-polio syndrome [4, 49]
- EFNS task force report criteria [50]
  - Prior episode of poliomyelitis with evidence of residual motor neuron loss

- ○ Period of ≥15 years after acute onset of polio with neurologic and functional stability
- ○ Gradual (rarely abrupt) onset of new weakness & abnormal muscle fatigability for ≥1 year
- ○ Rule out other medical conditions that cause similar symptoms

Other notes: Frequently have signs of chronic motor neuron loss in clinically normal areas (↑MUAP Amp and duration) [48].
Treatment: Primarily symptom mgmt. and supportive [48, 51, 52].
- Orthotic management for muscle weakness, pain and joint instability.
- Non-fatiguing strengthening exercises using low-intensity sessions with short reps lasting several seconds and alternating rest intervals [52].

Myopathy

CC: Weakness with muscle atrophy or hypertrophy, may also see: [4]
- Muscle stiffness, cramping, myalgias
- Decreased reflexes, hypotonia, paresthesias
- Myotonia—painless delay in muscle relaxation after voluntary contraction

Categories:
- Muscular dystrophies (Duchenne, Becker, Emery-Dreifuss, etc.)
- Inflammatory (polymyositis, dermatomyositis, inclusion body myositis)
- Infectious (HIV, toxoplasmosis, trichinosis)
- Endocrine-associated (thyroid, adrenal, parathyroid)
- Drug induced/Toxic (steroids, alcohol, colchicines, AZT, clofibrate, statins)
- Metabolic (glycogen or lipid storage, mitochondria metabolism, enzyme deficiency)
- Congenital (central core, nemaline rod, centronuclear myotubular, etc., based on bx)
- Periodic Paralysis (hypo/hyperkalemia, assoc. w/proximal vacuolar myopathy)

Pathophysiology: most genetic, autoimmune, or drug induced

Anatomy: Affects skeletal muscle fibers, some types affect cardiac muscle (mitochondrial), pathology affects different areas along pathway/feedback loops of energy breakdown to energy consumption/intracellular energy production

PE: Evaluate for:

- Proximal vs. distal weakness
- Myotonia, hypotonia
- Sensory loss, hyporeflexia
- Specific features:
    - *Dermatomyositis*: heliotrope sign (upper eyelid discoloration), Gottron papules (extensor MCPs/PIPs), alopecia, erythematous patch on face, chest
    - *Myotonic dystrophy*: hatchet facies, frontal balding, mental retardation
    - *Steroid*: cushingoid (buffalo hump, acanthosis nigricans, cataracts)
    - *Hypothyroidism*: myxedema, dry skin, loss of hair

Study Components: [2, 4]

- NCS: motor and sensory, upper and lower extremity
    - If ↓ CMAP, do 10 s max exercise & repeat 1 distal muscle
    - If h/o fatigability, do RNS of 1 proximal and distal muscle
- EMG:
    - At least 2 proximal and 2 distal muscles in the UE and LE (unilateral)
    - 1+ Paraspinal
- May consider:
    - Quantitative MUAP analysis: average 20 MUAPs from single muscle
    - Single-Fiber: To r/o NMJ d/o if EMG and RNS normal
- Leave one side untouched for biopsy (to avoid EMG myopathy)

Diagnostic Criteria: [2, 4, 53–55] see Table 16.18. Biopsy and genetic testing often required to define exact process. Biopsy should be taken from untested side to avoid needle artifact.

Other Notes:

- Differentials include motor neuron disease (MND), motor neuropathies (paraneoplastic), NMJ d/o, CNS lesions (i.e., ant. watershed zone "Man in a barrel")

Table 16.18 Myopathies [2, 4, 53–55]

Myopathy	Distribution	NCS sensory	NCS motor	EMG spontaneous	EMG myotonia	EMG recruitment	EMG MUAP	Labs
Inflammatory								
Polymyositis	P[a]	NL	NL	Fib/PSW, CRD	P	Early	↓D↓A	↑CK, LDH, aldolase
Dermatomyositis	P[a]	NL	NL	Fib/PSW, CRD	(+)	Early	↓D↓A	↑CK, LDH, aldolase
Inclusion body	D (quads, FDP)	NL/↓A	NL/↓A[b]	Fib/PSW, CRD	(−)	NL/Early/Reduced	↓D↓A or ↑D↑A	↑CK
Sarcoid m.	P>D (diaphragm)	NL[b]	NL[b]	Fib/PSW	(−)	Early	↓D↓A	↑CK
Infectious								
HIV-associated m.	P	NL/↓A[b]	NL/↓A[b]	Fib/PSW	(−)	Early	↓D↓A	NL
Dystrophies (non-myotonic)	P[a]	NL	NL/↓A	Fib/PSW, CRD (rare)	(−)	Early	NL/D↓A	↑CK, aldolase
Myotonic dystrophy	D[a]	NL	NL/↓A	Fib/PSW, CRD (rare)	D	Early	↓D↓A	NL/↑CK, ↑FSH
Myotonia congenita	P&D[a]	NL	NL	NL	P&D	NL	NL	NL CK
Drug/Toxic m.								
Alcohol m.	P[a] (quads, gastrocs)	NL[b]	NL[b]	Fib/PSW	(−)	Early	↓D↓A	↑CK, myoglobinuria
Statin m.	P	NL[b]	NL[b]	NL/Fib/PSW	(+/−)	Early	↓D↓A	↑CK
Steroid m.	P (hips)	NL	NL	NL/Fib/PSW	(−)	NL/Early	NL/D↓A	NL CK
Critical Illness m.	P (neck, face)	NL	↓Amp	Fib/PSW	(−)	NL/Early	↓D↓A	↑CK
Congenital	P	NL	NL	Fib/PSW	P&D	Early	NL/D↓A	NL CK
Pompe Dz	P (LE)	NL	NL	Fib/PSW, CRD	P (paraspinal)	Early	↓D↓A	↑CK
Endocrine								
Hypothyroid m.	P	NL[b]	NL[b]	NL[b]	(+)	NL/Early	NL/D↓A	↑CK, ↑TSH

NL normal, *D* distal, *P* proximal, *D↓A* short duration low amplitude polyphasic, *↑D↑A* long duration high amplitude polyphasic

[a]Possible cardiac involvement

[b]Possible concomitant neuropathy

- ↓D↓A MUAP may also be seen with NMJ d/o and terminal axon d/o's
- Nascent MUAP's units in non-myopathies are also polyphasic, ↓D↓A

Electrodiagnostic Reports

Example of the electrodiagnostic report:
1. List findings
2. Give your impression of the best fitting unifying diagnosis. Look for a pattern. Do not over diagnose. Sometimes there may be abnormal findings due to superimposed chronic problems or technical errors.
3. A patient may have more than one finding, i.e., a double crush syndrome.

Upper Extremity Report (Sample)

Motor Nerve Conduction Study:
The bilateral median and ulnar nerves displayed normal/prolonged distal latencies, normal/decreased amplitudes, and normal/slowed conduction velocities.
Sensory Nerve Conduction Study:
The bilateral median and ulnar nerves displayed normal/prolonged peak latencies and normal/low amplitudes.
Late Responses:
The median F-waves showed normal/prolonged latencies and did (not) display significant differences from side to side.
Needle Electromyography Exam:
Muscles tested innervated by roots C5–T1 displayed (no) abnormal electrical activity. Describe any abnormal electrical activities.
IMPRESSION:
(ESSENTIALLY) AB/NORMAL ELECTRICAL STUDY.
THERE IS
- NO ELECTRICAL EVIDENCE OF…
- ELECTRICAL EVIDENCE MOST CONSISTENT WITH…
- INSUFFICIENT ELECTRICAL EVIDENCE TO DIAGNOSE…

Example diagnoses:

- CERVICAL RADICULOPATHY (acute, chronic, subacute) (bilateral/unilateral) (multilevel)
- PERIPHERAL NEUROPATHY (diffuse vs. focal, axonal vs. demyelinating, primarily affecting the upper/lower limbs).
- ULNAR NEUROPATHY at the level of (the ulnar groove, consistent with cubital tunnel)
- RADIAL NEUROPATHY at or distal to the level of the (spiral groove)
- MEDIAN NEUROPATHY at the level of the wrist consistent with CTS

Lower Extremity Report (Sample)

Motor Nerve Conduction Study:
The bilateral tibial and fibular nerves displayed normal/prolonged distal latencies, normal/low amplitudes, and normal/slowed conduction velocities.

Sensory Nerve Conduction Study:
The bilateral superficial peroneal and sural nerves displayed normal/prolonged peak latencies and normal/low amplitudes.

Late Responses:
The tibial H-reflex performed bilaterally displayed normal/prolonged latencies with (no) significant side to side variability.

Needle Electromyography Exam:
The right/left-sided muscles tested innervated by the tibial, fibular, femoral, superior/inferior gluteal nerves and supplied by roots L2–S2 displayed (no) abnormal electrical activity.

IMPRESSION:
(ESSENTIALLY) AB/NORMAL ELECTRICAL STUDY.
THERE IS

- NO ELECTRICAL EVIDENCE OF…
- ELECTRICAL EVIDENCE MOST CONSISTENT WITH…
- INSUFFICIENT ELECTRICAL EVIDENCE TO DIAGNOSE…

Example diagnoses:

- LUMBOSACRAL RADICULOPATHY (acute, chronic, subacute) (bilateral/unilateral) (multilevel)

- PERIPHERAL NEUROPATHY-(diffuse vs. focal, axonal vs. demyelinating, primarily affecting the upper/lower limbs)
- SCIATIC/TIBIAL/FIBULAR NEUROPATHY at or distal to the level of ___

General rules:
- NCS/EMG is an extension of the physical exam
- If you have one abnormal finding that is not consistent with a diagnosis, you can state "the isolated finding of ___ may be consistent with ___"
- Remember NCV/EMG helps to rule *in* a diagnosis but if you obtain a negative study it does NOT rule out the diagnosis.
- Remember patients may have more than one finding, i.e., double crush.

Billing

Some physicians bill for a separate consultation for the history and physical examination. However, it should be noted that physicians billing that way may only be reimbursed for either the consultation or the procedure, but not both. Appeal letters from AANEM position statement may help [56–58] (Tables 16.19, 16.20, 16.21, 16.22, 16.23, 16.24, 16.25, 16.26).

Table 16.19 NCS–LIMB [57, 59]

CPT	Description/requirements
95907	1-2 nerve conduction studies
95908	3-4 nerve conduction studies
95909	5-6 nerve conduction studies
95910	7-8 nerve conduction studies
95911	9-10 nerve conduction studies
95912	11-12 nerve conduction studies
95913	13 or more nerve conduction studies

A single conduction study is defined as a sensory conduction test, a motor conduction test with or without an F- wave test, or with or without an H-reflex test. Each type of NCS is counted only once when multiple sites on the same nerve are stimulated or recorded.

The numbers, i.e., quantity of these separate tests should be summated to decide which code to use, as the unit of service in NCS codes is now equivalent to the *number of NCS performed*.

Table 16.20 Reflexes [57]

CPT	Description/requirements
95933	Orbicularis oculi (blink) reflex, by electrodiagnostic testing

It is assumed 95933 is always done bilaterally so there is no need for modifier

Table 16.21 Needle EMG (done on the same day as NCS) [56]

CPT	Description/requirements
95885	Limited extremity EMG, in combination with NCS
95886	Complete extremity EMG, in combination with NCS
	– Minimum 5 muscles (may count paraspinal(s) as one limb muscle)
	– 3+ peripheral nerves or 4+ spinal levels
95887	Non-extremity EMG, in combination with NCS

May bill multiple units for *limited* and/or *complete* extremity (max 4)
Each limb not meeting complete criteria count as 1 U of *limited* extremity

Table 16.22 Needle EMG (if not done on the same day as NCS) [57]

CPT	Description/requirements
95860	1 Extremity with or without related paraspinal areas
95861	2 Extremities with or without related paraspinal areas
95863	3 Extremities with or without related paraspinal areas
95864	4 Extremities with or without related paraspinal areas
95870	Limited study of muscles in one extremity or non-limb (axial) muscles (unilateral or bilateral), other than thoracic paraspinal, cranial nerve supplied muscles, or sphincters

Minimum 5 muscles per limb (may include paraspinal(s) as one limb muscle)
Must evaluate at least 3 peripheral nerves or four spinal levels per limb
Each limb not meeting these criteria count as 1 unit of 95870
Modifier 59 designates additional limbs as distinct extremities

Table 16.23 Needle EMG–OTHER [57]

CPT	Description/requirements
95867	Cranial nerve supplied muscle(s), unilateral
95868	Cranial nerve supplied muscle(s), bilateral
95869	Thoracic paraspinal muscles (excluding T1 or T12)

1 unit max

Table 16.24 Neuromuscular junction EMG [57]

95872	Needle electromyography using single fiber electrode, with quantitative measurement of jitter, blocking and/or fiber density, any/all sites of each muscle studied
95937	Neuromuscular junction testing (repetitive stimulation, paired stimuli), each nerve, any one method

Table 16.25 Chemodenervation guidance [57]

CPT	Description/requirements
95873	Electrical stimulation for guidance in conjunction with chemodenervation
95874	Needle electromyography for guidance in conjunction with chemodenervation

Bill multiple units if more than one contiguous body part is involved
List separately in addition to code(s) for chemodenervation (64612-64614)
Codes 95873 and 95874 should not be billed with EMG codes 95860-95870
Codes 95873 and 95874 should not be billed together

Table 16.26 Chemodenervation [57, 59]

CPT	Description/requirements
64612	Chemodenervation of muscle(s); innervated by facial nerve
64613	Chemodenervation of muscle(s); neck
64614	Chemodenervation of muscle(s); extremity and/or trunk
64615	Chemodenervation of muscle(s); muscle(s) innervated by facial, trigeminal, cervical spinal and accessory nerves, bilateral

Bill 1 unit per code regardless of number of injections or muscles
If bilateral, use Modifier 50
May bill more than one code, using Modifier 51 for 2nd and 3rd procedure(s)

References

1. Buschbacher RM. Manual of nerve conduction studies. New York, NY: Demos; 2000. p. 287. xiv.
2. Preston DC, Shapiro BE. Electromyography and neuromuscular disorders: clinical-electrophysiologic correlations. Boston: Butterworth-Heinemann; 1998. p. 581.
3. Wilbourn AJ, Aminoff MJ. AAEM minimonograph 32: the electrodiagnostic examination in patients with radiculopathies. American association of electrodiagnostic medicine. Muscle Nerve. 1998;21(12):1612–31.
4. Freeman TL, et al. Electrodiagnostic medicine and clinical neuromuscular physiology. In: Cuccurullo SJ, editor. Physical medicine and rehabilitation board review. New York: Demos Medical Pub; 2010. p. 337–456.
5. So YT. Guidelines in electrodiagnostic medicine. Practice parameter for needle electromyographic evaluation of patients with suspected cervical radiculopathy. Muscle Nerve Suppl. 1999;8:S209–21.
6. Dillingham TR, et al. Identification of cervical radiculopathies: optimizing the electromyographic screen. Am J Phys Med Rehabil. 2001;80(2):84–91.

7. Dumitru D, Amato AA, Zwarts MJ. Electrodiagnostic medicine. 2nd ed. Philadelphia: Hanley & Belfus; 2002. p. 1524.

8. Cho SC, et al. Utility of electrodiagnostic testing in evaluating patients with lumbosacral radiculopathy: an evidence-based review. Muscle Nerve. 2010;42(2):276–82.

9. Dillingham TR, et al. Identifying lumbosacral radiculopathies: an optimal electromyographic screen. Am J Phys Med Rehabil. 2000;79(6):496–503.

10. Whitman JM, et al. A comparison between two physical therapy treatment programs for patients with lumbar spinal stenosis: a randomized clinical trial. Spine (Phila Pa 1976). 2006;31(22):2541–9.

11. Werner RA, Andary M. Electrodiagnostic evaluation of carpal tunnel syndrome. Muscle Nerve. 2011;44(4):597–607.

12. Scott KR, Kothari MJ. Treatment of carpal tunnel syndrome. In: Basow DS, editor. UptoDate. Waltham, MA: UpToDate; 2011.

13. Chorley J. Elbow injuries in the young athlete. In: Basow DS, editor. UpToDate. Waltham, MA: UpToDate; 2011.

14. Posner MA. Compressive neuropathies of the median and radial nerves at the elbow. Clin Sports Med. 1990;9(2):343.

15. Hunter JM, Mackin E, Callahan AD. Rehabilitation of the hand: surgery and therapy. 4th ed. St. Louis: Mosby; 1995.

16. Rutkove SB. Overview of upper extremity. In: Basow DS, editor. UpToDate. Waltham, MA: UpToDate; 2011.

17. Campbell WW. Guidelines in electrodiagnostic medicine. Practice parameter for electrodiagnostic studies in ulnar neuropathy at the elbow. Muscle Nerve Suppl. 1999;8:171–205.

18. Doherty TJ. Ulnar neuropathy at the elbow and wrist. In: Basow DS, editor. UpToDate. Waltham, MA: UpToDate; 2011.

19. Sechrest RC. Guyon's canal syndrome. In: eORTHOPOD. Medical Multimedia Group, L.L.C; 2009–2011. http://www.eorthopod.com/content/guyons-canal-syndrome. Accessed 15 Feb 2011.

20. Anderson BC. Meralgia paresthetica. In: Basow DS, editor. UpToDate. Waltham, MA: UpToDate; 2011.

21. Wheeler SG, et al. Approach to the diagnosis and evaluation of low back pain in adults. In: Basow DS, editor. UpToDate. Waltham, MA: UpToDate; 2011.

22. Marciniak C, et al. Practice parameter: utility of electrodiagnostic techniques in evaluating patients with suspected peroneal neuropathy: an evidence-based review. Muscle Nerve. 2005;31(4):520–7.

23. Rutkove SB. Overview of lower extremity peripheral nerve syndromes. In: Basow DS, editor. UpToDate. Waltham, MA: UpToDate; 2011.

24. Patel AT, et al. Usefulness of electrodiagnostic techniques in the evaluation of suspected tarsal tunnel syndrome: an evidence-based review. Muscle Nerve. 2005;32(2):236–40.

25. Dyck PJ, Carter RE, Litchy WJ. Modeling nerve conduction criteria for diagnosis of diabetic polyneuropathy. Muscle Nerve. 2011;44(3):340–5.

26. England JD, et al. Evaluation of distal symmetric polyneuropathy: the role of autonomic testing, nerve biopsy, and skin biopsy (an evidence-based review). Muscle Nerve. 2009;39(1):106–15.

27. England JD, et al. Evaluation of distal symmetric polyneuropathy: the role of laboratory and genetic testing (an evidence-based review). Muscle Nerve. 2009;39(1):116–25.

28. Ferrante MA. Brachial plexopathies: classification, causes, and consequences. Muscle Nerve. 2004;30(5):547–68.

29. Visco CJ, Chimes GP. McLean course in electrodiagnostic medicine. New York: Demos Medical; 2011.

30. Kavanagh B. Complications of peripheral nerve irradiation. In: Basow DS, editor. UpToDate. Waltham, MA: UpToDate; 2011.

31. Soto O. Radiation-induced conduction block: resolution following anticoagulant therapy. Muscle Nerve. 2005;31(5):642–5.

32. Glantz MJ, et al. Treatment of radiation-induced nervous system injury with heparin and warfarin. Neurology. 1994;44(11):2020.

33. Schierle C, Winograd JM. Radiation-induced brachial plexopathy: review. Complication without a cure. J Reconstr Microsurg. 2004;20(2):149–52.

34. Malanga GA, Nadler SF. Musculoskeletal physical examination: an evidence-based approach. USA: Elsevier; 2006.

35. Bromberg MB. Brachial plexus syndromes. In: Basow DS, editor. UpToDate. Waltham, MA: UpToDate; 2011.

36. Cuetter AC, Bartoszek DM. The thoracic outlet syndrome: controversies, overdiagnosis, overtreatment, and recommendations for management. Muscle Nerve. 1989;12(5):410–9.

37. Watkins PJ. Clinical observations and experiments in diabetic neuropathy. Diabetologia. 1992;35(1):2–11.

38. Twydell PT. Diabetic amyotrophy and idiopathic lumbosacral radiculoplexus neuropathy. In: Basow DS, editor. UpToDate. Waltham, MA: UpToDate; 2011.

39. Dyck P, James B, Windebank AJ. Diabetic and nondiabetic lumbosacral radiculoplexus neuropathies: new insights into pathophysiology and treatment. Muscle Nerve. 2002;25(4):477–91.

40. Dyck PJ, Norell JE, Dyck PJ. Microvasculitis and ischemia in diabetic lumbosacral radiculoplexus neuropathy. Neurology. 1999;53(9):2113–21.

41. Chen JT, et al. Botulism: heart rate variation, sympathetic skin responses, and plasma norepinephrine. Can J Neurol Sci. 1999;26(2):123–6.

42. Costa J, et al. Repetitive nerve stimulation in myasthenia gravis—relative sensitivity of different muscles. Clin Neurophysiol. 2004;115(12):2776–82.

43. Zambelis T, Kokotis P, Karandreas N. Repetitive nerve stimulation of facial and hypothenar muscles: relative sensitivity in different myasthenia gravis subgroups. Eur Neurol. 2011;65(4):203–7. Epub 2011 Mar 17.

44. Chiou-Tan FY, Tim RW, Gilchrist JM. Practice parameter for repetitive nerve stimulation and single fiber EMG evaluation of adults with suspected myasthenia gravis or Lambert-Eaton myasthenic syndrome: summary statement. Muscle Nerve. 2001;24(9):1236–8.

45. Brooks BR, et al. El escorial revisited: revised criteria for the diagnosis of amyotrophic lateral sclerosis. Amyotroph Lateral Scler Other Motor Neuron Disord. 2000;1:293–9.

46. Miller RG, et al. Riluzole for amyotrophic lateral sclerosis (ALS)/motor neuron disease (MND). Cochrane Database Syst Rev. 2012 Mar 14; 3: CD 0001447.

47. Galvez-Jimenez N. Symptom-based management of amyotrophic lateral sclerosis. In: Basow DS, editor. UpToDate. Waltham, MA: UpToDate; 2011.

48. Simionescu L, Jubelt B. Post-polio syndrome. In: Basow DS, editor. UpToDate. Waltham, MA: UpToDate; 2011.

49. Trojan DA, Cashman NR. Post-poliomyelitis syndrome. Muscle Nerve. 2005;31(1):6–19.

50. Farbu E, et al. EFNS guideline on diagnosis and management of post-polio syndrome. Report of an EFNS task force. Eur J Neurol. 2006;13(8):795–801.

51. Gonzalez H, Olsson T, Borg K. Management of postpolio syndrome. Lancet Neurol. 2010;9(6):634–42.

52. Jubelt B. Post-polio syndrome. Curr Treat Options Neurol. 2004;6(2):87–93.

53. McDonald CM, et al. Myopathic disorders. In: Braddom RL, editor. Physical medicine & rehabilitation. Philadelphia: Saunders; 2007. p. 1099–131.

54. Radcliffe KA, Campbell WW. Statin myopathy. Curr Neurol Neurosci Rep. 2008;8(1):66–72.

55. Pestronk A. Myopathy. Neuromuscular disease center. 2011. http://neuro-muscular.wustl.edu/index.html. Accessed 31 Aug 2011, 16 Dec 2011.

56. American_Association_of_Neuromuscular_and_Electrodiagnostic_Medicine. Coding Updates. 2011. http://www.aanem.org/Practice/Coding/Coding-Resources/Coding-Updates.aspx. Accessed 31 Dec 2011.

57. AANEM. Guidelines in electrodiagnostic medicine. Recommended policy for electrodiagnostic medicine. Muscle Nerve Suppl. 1999;8:S91–105.

58. AANEM. Billing for same day evaluation and management and electrodiagnostic testing: position statement. 1999. http://www.aanem.org/getmedia/daeab80f-7454-4222-838f-2ed91437c201/billing_for_same_day.pdf.aspx. Accessed 31 Dec 2011.

59. AANEM. CPT Changes Every EDX Provider Should Prepare For. 2012. Available from: http://www.aanem.org.

Chapter 17
Medical Acupuncture

Shan Babeendran, John-Ross Rizzo, and Alex Moroz

Introduction (Fig. 17.1)

- Origin: China
- Branch: CAM (Complementary and Alternative Medicine)
- Technique:
  - Insert solid, thin, and pliable needles into the body at various defined points
  - Varying depths, angles, and rotations are utilized for needle manipulation
  - Combining with electrical stimulation or moxibustion is common
- Uses: pain relief, decreasing symptoms of: asthma, fatigue, or GI issues

The Facts

- In 1965, human and animal trials began in China to evaluate acupuncture analgesia.
- By 1980, a connection was noted between the endogenous opioid peptide system and analgesic events observed with electrical acupuncture stimulation.

S. Babeendran, D.O. (✉) • J.R. Rizzo, M.D. • A. Moroz, M.D.
Department of Rehabilitation Medicine, New York University Langone
Medical Center, New York, NY, USA
e-mail: ShanBabeendran@gmail.com

K.A. Sackheim (ed.), *Rehab Clinical Pocket Guide:*
Rehabilitation Medicine, DOI 10.1007/978-1-4614-5419-9_17,
© Springer Science+Business Media, LLC 2013

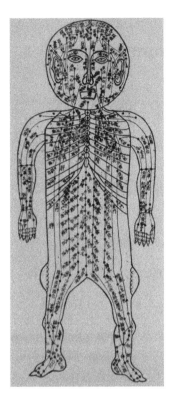

Fig. 17.1 Postulated representation of the electrical charges transmitted through fluid bathing the organs and muscles, which are projected to the surface of the body as acupuncture points

- The connection was later reproduced in a variety of animal studies including mice, monkeys, rats, and rabbits, which led to the suggestion that acupuncture analgesia can be thought of as a general phenomenon in the mammalian world.
- Acupuncture seems to provide a mechanism to activate the human bodies pain modulation system, changing the processing of noxious stimuli.
- There are many theories of how exactly acupuncture works; the following is one commonly accepted **physiological** explanation [1]:
  - Every organ has its own encompassing electrical field.
  - This electrical field results from the sum of individual cellular electrical fields.
  - Each organ produces a distinct field and transmits that field to the surface.

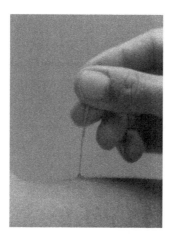

Fig. 17.2 Example of needle inserted into skin

- The electromagnetic mediums are the fascia and interstitial fluid.
- Electrical charges transmitted through the fluid bathing the organs/muscle are projected onto the body's surface as channels or meridians.
- On the surface of the body, traditionally described meridians are usually located between muscle groups and allow direct access to the fascia and ionic flow.

- The **hardware**: (Fig. 17.2)
  - The needle electrode is an instrument used to influence the electrical flow through the acupuncture circulation network.
  - The design is carefully crafted and follows principles of the thermoelectric effect of Thomas Kelvin, the Bimetallic effect, and the Electron Transfer effect.
  - The needle itself consists of two separate spiraled portions of metal:
    - The first spiral → needle shaft
    - The second spiral → needle handle
  - When inserted into the body, the tip of the needle is warmer than the handle.
  - The spiral handle of the needle acts as a radiator, which maintains a rather large surface area of metal in contact with air, and in turn allows the temperature gradient to be preserved for a longer period of time.

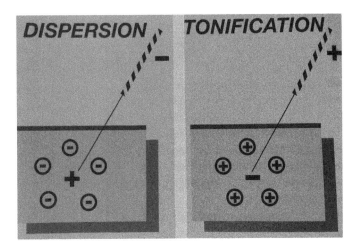

Fig. 17.3 Illustration of dispersion and tonification

- The electrical gradient along the shaft is reinforced by the electromagnetic effect of the second metal spiral, which is in close contact with the first, creating a sort of bimetallic battery.
- The positive electrode (needle tip), which is inserted into the interstitial medium, the meridian, attracts negative ions until equilibrium is reached.
- It takes approximately 10–15 min to reach electrical equilibrium after insertion, a needling technique known as *dispersion* (Fig. 17.3).
- If the needle handle is heated or manipulated manually, the polarity of the needle tip is altered to become a positive electrode, attracting positive ions.
- A heated needle can take up to 60 min to reach equilibrium, an acupuncture technique known as *tonification*.
- The needle-electrode placed in tonification stimulates a flow of electrons toward a second needle placed in dispersion along the same flow pathway. If this sequence is repeated, an acupuncturist is thought to be able to influence the ionic flow. This is achieved by provoking an electron wave that is capable of propagating itself in a specific trajectory along the acupuncture channel.

Overview

- Acupuncture is a CAM treatment that is generally safe, with grow-
  ing evidence for applications in a variety of medical conditions.
- *Risks:* bleeding, infection, and organ puncture including
  pneumothorax
  - A phenomenon known as *needle shock* is also a rare side effect
    that typically occurs during the first acupuncture treatment.
    This is a type of vasovagal reaction, which involves symptoms
    of sweating, flushing, tunnel vision, and can progress to
    syncope.
  - Per a study conducted by Macpherson et al. in 2004 which
    surveyed **6,348** patients in the UK, 11% of patients experienced
    side effects including fatigue, local pain, headache [2].
  - Per another study conducted by Witt et al., which surveyed
    229,230 patients in Germany, 9% of patients experienced adverse
    effects of bleeding/hematoma, pain, or vegetative symptoms [3].

Evaluation of the patient
  - **The Diagnostic Evaluation**
    ○ Open-ended history and physical
    ○ Focused questions regarding symptoms related to specific
      energy axis
    ○ Expedited review of symptoms
    ○ General strengths and weaknesses in family health
    ○ Acupuncture evaluation initially considers all symptoms
      equally. The goal of this evaluation is to determine the
      energy circulation network level that is disturbed in the
      patient, the level of intensity of this disturbance, and the
      subsystems and axis, which give access to that disturbance.

The Initial Interview
- The initial interview forms a diagnostic impression and will aide
  construction of a provisional therapeutic input.
- The level of a manifested issue should be determined, as well as
  the disturbed energy axes or meridian segments.
- Symptoms may be associated with synergistic and coupled meridians within the energetic sub circuit.
- Investigate for patterns of symptoms, particularly if daily recurrence occurs, warranting investigation into organ midday–mid-
  night relationships.

- The acupuncturist may label the symptoms noted in the history via energy axis, elemental term, or even by the trigram of the energy axis. This is important as labels may lead to the recognition of clustering of symptoms and a predominant energy axis.
- If a patient has multiple complaints, it is often found that when treating the most distressful issues first, secondary and tertiary issues often achieve relief as well.

Physical Exam
- The physical exam begins at first contact with the patient. The strength of a handshake, gait, posture, skin color, liveliness of the voice all give clues to the overall well-being of a person.
- It is also important to examine the diagnostic somatotopic systems that microcosmically depict the energy of various organs. Commonly used somatotopic systems are the tongue, radial pulse, and external ear.
  - **Tongue Inspection** [1]
    - ○ Through its color, body, coating, and surface irregularities, the tongue is thought to reflect the condition and underlying problem of a patient.
    - ○ Meridian branches of the kidney, heart, liver, spleen, lung, and stomach all pass through the oropharynx or tongue.
    - ○ Changes in tongue quality can be followed daily or weekly, and may serve as an indicator of illness evolution.
    - ○ The surface reflex system of the tongue has many different documented configurations. Although most have accepted that the anterior, middle, and posterior thirds of the tongue can be described as upper, middle, and lower heaters.
  - **Radial Pulse** (Fig. 17.4)
    - ○ Provides a means of evaluating the patient's overall well-being
    - ○ Due to its constant change, the pulse can be used to monitor whether an input has had the desired effect.
    - ○ The pulse is palpated at three contiguous areas overlyi ng the radial artery. It is believed that the width of each position is equal to the width of the patient's fingertip. The pulse gives the physician a view of the internal balance among the organs.
    - ○ The styloid process is the bony landmark used to identify the middle position. The other two positions are immediately proximal and distal to the middle. Thus, the following

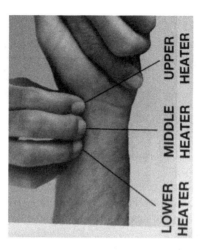

UPPER
HEATER

MIDDLE
HEATER

LOWER
HEATER

Fig. 17.4 Radial pulse being palpated, while practitioner's opposite hand slides over the edge of the radius from the dorsal surface of the forearm

terminology is used, distal pulse = upper heater, middle pulse = middle heater, and proximal pulse = lower heater.
  ○ A radial artery diagnostic somatotopic system has also been mapped and can be found in various acupuncture texts.
- Temperature: during evaluation, notation should be made of any region that appears unusually warm or cool. The musculoskeletal evaluation should include identification of muscle knots, trigger points, and any subcutaneous bands or nodules overlying musculature. Each painful point should be taken into consideration when designing a treatment plan.

The Acupuncture Treatment (Fig. 17.5)
- Location of acupuncture points demand a refined sensitivity to palpation, as each patient's acupuncture sites are unique. Acupuncture points may be described at a fixed distance of inches or "cun," from an anatomic landmark.
- Needle insertion, similar to locating an acupuncture point, is a skill that is acquired with experience. The needles must be sterile, and the use of isopropyl alcohol can be used to alleviate the patient's fear of infection, although an aseptic technique is adequate unless the skin is grossly soiled.

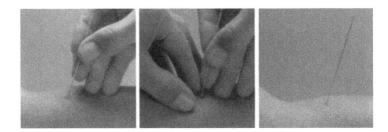

Fig. 17.5 Example of needling technique

- The most important consideration in needle insertion is the minimization of discomfort. Pain with needle insertion is mostly associated with the initial piercing of skin and then again as adequate depth is achieved.
- When the needle achieves a depth that supports its upright posture, it must be advanced by simultaneously rotating and progressing until the "De Qi" is felt.
  - "De Qi" also known as "the arrival of Qi" is a term used when contact is made with energy of a channel. The patient may describe this sensation as an electrical sensation or even as a dull ache. It is vital to the effectiveness of treatment that each needle achieve "De Qi" [1].
- There are many techniques for manipulating the needle for tonification and sedation. The most widely accepted method to achieve tonification is by angling the needle in the direction of channel's energy flow, and advancing the needle slowly, and with slow, firm clockwise rotation. Sedation needle technique contrasts tonification technique.
- Positioning of the patient is also very important. Both the patient and the acupuncturist should be as comfortable as possible prior to beginning treatment.
- Following treatment, patients should be made aware that they may feel somewhat lightheaded or disoriented for ≥30 min. As further treatments are provided, this sensation should subside. Patients should also be made aware that after initial treatment one of several phenomena may happen:
  - Gradual and progressive improvement
  - Marked amelioration of symptoms
  - Marked exacerbation of symptoms
  - No change at all in the symptoms

Acupuncture In Practice

- **Headache/migraine**—Various studies have been conducted with regard to acupuncture and headache; the results are conflicting. Some studies have found evidence to support the use of acupuncture for headache, while others have found that most of the studies were of poor quality. Several studies have demonstrated that acupuncture reduces migraine symptoms and is as effective as certain pharmaceutical treatments for headache. In 2009, Linde et al. found that acupuncture might help to relieve tension headaches [4]. However, two large trials that looked at acupuncture for migraines found no difference between actual and simulated acupuncture.
- **Neck pain**—Studies aimed at acupuncture and its ability to relieve chronic neck pain, as demonstrated by Trinh et al. in 2006, have more consistently revealed that acupuncture provided better pain relief than some simulated treatments [5]. It is important to note that stronger studies are needed, as the previous studies varied in terms of design and most had small sample sizes.
- **Low-back pain**—According to clinical practice guidelines issued by the American Pain Society and the American College of Physicians in 2007, acupuncture is one of several complementary and alternative medicine therapies physicians are encouraged to consider when patients with chronic low-back pain do not respond to conventional treatment. Early studies, have demonstrated that combining acupuncture with conventional treatment was more effective than conventional treatment alone for relieving chronic low-back pain.

Sample Acupuncture Referral

Patient Name:
DOB:
Referring Physician:
Referring Physician Phone #: (Fig. 17.6)
Primary Dx:
Brief Hx:
Significant Past medical Hx:

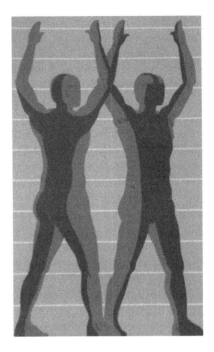

Fig. 17.6 Image should be used to notate areas of discomfort

Allergies:

Regions of discomfort listed from most significant to least significant

    1.

    2.

    3.

Patient's expectation of treatment:

Restrictions or conditions of treatment:

Has patient had acupuncture treatments in the past?

History of needle-phobia? Relative contraindications to treatment (please circle all that apply). Extreme frailty—Concurrent febrile illness—Local skin infection—First trimester of pregnancy—Use of anticoagulants—Hx of bleeding disorders—Cardiac pacemaker (when electrical stimulation used)

References

1. Helms JM. Acupuncture energetics a clinical approach for physicians. 1st ed. Berkely, CA: Medical Acupuncture Publishers; 1995.
2. MacPherson H, Scullion T, Thomas K, Walters S. Patient reports of adverse events associated with acupuncture: a large scale prospective survey. Qual Saf Health Care. 2004;13:349–55.
3. Witt CM, Pach D, Brinkhaus B, et al. Safety of acupuncture: results of a prospective observational study with 229,230 patients and introduction of a medical information consent form. Forsch Komplementmed. 2009; 16(2):91–7.
4. Linde K, Allais G, Brinkhaus B, et al. Acupuncture for tension-type headache. Cochrane Database Syst Rev. 2009;(1):CD007587.
5. Trinh KV, Graham N, Gross AR, et al. Cervical overview group acupuncture for neck disorders. Cochrane Database Syst Rev. 2006;3:CD004870.

Chapter 18
Common Medications Used in Rehabilitation Medicine

Christopher Sahler

This chapter covers some of the commonly used medications in rehabilitation medicine. Although we have dosing recommendations below, all doses should be verified and adjusted according to your patient's co-morbidities and needs.

C. Sahler, M.D. (✉)
Department of Physical Medicine and Rehabilitation,
Mt. Sinai Hospital, 5 E 98th St, New York, NY 10029, USA
e-mail: christophersahler@gmail.com

K.A. Sackheim (ed.), *Rehab Clinical Pocket Guide:*
Rehabilitation Medicine, DOI 10.1007/978-1-4614-5419-9_18,
© Springer Science+Business Media, LLC 2013

SPASTICITY MEDICATIONS [1, 2]

Medication	Mode of Action	Dosing	Side Effects/Cautions
Baclofen (Lioresal)	– Acts Pre- and Post-synaptically as an agonist at the **GABA-b** receptor in CNS – Decreases the release of excitatory neurotransmitters	Available doses: 10, 20 mg tablets – Start 5 mg qd-tid (usually tid) – May be increased by 5-15 mg/day increments every 3 days if tolerated *Max daily dose:* 80 mg/day (20 mg tid)	**Side Effects:** Weakness, vertigo, urinary frequency, fatigue, insomnia, confusion, nausea, constipation, sedation, headache, seizures, impaired vision *Precautions:* – May lower seizure threshold – Caution with renal patients as drug is excreted renally, may require reduced dose – Pregnancy- teratogenic Baclofen withdrawal Syndrome: – Abrupt withdrawal may precipitate seizure, hallucinations, and/or rebound spasticity – Can be avoided by tapering dose

Baclofen Intrathecal (ITB)	– Acts as an agonist at the **GABA-b** receptors in CNS – Decreases release of excitatory neurotransmitters	Patients are candidates for ITB if suffering from severe spasticity refractory to conservative treatments Starting dose is 25 mg per day, with titration to efficacy, up to a maximum dose of 200 mg per day depending on patient needs and tolerability of medication With ITB, less baclofen is needed compared to oral doses. This can help to minimize adverse side effects such as drowsiness and sedation	**Side Effects:** Weakness, fatigue, confusion, constipation, sedation, cardio-respiratory depression *Precautions:* May lower seizure threshold, abrupt withdrawal may precipitate seizure, hallucinations, rebound spasticity, cardio-respiratory arrest
Dantrolene	– Intrafusal and extrafusal muscle fibers – Decrease release of calcium from sarcoplasmic reticulum	Available doses: 25, 50, 100 mg – Start 25 mg qday x 7 days, if needed can then increase to 25 mg tid x 7 days, then 50 mg tid x 7 days, then 100 mg tid *Max daily dose:* 400 mg in divided doses	**Side Effects:** Weakness, fatigue, drowsiness, dizziness, diarrhea *Precautions:* Hepatotoxicity – Check baseline **LFTs** and monitor frequently Note: – Drug of choice for spasticity of cerebral origin – Less sedating than CNS acting agents

(continued)

Medication	Mode of Action	Dosing	Side Effects/Cautions
Benzodiazepines Diazepam (Valium) Klonopin (Clonazepam)	– **GABA-a** receptors of brain stem, reticular formation, spinal cord – Increase GABA binding, potentiating presynaptic inhibition	**Diazepam** Available doses: 2, 5, 10 mg – Start 2-5 mg bid doses can range from 2 to 10 mg, tid – qid – Geriatric start at 2.0 to 2.5 mg qd **Klonopin** Available doses: 0.5, 1, 2 mg Start 0.5-1 mg qhs Note: Used to decrease nocturnal spasms, hyper-reflexia, and ROM resistance	**Side Effects:** Drowsiness, fatigue, ataxia, weakness, hypotension, sedation, and memory impairment *Precautions:* Tolerance and dependence, potential for abuse and dependence, CNS depression Caution with elderly as they may be more susceptible to the adverse side effects Caution with renal and hepatic impairment

Clonidine (Catapress)	– Agonist in brain, brain stem, substantia gelatinosa of spinal cord	*Available doses:* PO- 0.1, 0.2, 0.3 mg Transdermal patch- 0.1, 0.2, 0.3 mg	**Side Effects:** Bradycardia, hypotension, depression sedation, somnolence
	– Inhibits short latency of motor neurons; augmentation of presynaptic inhibition	**PO:** Start 0.1 mg bid, can titrate up to 0.2 to 0.6 mg bid if tolerated *Max daily dose:* 2.4 mg in divided doses	*Precautions:* Blood pressure and pulse monitoring
		Transdermal patch- Start with 1 patch (equivalent to 0.1 mg per 24 hours) q 7 days, can increase up to 0.3 mg q 7 days if needed	*Note:* May cause rebound hypertension upon discontinuation
		Note: Patch takes 2-3 days for the patch to have affect, may need overlap with po medication during that time	

(continued)

Medication	Mode of Action	Dosing	Side Effects/Cautions
Tizanidine (Zanaflex)	– Adrenergic receptors in spinal cord and brain – Prevents release of excitatory amino acids from presynaptic terminal of spinal interneurons; may facilitate glycine which is an inhibitory neurotransmitter	Available doses: 2, 4, 6 mg – Start with 2-4 mg qhs – Increase by 2 mg q 2-4 days if tolerated – Frequency can be up to 6- to 8-hrs as needed up to 3 doses per day *Max daily dose:* up to 36 mg if no renal issues (usual doses 18 mg max)	**Side Effects:** Dry mouth, sedation, dizziness, Dystonia *Precautions:* Orthostatic hypotension, hallucination. Hepatotoxicity (Check baseline LFTs and monitor frequently) Note: Tablet vs capsule tablet is absorbed 80x faster than capsule
Metaxalone (Skelaxin)	– General CNS depressant	Available doses: 800 mg Start 800 mg ½ -1 pill po qd-qid prn *Max daily dose: 800 tid*	**Side Effects:** Drowsiness, dizziness, headache, Nausea, hemolytic anemia, Jaundice *Precautions:* h/o drug induced, hemolytic, or other anemias Caution with renal and hepatic insufficiency as this has not been fully studied Consider monitoring LFTs Do not use in pregnancy

INJECTABLE SPASTICITY MEDICATONS

Medication	Mode of Action	Dosing	Side Effects/Cautions
Botulinum Toxin	– Irreversibly prevents the pre-synaptic release of Acetylcholine at the neuromuscular junction – Type A (Botox): cleaves SNAP-25 – Type B (Myobloc): acts on Synaptobrevin	– 1-1 2 units/kg depending on size of muscle – No more often than every 3 months **Per Muscle Dose Ranges** FDP 30-50 U FDS 30-50 U FCR 12.5-50 U FCU 12.5-50 U Biceps 100-200 U *Max dose in a 3 month time frame:* 360 units in 3 month time frame, usual dose is 100-200 units *Note:* Toxin is usually dissolved in 2 ml NS for 100 units and 4 ml of NS for 200	**Side Effects:** Weakness, allergic reaction, difficulty breathing, burning, numbness, difficulty swallowing *Precautions:* Antibody formation with repeated use which can decrease efficacy, respiratory arrest (more commonly in patients with pre-excising respiratory issues) **RULE OF 3s:** – Onset = 3 days (24 to 72 hrs) – Max effectiveness = 2-3 weeks – Duration = up to 3 months Note: Used in UMN spasticity found mostly in SCI, TBI, and MS patients

(continued)

Medication	Mode of Action	Dosing	Side Effects/Cautions
Phenol	– Proteolytic agent – Works at the peripheral nerve and motor end plate to denature the protein and disrupt the myoneural junction	Solutions: 5% solution contains 50 mg of phenol/ml 7% solution contains 70 mg of phenol/ml Recommended max dose 30 mg/kg	**Side Effects:** Pain, skin irritation, transient dysesthesias and/or numbness, hematoma, peripheral neuropathy, weakness *Precautions:* Cardiac arrhythmia, Thrombophlebitis Note: May have non reversible effects lasting 6-12 mos, possibly permanent Systemic affects with intravascular injection

BOWEL MEDICATIONS (PO) [3]

Medication	Mode of Action	Dosing	Side Effects/Cautions
Colace	– Stool softener – Reduces surface tension of oil and water interface of stool	Available doses: 50, 100 mg Start 100 mg PO bid- tid, can increase as needed *Max daily dose:* 50–300 mg in divided doses	**Side Effects:** Cramping, Rash, low magnesium Onset: 12–72 hours
Senna Senna S (Senna + Colace)	– Irritant to the lining of the bowel – Acts at the myenteric plexus and increases peristalsis	Available doses: 8.6 mg Start 1-2 tabs po qhs (or Qam depending on when you want BM); Increase for refractory cases if tolerated, can also do bid dosing if needed *Max daily dose:* 4 tablets bid	**Side Effects:** electrolyte imbalances, cramping, abdominal pain, nausea, vomiting Onset: 8 hours *Caution:* Extended use can irritate the colon Note: qhs dosing should result in Bowel movement the next morning

(continued)

Medication	Mode of Action	Dosing	Side Effects/Cautions
Bisacodyl (Dulcolax)	Stimulates Peristalsis; Laxative (Promotes increase H20 and electrolyte secrection)	Available doses: **PO:** 5 mg **PR:** 10 mg	**Side Effects:** abdominal pain, nausea, May cause cramping
		PO: Start at 5-15 mg po qday	PO Onset: 8 hours PR Onset: 0.5-1 hours
	Direct irritation of smooth muscle, possibly colonic intramural plexus	*Max daily dose:* up to 30 mg PR: Start at 10 mg pr qday	**PO Notes:** Bowel movement should occur within 15 to 60 min, although it may take up to 6-12 hrs
			Swallow this medication whole. Do not crush, chew, or alter tablet
			Do not take within 1 hr of antacids or milk products as this can alter the coating on the tablet and lead to GI upset and/or nausea
Lactulose	– Colonic acidifier – Bacterial inhibition of lactulose resulting in acidic pH which inhibits diffusion of NH3 into the blood – Increases Peristalsis	Available doses: 10 g/15 mL Start 15-30 ml PO x 1 Can be repeated tid in severe cases *Max daily dose:* 60 ml	**Side Effects:** allergic reaction, bloating, gas, stomach pain, diarrhea, nausea and/ or vomiting Onset: 4 hours Note: This medication is also used in hepatic encephalopathy patients

| Polyethylene glycol (Miralax, GoLytely) | – Osmotic dieresis (draws water into intestines)
– Decreases stool consistency and increases stool frequency | Start with 17 g (1 heaping tablespoon) of powder qday mixed in 4-8 ounces of water, juice, soda, coffee, or tea | **Side Effects:** Nausea, abdominal bloating, cramping and flatulence

Note: It may take up to 2-4 days for Bowel movement to occur |
| Magnesium Citrate | – Osmotic dieresis (draws water into intestines) | Start with 150-240 mL po x 1, Can be repeated if needed

Max daily dose: 300-350 mg in divided doses | **Side Effects:**
Slow heart beat, low blood pressure, nausea, drowsiness

Onset: 2 hours

Caution with renal patients, may cause low magnesium
Patients should take on an empty stomach with a full glass of water or juice to facilitate absorption and prevent complications
Bowel movement in ≤ 6 hrs |

(continued)

Medication	Mode of Action	Dosing	Side Effects/Cautions
Milk of Magnesia (MOM)	Osmotic laxative (draws water into intestines)	Start 15-30mL po qdaily prn (can be dosed up to qid if needed) *Max daily dose:* 30-60 mL per day (depending on concentration)	**Side Effects:** Diarrhea, dehydration, electrolyte imbalances Onset: 2 hours Note: Take with full glass of water 30 min - 6 hrs prior to time of desired bowel movement
Psyllium (Metamucil)	Increases stool bulk by providing additional fiber	Start 1 tablespoons/packet po qday-tid	**Side Effects:** Abdominal fullness/bloating, allergic reaction, nausea, vomiting Onset of action: 12-24 hours Note: Dosing should be followed by a full glass of water
Methylcellulose (Citrucel)	Increases stool bulk by providing additional fiber	Start with 1 heaping tablespoon dissolved in 8 ounces of water qday – tid	**Side Effects:** Allergic reaction, abdominal pain, nausea or vomiting Note: Bowel movement should occur in 12 -72 hrs

BLADDER MEDICATIONS [3]

Medication	Mode Of Action	Dosing	Side Effects/Cautions
Bethanechol (Urecholine)	Acts at Cholinergic muscarinic (M2 and M3) receptors as an **agonist**→ increasing detrusor activity (contracting the bladder)	Available doses: 5, 10, 25, 50 mg – Start 5-10 mg can increase till desired effect reached, up to 50 mg tid-qid	**Side Effects:** Abdominal cramps, diarrhea, flushing, headache, hypotension, nausea, vomiting, urinary urgency *Precautions:* Contraindicated in patients with Asthma, coronary pathology, peptic ulcers, intestinal obstruction, hyperthyroidism, epilepsy, or parkinsonism Note: Used to treat urinary retention

(continued)

Medication	Mode Of Action	Dosing	Side Effects/Cautions
Oxybutynin (Ditropan)	Anticholinergic effects at the CNS	Available doses: 5 mg	**Side Effects:** Dry mouth, dry eye, headache, blurred vision, constipation, agitation, confusion and somnolence
	Inhibits muscarinic activity (Receptor **antagonist**) and relaxes the detrusor muscle	**Immediate release dosing (IR):** 5 mg bid-tid	*Precautions:* Contraindicated in patients with glaucoma
		Long acting dosing (LA): 5 mg qday	Caution to avoid urinary retention with use of this medications
		Max daily dose: 5 mg qid	Note: Used to treat urinary incontinence or frequency (neurogenic bladder)

Tolterodine (*Detrol*)	Anticholinergic effects at the CNS	Available doses: **Immediate release (IR):** 1, 2, 4 mg	**Side Effects:** Dry mouth, dry eye, headache, blurred vision, constipation, agitation, confusion and somnolence
Detrol LA (long acting)	Inhibits muscarinic activity (Receptor **antagonist**) and relaxes the detrusor muscle	**Long acting (LA):** 2, 4 mg	Contraindicated in patients with urinary or gastric retention, and narrow-angle glaucoma
		IR dosing: 2 mg bid, if not tolerated can decrease to 1 mg	
			Caution with hepatic or renal pathology
		LA dosing: 2 mg qday, if tolerated can increase to 4 mg qday	Can use IR 1 mg bid or LA 2 mg bid
			Note: Used for treatment of urinary incontinence
Tamsulosin (Flomax)	Alpha 1 Adrenergic receptor **antagonist** smooth muscle relaxation of prostate and bladder neck resulting in an improvement in urine flow rate	Available doses: 0.4 mg	**Side Effects:** Orthostatic hypotension, retrograde ejaculation
		Start 0.4 mg po qhs, can increase after 2-4 weeks to 0.8 mg if needed	*Precautions:*
			– Don't use with Nitro
			– Contains Sulfa (allergies)
			– Can predispose to floppy iris syndrome
			Note: Used to treat bladder outlet obstruction

(continued)

Medication	Mode Of Action	Dosing	Side Effects/Cautions
Doxazosin (Cardura)	Alpha 1 Adrenergic receptor **antagonist**→ smooth muscle relaxation of prostate and bladder neck resulting in an improvement in urine flow rate	Available doses: 1, 2, 4, 8 mg Start 1 po qday, can increase over a few weeks till desired affect obtained *Max daily dose:* 8 mg	**Side Effects:** Nausea, headache, dizziness, orthostatic hypotension

AROUSAL/COGNITION MEDICATIONS [4]

Medication	Mode Of Action	Dosing	Side Effects/Cautions
Methylphenidate (Ritalin)	Norepinephrine and dopamine reuptake inhibiter Sympathomimetic agent	Available doses: 5, 10, 20 Start 5 mg po bid, can increase as needed if tolerated *Max daily dose:* 60 mg divided in bid-tid dosing	**Side Effects:** Insomnia, headache, anorexia, tachycardia, seizure, blurred vision, nervousness, anxiety, nausea, dizziness, palpitations *Precautions:* – Psychotic/manic manifestations – Cardiovascular precautions – Physiologic dependence – Rhabdomyolysis Note: Can avoid insomnia with earlier dosing before breakfast, and before lunch Used to treat inattention

(continued)

Medication	Mode Of Action	Dosing	Side Effects/Cautions
Amantadine	Dopaminergic Noradrenergic Serotonergic	Available doses: 100 mg Start 50-150 mg po bid	**Side Effects:** Insomnia, seizure, nausea, livedo reticularis *Precautions:*
	Weak NMDA receptor antagonist, anticholinergic	*Max daily dose:* 400 mg in divided doses	– Neuroleptic malignant syndrome associated with dose reduction/withdrawal – *Caution with cardiac pathology* – Caution with renal or hepatic impairment Note: Used to treat apathy in brain injury patients
Modafinil (Provigil)	Dopaminergic Noradrenergic	Available doses: 100, 200 mg Start 100-200 mg daily *Max daily dose:* 400 mg qd	**Side Effects:** Erythema multiforme, SJS, toxic epidermal necrolysis (TEN), Allergic reaction, fever, sore throat, headache, and vomiting *Caution with cardiac pathology* Note: Used to promote wakefulness

Dextroamphetamine (Dexedrine)	Dopaminergic Noradrenergic Dopamine 1 and 2 receptor agonist; stimulates release	Available doses: 5, 10, 15 mg Start at 5 mg qd to bid, increase as needed for desired affect *Max daily dose:* 40 mg in divided doses bid	**Side Effects:** Anorexia, tachycardia, hyperthermia, psychosis, light headedness, hypertension, headache, blurred vision, anxiety *Precautions:* Contraindicated in HTN, glaucoma, seizure, hyperthyroid, symptomatic CV disease *Caution with cardiac pathology*
Atomoxetine (Strattera)	Selective norepinephrine reuptake inhibitor	Available doses: 10, 18, 25, 40, 60, 80, 100 mg Start 40 mg qday or 20 mg bid *Max daily dose:* 80 mg in divided doses	**Side Effects:** Dry mouth, insomnia, abdominal pain, irritability, nausea, urinary retention/hesitancy, anxiety, priapism *Precautions:* – increased risk of suicidal thoughts – Caution when using SSRIs *Caution with cardiac pathology*
Donepezil (Aricept)	Cholinergic Central acetylcholinesterase inhibitor	Available doses: 5, 10 mg Start 5 mg qhs After 4-6 weeks can increase dose to 10 mg *Max daily dose:* 10 mg	**Side Effects:** Bradycardia, nausea, vomiting, diarrhea, loss of appetite, muscle cramps, fatigue, insomnia *Precautions:* Can cause drowsiness so dose qhs

(continued)

Medication	Mode Of Action	Dosing	Side Effects/Cautions
Memantine (Namenda)	NMDA (N-methyl-D-aspartate) receptor **antagonist**	Available doses: 5, 10 mg Start 5 mg qday x 1 week, if tolerated, increase to 5 mg bid for 1 week, if needed can increase by 5 mg q week Usual dose is 10 mg bid *Max daily dose:* 30 mg in divided doses	**Side Effects:** Confusion, headache, insomnia dizziness, constipation, coughing, hypertension, somnolence, fatigue *Precautions:* – Extra-pyramidal side effects may occur in younger population *Caution with renal and hepatic impairment*

AGITATION MEDICATIONS [4]

Medication	Mode Of Action	Dosing	Side Effects/Cautions
Typical Antipsychotics Haldoperidol (Haldol)	Dopamine receptor **antagonist** (post-synaptically blocks D1 and D2 receptors) to decrease the release of hormones	Start with 2 mg IM x 1 dose for severe agitation Can be given 2-10 mg IM every 30min-6 hrs prn acute agitation	**Side Effects:** Akathisia, hypotension, constipation, dry mouth, tardive dyskinesia, neuroleptic malignant syndrome *Precaution:* Cardiovascular (can prolong QT) Caution with renal or hepatic impairment **Caution with brain injury patients:** it can severely impair their cognitive performance

(continued)

Medication	Mode Of Action	Dosing	Side Effects/Cautions
Atypical Antipsychotics	Dopamine receptor **antagonist** Each drug may have varying mechanisms		**Side Effects:** Sedation, weight gain, QTc interval prolongation, myocarditis, sexual side effects, akathisia, extrapyramidal side effects and cataract, neuroleptic malignant syndrome, hyperglycemia
Olanzapine (Zyprexa)		**Olanzapine** Start 2.5 mg po qday *Max daily dose:* 20 mg	
Risperidone		**Risperidone** Start 0.25 mg daily *Max daily dose:* 8 mg	*Precaution:* Zyprexa: black box warning; increased mortality in elderly with dementia-related psychosis
Ziprasidone (Geodon)		**Ziprasidone** Start 20 mg daily *Max daily dose:* 160 mg	*Precaution:* Cardiovascular (can prolong QT)
Quetiapine (Seroquel)		**Quetiapine** Start 12.5-50 mg q12 prn *Max daily dose:* 800 mg	
Beta Blockers Propranolol	Acts at β1 and β2 adrenergic receptors Non-selective blocker	Available doses: 10, 20, 40 Start 10-20 mg bid-tid *Usual Max daily dose:* 240 mg	**Side Effects:** Nausea/diarrhea, bronchospasm, bradycardia, hypotension *Precaution:* Hypoglycemia can occur (B2 activity stimulates glycogenolysis) Note: – Crosses BBB – May be used as treatment for Tachycardia secondary to dysautonomia from TBI Used to treat agitation in brain injury patients

| Antiepileptics
Carbamazepine
Valproate | **Carbamazepine**
Available doses: 100, 200, 300 mg

400-1600 mg daily
Reduces agitation

Valproate
Available doses: 250, 500 mg

May decrease agitation and improve
behavior | **Side Effects**: Dizziness, drowsiness, weight gain, glaucoma, skin rash, hepatotoxicity, colitis, and movement disorders |

INSOMNIA MEDICATIONS [3]

Medication	Mode Of Action	Dosing	Side Effects/Cautions
Trazadone	Serotonin **antagonist** and reuptake inhibitor	Available doses: 50, 100, 150, 300 mg Start 50 mg qhs If tolerated can increase for desired affects *Max daily dose:* 200 mg for sleep	**Side Effects:** Cardiac arrhythmia, blurred vision, priapism, headache, dry, mouth, constipation, syncope, QT prolongation *Precaution:* – Cannot be abruptly stopped – Metabolized by CYP3A4; may accumulate with substances that inhibit CY3A4 (ex. grape juice) *Caution with concurrent SSRIs or SNRIs* *Do not use in patients with renal impairment* *Caution in patients with hepatic impairment*

| Zolpidem (Ambien) | GABAA receptor agonist → potentiates GABA | Available doses: 5, 10 mg

Start 5 mg po qhs, can increase as needed | **Side Effects:** Nausea/vomiting, hallucinations, headache, dizziness, drowsiness, diarrhea, constipation, unusual dreams, dry mouth, unsteady balance

Note:
– Associated with tolerance, dependence, and rebound insomnia

Caution with elderly, increased risk with fractures and falls from unsteady gait (If needed only use 5 mg) |
| Eszopiclone (Lunesta) | Nonbenzodiazepine hypnotic agent | Available doses: 1, 2, 3 mg

Start 2 mg po qhs, increase/decrease as needed | **Side Effects:** Unpleasant taste, headache, aggression, agitation, changes in behavior; hallucinations, change in memory or concentration, nausea, dry mouth |

(continued)

Medication	Mode Of Action	Dosing	Side Effects/Cautions
Mirtazapine (Remeron)	Alpha 2 adrenergic and serotonin 5-HT **antagonist**	Available doses: 15, 30, 45 mg Start 15 mg po qhs *Max daily dose:* 45 mg	**Side Effects:** Drowsiness, dizziness, increased appetite, weight gain, agitation, hallucinations, tachycardia, nausea, vomiting, diarrhea, loss of coordination, confusion, headache Consider in elderly patients as appetite increases as well Not with MAOI *Precautions:* Has been associated with increased suicidality *Caution with hepatic impairment*

Quetiapine (Seroquel)	Dopamine and 5HT receptor **antagonist**	Available doses: 25, 100, 150, 200, 300 mg Start 12.5-50 mg po qhs prn	**Side Effects:** Sedation, weight gain, QTc interval prolongation, myocarditis, sexual side effects, akathisia, extrapyramidal side effects and cataract, neuroleptic malignant syndrome
			Hyperglycemia as increases glucose intolerance
			Caution when used for sleep as there is a high side effect profile
			Caution with hepatic impairment
			Precaution: Cardiovascular (can prolong QT)
			Sleep is an off label use

SEIZURE MEDICATIONS [3]

Consultation from neurology is recommended when managing patients who have seizure disorders. These medications should not be started unless approved by the neurologist.

Medication	Mode Of Action	Dosing	Side Effects/Cautions
Levetiracetam (Keppra)	Inhibits nerve conduction across synapses	Available doses: 250, 500, 750 mg Start 500 mg po bid, can increase every 2 weeks if needed *Max daily dose:* 1500 mg bid	**Side Effects:** Headache, nausea, dizziness, ataxia, diplopia, agitation, amnesia, depression *Caution with renal impairment* Avoid in pregnancy
Phenytoin (Dilantin)	Stabilizes the inactive state of voltage gated sodium channels	Available doses: 100 mg Start 100 mg tid	**Side Effects:** Horizontal gaze nystagmus, sedation, ataxia, hypotension Contraindicated in pregnancy- Teratogenetic Contraindicated with heart bock and sinjus bradycardia Caution with cardiovascular disease and elderly – May cause drug induced lupus – Monitoring of levels is required

Medication	Mode Of Action	Dosing	Side Effects/Cautions
Valproic Acid (Depakote)	Inhibits GABA transaminase which increases GABA concentrations	Available doses: 125, 250, 500 mg Start 10-15 mg/kg/day divided bid-tid	**Side Effects:** Nausea/vomiting/diarrhea, hallucinations, dizziness, weight gain, headache *Contraindication:* – Hepatic toxicity – Teratogenic: Do not give women who plan to become pregnant or are pregnant – Can cause pancreatitis – Monitoring of levels is required
Phenobarbital	Increases GABA concentration	Available doses: 15, 30, 60, 100 mg Start 60 mg po qd-tid, can increase by 30 mg q2-4 weeks to a target dose of 90-120 mg/day Maintenance: 1-3 mg/kg/day in divided doses	**Side Effects:** -Drowsiness, dizziness, lethargy, respiratory depression, changes in memory, Stevens-johnson syndrome, bradycardia, confusion *Precaution:* – Potential withdrawal *Caution with renal and hepatic impairment*

(continued)

Medication	Mode Of Action	Dosing	Side Effects/Cautions
Lamotrigine (Lamictal)	Acts at voltage gated sodium channels, decreases glutamate release	Available doses: 25, 50, 100, 200 mg Start 25 mg po qday, can increase q 1-2 weeks by 25-50 mg if needed Maintenance: 100-500 mg/day in divided doses (bid)	**Side Effects:** Rash, myalgias, easy bruising, abdominal pain, nausea, confusion. dizziness, loss of coordination, fatigue *Precaution:* Stephens-Johnson Syndrome- life threatening rash *Caution with use in pregnancy*
Oxcarbazepine (Trileptal)	Blocks voltage gated sodium channels, stabilizes neural membranes	Available doses: 150, 300, 600 mg Start 300 mg bid, if needed can increase qweek by 600 mg till effective results obtained *Max daily dose:* 2400 mg	**Side Effects:** Hyponatremia, pancytopenia, allergic reaction, dizziness, drowsiness, headache, gastric upset, nausea, vomiting, diarrhea *Precaution:* Teratogenic *Caution in patients with renal impairment* *Monitor for hyponatremia* (signs include headache, difficulty concentrating, confusion, loss of appetite, unsteadiness, hallucinations, seizure)

| Carbamazepine (Tegretol) | Stabilizes the inactivated voltage gated sodium channels | Available doses: Tablet- 200 mg
Chewable tablet- 100 mg

Start 200 mg bid, can increase by 200 mg weekly till desired effect achieved

Usual dose: 800-1200 mg divided tid-qid

Max daily dose: 1600 mg in divided doses | **Side Effects:** Allergic reaction, headache, confusion, agitation, dizziness, drowsiness, sedation, Nausea, vomiting, diarrhea, constipation, TEN, Syndrome Johnson Syndrome

Associated with:
Aplastic anemia, Agranulocystosis, SIADH |

NEUROPATHIC PAIN MEDICATIONS

Medication	Dosing	Side Effects/Cautions
Gabapentin (Neurontin)	Not fully understood, Acts to decrease excessive neuronal firing	Available doses: 100, 300, 400, 600, 800 mg	**Side Effects:** Somnolence, dizziness, GI upset, diarrhea, lower extremity edema, weight gain
	Start at 100-300 mg 1 po qhs or tid	Caution with renal impairment and elderly
	Depending on patients co-morbidities, age and ability to tolerate medications	Note: If discontinuing may require a taper to prevent adverse affects
	Max daily dose: 3600 mg in divided doses???	
	Caution with renal pathology and elderly	

Pregabalin (Lyrica)	Acts centrally at the dorsal horn at the voltage gated calcium channels, by modulating the amount of calcium to decrease excessive neuronal firing	Available doses: 25, 50, 75, 100, 150, 200, 225, 300 mg	**Side Effects:** Somnolence, dizziness, lower extremity edema, angioedema, weight gain, blurry vision, confusion
		Start 25-50 mg bid or tid depending on patient	Renal patients may need to start at lower dose
		Effective dose is 150 mg	
		Max daily dose: 450-600 mg depending on diagnosis (see below)	*Caution with elderly as they are more susceptible to adverse side effects*
		Fibromyalgia: 450 mg divided bid	Note: If discontinuing may require a taper to prevent adverse affects
		Diabetic peripheral neuropathy: 300 mg divide tid	
		Other neuropathies: 600 mg in divided doses	

(continued)

Medication	Dosing	Side Effects/Cautions
Cymbalta (Duloxetine)	Available doses: 20, 30, 60 mg	**Side Effects:** Gastric upset, weight gain, weight loss, decreased appetite, orthostatic hypotension, sexual side effects
Serotonin (SE) and norepinephrine (NE) reuptake inhibitor	Start at 30 mg qday in middle of largest meal	
	If needed can increase after a month to 60 qday	Caution when used with coumadin
	After 14 days of initiation, should have some benefits	May require renal dosing
		Monitor LFTs
	Elderly can start at 20 mg	*Caution with concurrent use of SSRI, SNRI, triptans or other medications that may affect serotonin* (to avoid causing Serotonin syndrome)
	Max daily dose: **Chronic pain:** 60 mg qday or 30 g bid **Anxiety/depression:** 120 mg qday in divided doses	Note:
	Discontinuing medications: Taper every 4 days Can get rebound effect if taper too fast	– Best to instruct patients to take this medication in the middle of their largest meal as it can cause gastric upset

Savella (Milnacipran)	Serotonin (SE) and norepinephrine (NE) reuptake inhibitor	Available doses: 12.5, 25, 50, 100 mg Start with 12.5 mg qday x 1 week if tolerated can increase to12.5 mg bid 1 week, then 25 mg in am and 12.5 mg in pm, then 25 mg bid, goal 50 mg bid if tolerated Although, some patients do well with 25 mg po bid	**Side effects:** Transient over 1st few weeks, nausea, constipation, hot flush, hyperhidrosis, palpitations, hypertension, vomiting, dry mouth, increased HR Note: Instruct patients to take medications in the middle of the largest meal (nausea is most common complication) Cardiovascular warnings
Tricyclic Antidepressants (TCAs) Elavil (Amitriptyline) Pamelor (Nortriptyline)		Available doses: Elavil- 10, 25, 50, 75, 100, 150 mg Pamelor- 10, 25, 50, 75 mg Elavil and Pamelor: Start 25 mg qhs, can increase if needed *Elavil Max daily dose:* 100-150 mg	**Side effects:** Nausea, vomiting, drowsiness, headache, dry mouth, constipation, difficulty urinating, blurred vision, confusion, unsteadiness *Caution with cardiovascular patients and patients with hepatic impairment* **Do not use with MAOI** Note: May take 4 weeks to see clinical effect

PAIN MEDICATIONS (SHORT ACTING OPIATES)

Opiate Mode of Action: mu receptor opioid agonist

Opiate Side Effects: All medications above can cause sedation, dizziness, constipation, gastric upset, nausea, vomiting, pruritis, sweating, miosis, orthostatic hypotenion

Opioids affect Hypothalamic Pituitary
Males: Low testosterone, libido, gynecomastia
Females: Low hormone output → amenorrhea, anovulation, reduced milk production

Caution in patients with respiratory disease
If patients experience pain while on opiates, consider increasing the dose or frequency depending on patient's response to the medications.
All patients on opiates should be monitored to avoid side effects, overdose, and misuse.

Medication	Dosing	Dosing/Cautions
Tramadol (Ultram)	Available doses: **Ultram** 50 mg **Ultracet** 37.5/325, 50/500 mg (other doses may exist) *Long acting formulations available as well*	Start at 50 mg, can be given 1-2 pills q4-6 prn pain *Max daily dose:* 400 mg in divided doses Combination products are also limited by the amount of acetaminophen *Caution with concurrent use of SSRI, SNRI or other medications that may affect serotonin* *Can lower seizure threshold* *Note: Additional mechanism - inhibiting serotonin reuptake*
Codeine (Tylenol #3, Tylenol #4)	Available doses: **Tylenol #3** 300/30 mg **Tylenol #4** 300/60 mg **Codeine** 15, 30, 60 mg	Start Tylenol #3 1pill po q4-6 prn pain , can change to Tylenol #4 if higher dose of codeine required for adequate pain control *Max daily dose:* Limiting factor products combined with Acetaminophen No ceiling dose for non combination codeine products

(continued)

Medication	Dosing	Dosing/Cautions
Morphine	Available doses: 15, 30 mg	Start 15 mg po q4-6 prn pain
	Long acting formulations available as well	*Max daily dose*: No ceiling dose , titrate according to tolerance and adequate pain control
Hydrocodone (Vicodin, Norco)	Available doses: **Norco** 5/325, 7.5/325, 10/325 mg **Vicodin** 5/500, 7.5/500, 10/500 mg	Start 5/325 mg 1 po q4-6 prn pain , increase as needed
		Max daily dose: Limiting factor products combined with Acetaminophen
		Note: Some patients do experience a "high" like feeling with this medication
		Caution with Tylenol dose in patients with hepatic impairment
Oxycodone (Percocet)	Available doses: **Percocet** 5/325, 7.5/325, 10/325 mg **Oxycodone** 5, 10, 15, 30 mg	Start 5/325 mg q4-6 prn pain
	Long acting formulations available as well	*Max daily dose:* Limiting factor products combined with Acetaminophen No ceiling dose for non combination oxycodone products
		Note: *Oxycodone 30 mg should only be written on rare occasion when absolutely needed for proper pain control. Not to be used in patients who may misuse.*

Tapentadol (Nucynta)	Available doses: 50, 75, 100 mg	Start at 50 mg 1 po q4-6 prn pain, if tolerated and not strong enough can increase to higher dose
	Long acting formulations available as well	*Max daily dose:* 600 mg in divided doses
		Note: Increased tolerability if started at lower dose first, this can avoid the side effect of headache. If titrated up slowly side effects are less likely to develop
		Caution with concurrent use of SSRI, SNRI or other medications that may affect serotonin (to avoid causing Serotonin syndrome)
		Do not use with respiratory issues, hypotension, h/o seizures, renal (not dialyzable) or hepatic impairment
		Side effects: Constipation, pruritis, hyperhydrosis, pyrexia, nausea, headache, dizziness, somnolence
		Note: Additional mechanism- Norepinephrine reuptake inhibitor
Oxymorphone (Opana)	Available doses: 5, 10 mg	Start 5 mg q 4-6 prn pain
	Long acting formulations available as well	
		(continued)

Medication	Dosing	Dosing/Cautions
Hydromorphone (Dilaudid)	Available doses: 4, 8, 16 mg	Start 4 mg q 4-6 prn pain
		Max daily dose: No ceiling dose , titrate according to tolerance and adequate pain control
	Long acting formulation available as well	Note: *Do not use in opiate naïve patients or patients at high risk of misuse/abuse*

References

1. Movement Disorder Virtual University http://www.mdvu.org/library/disease/spasticity/spa_mtop.asp.
2. Cuccurullo, Sara J, M.D. (2004). Physical Medicine and Rehabilitation Board Review. New York, NY: Demos Medical Publishing.
3. Epocrates Online Drugs [Internet]. San Mateo (CA): Epocrates, Inc. ©2011. [continuously updated; cited 2011 Jan 12]. Available from: http://www.epocrates.com.
4. The Journal of Family medicine Practice: Traumatic Brain Injury: Choosing Drugs to Assist Recovery. John Daniels. *Vol. 5, No. 5/May 2006*. http://www.jfponline.com/Pages.asp?AID=4135.

Index

Lightning Source UK Ltd.
Milton Keynes UK
UKHW02f1257050118
315547UK00007B/54/P